The Game-Changers Series

The Game-Changers Series

A compilation of books inspired by
four great historical thinkers

Tham Trong Ma

The Game-Changers Series

ISBN 978-1-954891-93-7 (eBook)

ISBN 978-1-954891-94-4 (Paperback)

ISBN 978-1-954891-95-1 (Hard Cover)

CONTENTS

INTRODUCTION

T he *Game-Changers Series* is a compilation of books that examines the writings of four figures from classic history: Lao Tzu, Sun Vu, Niccolo Machiavelli, and Musashi Miyamoto. These four historical figures are well-known for having significantly impacted society through their contributions to their respective fields of endeavor. They paved the way for new ways of thinking and acting by challenging accepted wisdom. They were able to alter the rules in their respective fields through their creativity, tenacity, and sheer force of will, and they served as an example for others to follow.

"Game-changer" is a term that has become popular in the last few years. Prominent people, such as athletes, scientists, and businesspeople, are called 'game changers.' What they all have in common is that they changed their respective fields. They may have changed them a little or a lot; they may have changed them for the better or, in varying degrees, for the worse, but their input was crucial to giving new shape to the world around them. Game-changers have a different functioning mechanism than the majority of people. They have learned to take advantage of changing circumstances and control their lives the way they want to. Whether they are visionaries, thought leaders or rebels, the individuals who inspired the books in this series have all made a lasting impact on the world and have left a lasting legacy that will continue to inspire and influence future generations.

When people ask, "What does it take to be a game-changer?" The traditional answer is usually along the lines of "a strong sense of ambition and motivation" or "striving for success and making one's mark in the world." But there's more to being a game-changer than this. In today's rapidly changing world, it is more important than ever for individuals to be innovative and forward-thinking in order to stay relevant and competitive. Changing the game requires more than just having a good idea or the desire to make a difference. It will take the efforts of game changers to find original and practical solutions to the numerous complex challenges and issues the world is currently facing, such as perpetual conflicts and wars, climate change, inequality, and pandemics. People must step up and change the world because, without game changers, progress may be slow or even stop.

Game-changers can embrace new ideas, technologies, and methods of doing things, and they inspire and motivate others to follow in their footsteps. It also requires careful planning, strategy, a solid mindset to turn those ideas into reality, and, most importantly, a balanced life. A balanced life is critical for game-changers because it ensures they have the energy and resources to change an industry or create something new.

You encounter difficult situations every day, whether you're an entrepreneur, a politician, a teacher, a student, an engineer, an accountant, or even a stay-at-home mom. Each book in this series dissects these central issues while applying age-old precepts and lessons adapted to address our modern-day challenges. These books contain the knowledge necessary to improve one's mindset, teach how to plan and strategize, and assist you in finding a healthy balance in life, thereby enabling you to perform at your best in both your personal and professional lives, as well as in society and the world at large. These books are a must-read for anyone looking to make a difference in their lives and the world around them.

On The Soldier's Path

Miyamoto Musashi is considered by many to be the greatest swordsman and one of the most influential strategists in history. Trained from infancy to be the best, his skills were so excellent that even those who could beat him could not match him. Musashi's philosophy laid the foundation for training in martial arts and influenced other fields, such as business and sports. Musashi Miyamoto was a samurai, yet he was also an artist, a philosopher, and a man of letters. As a swordsman, He wrote a classic book on strategy, tactics, and philosophy named *The Five Spheres*. It contains principles that can be applied to most forms of combat and have become required reading for business people and managers in Japan. Musashi's life and teachings have had a lasting influence on martial arts and military strategy, which is why *On the Soldier's Path* is heavily influenced by Musashi's writings as well as by Sun Vu's *The Law of War*, Lao Tzu's *The Book of Ethics*, and Niccolo Machiavelli's *The Prince*.

We have reached heights that most people could only have imagined a few decades ago because we presently live in one of the most technologically advanced eras in human history. However, our progress has turned out to be a double-edged sword that has also hurt us in terms of the destructive nature of the global military environment. We have reached a turning point where we understand that a paradigm shift is necessary.

The definition of the military is a strong organization that uses force to defend its country from foreign adversaries. The path to war is long, and the way to peace is even longer because the struggle for peace is ongoing, and we live in a world with failing systems. Currently, there cannot be peace without war. Many battles have taken place in the world in which we now live in an effort to end ongoing conflicts. International conflicts continue to occur despite an arms race reaching its peak. The numerous wars the world has experienced should demonstrate that the true enemy is not the person next to you or your neighboring country; the true enemy is our own self-centered individual interests, which divert us from working for peace.

On the Soldier's Path analyzes what it means to be a soldier. What responsibilities does he shoulder? What characteristics and qualities must he have? The warrior's path, according to Musashi, is paved with discipline, focus, restraint, and honor and is upheld by moral and ethical standards. A soldier's mind is his greatest weapon, and the ability to control and utilize it effectively can mean the difference between being a casualty of war or living to share war stories as a veteran in his later years. The key to this lies in the codes and principles that the soldier holds dear and believes in.

With so much turmoil, there is no time to waste. Adversaries of peace are constantly devising new ways to disturb stability for their gain; unfortunately, they often have the resources to do so. This means that the soldier must be strategic to outmaneuver them. *On the Soldier's*

Path offers several strategies for achieving this, including in-depth chapters on alternative methods of winning wars without resorting to combat. This book is a game changer, and a transformative guide for soldiers, diplomats, and anyone who loves their country desires a peaceful world, and wants to protect the future of our planet.

The Entrepreneur's Battle Plan

Making your money work for you is the first step toward financial freedom. Do you frequently feel your finances are working against you and want to take charge of your money so that it works for you? There are many ways to achieve this, but starting your own business and becoming an entrepreneur is at the top of the list.

A good entrepreneur is aware of how competitive the business world is. You would always be at odds with yourself, trying to improve yesterday's version of yourself. The struggle to get your team to share the vision would continue, and you would constantly be attempting to outpace your rivals.

Every day brings a fresh challenge, but the benefits are priceless. You may encounter obstacles such as established companies, new businesses entering the market, economic policies, and global economic conditions. However, the most significant hurdle is self-doubt and the temptation to give up. Faced with these internal and external factors, you can either retreat or strive for success.

While entrepreneurship can be challenging, some individuals and companies have a history of consistently coming out on top. Sun Vu, who never lost a battle during his career as a military strategist and General, is a prime example of this principle. This is why The Entrepreneur's Battle Plan examines effective methods for success in the business world, drawing inspiration from Sun Vu's *The Law of War*, a classic text on military strategy.

Sun Vu achieved his record of never losing a battle, not because he had the strongest soldiers but because he understood that each battle is unique and must be approached accordingly. His ideas on warfare and those of Miyamoto Musashi, whose principles on military strategy formed the foundation of *On The Soldier's Path*, share a similar approach. Both men believed that warfare goes beyond just weapons.

They understood that battles are as much mental as they are physical and therefore developed their own strategies.

The Entrepreneur's Battleplan is a comprehensive guide for successfully navigating the challenges of the business world. It outlines the essential tactics, resources, and qualities necessary for achieving success, from the initial planning stages to overcoming potential obstacles. To be successful, entrepreneurs must have a clear understanding of the market and be able to develop strategic plans. Much like a General preparing for war, creating a solid business plan is crucial for success and should not be underestimated. Experience is important, but having a well-defined strategy in place is essential for avoiding failure in business.

For entrepreneurs looking to take their businesses to the next level, The Entrepreneur's Battleplan is a must-have. The ideas in this book are all you need to change the game and be on a constant victory march. It is the guide to success with age-old strategies that have worked time and time again. This book will give you the knowledge and confidence you need to succeed in the challenging and ever-changing business world. Imagine yourself as a soldier fighting a financial war for your freedom and success. With The Entrepreneur's Battleplan in your hands, you can be assured of victory.

Inside The War Room

If there was one quality that these three men, Niccolo Machiavelli, Sun Vu, and Miyamoto Musashi, shared, it was a similar understanding of the concept of victory, and they achieved this by any means necessary. Inside the war room combines three books, *The Book of Five Spheres*, *The Prince*, and *The Law of War*, to create a brilliant book about 25 winning strategies for political power. Don't let the title fool you; these strategies go much deeper and can be applied to any aspect of life, including business and personal relationships.

Every day in life can be likened to a new battleground where you must confront a different foe or a challenge. To defeat your adversary, you would need a war strategy that would guarantee victory at all costs. By analyzing the tactics outlined in each book, you can glean enough information to construct a viable winning plan for your entire life.

One of the main points in this book is the vital role strategy plays in planning. Strategy is a way of thinking and acting that allows one to navigate challenging situations and achieve goals. The ability to respond appropriately in the face of pressure to handle the most trying circumstances is an art. It involves adapting and modifying existing principles to fit changing circumstances and involves careful planning and proactive decision-making. Those skilled at strategy can anticipate challenges and make calculated decisions rather than reacting impulsively. Your ultimate objective is something you already have in mind. The only things left are the calculated actions leading you to your goal. Strategy is a vital tool for navigating the complexities of life and is crucial to achieving success.

While the book examines conflict and its resolution, it is crucial to recognize that conflict is not necessarily an opposing force. Properly managed conflict can serve as a valuable tool for resolving issues and reconciling differences. The key is approaching conflict with a mindset of finding a solution rather than seeing it as a hindrance. The ability to effectively navigate and resolve conflicts can significantly impact the success of one's efforts.

The purpose of the knowledge imparted in this book is to empower readers to effect change within the political realm. It is not about achieving personal gain through coercion or self-defense but rather about learning how to approach political situations with strategy and reason. This includes effectively managing conflicts, people, and opposition, as well as using one's instincts to positively impact the world. By adopting this approach, readers can become game-changers in the political sphere.

Insights To Better Living

Insights to Better Living is written based largely on Lao Tzu's *The Book of Ethics*, which was inspired by philosophies birthed from his spiritual experiences. *The Book of Ethics* is considered a fundamental philosophical and religious Taoism text. However, its precept spans beyond the boundaries of religion, philosophy, and politics. Professionals like poets, artists, calligraphers, and gardeners have read and applied principles from the book to their professions.

A chaotic world is the product of the imbalance between good and evil, right and wrong. Lao Tzu taught the principles of living in harmony with nature and the universe. He advised people to transform themselves, and, like Musashi, he taught them to embrace asceticism by giving up their desires. According to Lao Tzu, "If people and things were in harmony, they would all be inanimate and desireless, so there would be no need to fight and conquer. Therefore, humans will have peace, well-being, and happiness."

Insights to Better Living teaches how to seek ways to find peace and harmony in a chaotic world. The book is divided into three parts; The Body, The Spirit, and The Harmony between the Body and The spirit. The book comprehensively explores each aspect of the human being, the relationship between these aspects, and how to achieve a balance to live harmoniously with our environment. It delves into a variety of profound topics related to the human experience. These include the nature of the body and mind, achieving longevity, self-discovery, and finding happiness. At its core, however, the book focuses on the importance of balance and harmony in achieving a fulfilling life. Drawing on ancient wisdom, it offers practical guidance for applying these timeless lessons to modern living. The value of this book lies in its ability to impart invaluable insights into healthy living, manifesting one's desires, and living in peace and harmony.

One of society's most significant challenges is the lack of balance in people's lives. Many of us lead hectic and fast-paced lifestyles, which can lead to emotional burnout and physical stress. The constant rush to keep up with demands can leave the mind and body fatigued, leading to negative emotional states such as anger, apathy, and a lack of motivation. The root of this issue is that the body and mind are not in harmony.

Insights to Better Living is an essential guide for any game-changer looking to perform at their best. The book provides valuable strategies and techniques for optimizing mental and physical well-being, allowing you to rise above the challenges of the fast-paced and demanding environment. It delves into understanding the mind and body and guides how to work on them for improvement. Whether you're an entrepreneur, leader, or innovator, mastering your own well-being is key to reaching your full potential and achieving success. It's not just about reading but also implementing techniques that work best for you; this book will be a great starting point.

****

These four books are a treasure trove of wisdom and guidance, essential for anyone looking to cultivate themselves, achieve financial freedom, lead their family, govern their nation, and strive for world peace and a balanced life. These timeless principles have been effective in countless situations across all aspects of life. These ideas can transform your life from mastering the art of war and navigating the complexities of politics and business to improving your relationships and overall well-being. But it is not enough just to read these books; you must also put the ideas into practice. By doing so, you will gain a broader perspective and an increased resilience that will help you make better decisions, navigate challenges and achieve your goals. You will gain a deeper understanding of yourself and the world around you and be well on your way to a fulfilling and successful life. *The Game-Changers Series* will be a valuable companion throughout your journey, providing guidance and inspiration when you need it the most.

ON THE SOLDIER'S PATH

The Way Of Warrior

INTRODUCTION

Dear Soldier,

For the love of country: This was your motivation when you set out on this journey, donned your uniform, and picked up your gun. You were not deterred by the rigorous training nor the fact that you would be separated from those you love most of the time. In our current world, peace has become a scarce resource, so you need to understand how valuable you are.

A country is a slice of humanity. Therefore, the moment you decided and followed through on becoming a soldier, you became a vital thread stitching a semblance of peace into humanity's fabric of chaos. It may seem that you are unseen, unknown, and unsung but always know that your blood and sweat are indelible imprints. And the earth—humanity—will never forget.

Only a few understand and appreciate the depth of your vocation. Even some soldiers get into the military for the wrong reasons. There are those who join because of the paycheck and benefits of being in the armed forces. Some join because it is a family tradition. Others want the prestige and respect that come with wearing a military uniform. Such reasons have made many soldiers stray from the true path of dedication and service. But just like everything else in the world, deviating from the true path is not new. And this is why I want to tell you the story of Miyamoto Musashi.

Miyamoto Musashi was a Japanese warrior who lived between the 16th and 17th centuries. Born on March 12, 1584, in Miyamoto-Sanomo village, Harima province, Japan, Miyamoto was respected as a *Kensei*—a sword saint of Japan because between when he was 13 and

29 years old, he fought in more than sixty to-the-death sword fights and was never defeated.

His fame spread through Japan when at 21, he defeated three in-structors of a renowned swordsman school. In that fight, it was re-corded that he fought against sixty opponents simultaneously, all armed with swords, muskets, spears, bows, and arrows. After that, he traveled and had one-on-one duels with many masters.

When he turned 30, he determined to train himself to gain deeper principles of swordsmanship. He practiced hard until the age of 50, when he discovered the Way of the Warrior and applied it to every-thing he did without needing a teacher.

Like what we see today, Musashi knew that many warriors stray from the true path of martial arts; thus, he decided to do two things: He founded a school of swordsmanship called Hyōhō Niten Ichi-ryū; and wrote books on the principles of swordsmanship he had gained. Musashi did these things to achieve one goal: steer the warrior's mind back to the true way. His most famous book, *The Five Spheres*, taught the principles and strategic significance of martial art based on his own principles. And it is on the foundation of Musashi's prin-ciples that this book, *On The Soldier's Path*, is birthed.

Miyamoto Musashi, who died on June 13, 1645, at the age of 61, may be long gone, but the principles of his martial art are relevant in the modern world. It is not surprising that Musashi's voice still reso-nates till today because if he could win more than sixty fights where his life was on the line, he definitely did many things right.

His ideas are simple yet laced with depth. They are like calm waters that run deep. For Musashi, a true warrior must master the Way of Strategy. This Way, practical and straightforward in its approach, is founded on one notion: defeat the enemy. Musashi teaches that de-feating the enemy goes beyond fighting against the enemy's weapon; the true warrior must understand the enemy's psychology and cir-cumstances and strategically employ them to his favor.

The book, *The Five Spheres* is a discourse on the Way of Strategy sectioned into five scrolls: Earth, Water, Fire, Wind, and Emptiness. In the Earth or Ground scroll, Musashi compares the Way to carpentry. Just like a carpenter who follows a plan to build a house, the warrior must also be methodical in fighting the enemy. The scroll also emphasizes timing and the importance of perception. The Water scroll is a guide to sword fighting. It teaches the warrior the right stance and gaze when facing an adversary. The Fire scroll deals with actual strategy—how the warrior can gain advantage and exploit the adversary's weaknesses. In the Wind scroll, Musashi criticizes the techniques of other schools of swordsmanship. Finally, he summarizes his principles with the Emptiness scroll or the Scroll of the Void, which lives a striking lesson: the more knowledge we gain, the more we realize how little we know.

For this book, *On The Soldier's Path*, these five scrolls are metaphors for the characters a soldier should possess. Just like Musashi taught, defeating the enemy is more about psychology and circumstances than engaging the enemy's weapon. The world we live in has seen many battles, all in a bid to resolve lingering conflicts. But the many wars the world has seen should show that the real enemy is not the next individual or the neighboring nation; the real enemy is our selfish individual interests that distract us from seeking peace.

Therefore, each chapter, each scroll in this book, will represent the different qualities a soldier can and should possess as he journeys on this long road to peace. Some of these qualities are opposites, but they make him complete when fused together in a soldier. Completeness is a crucial requirement for a soldier—because a broken soldier cannot restore order to a broken world.

So I consider myself, dear soldier, privileged to communicate Musashi's principles to you through this book. By reading this book and putting it to practice, the world will be a better place. This is the way I see it: I am leaning on the back of Musashi, while you are leaning on mine—and together we are gifting peace to the world. Our efforts are connected by different times and events and fused into a synergy for the world to enjoy a semblance of peace.

May this synergy never be in vain.

PART I

THE FIVE SPHERES

CHAPTER ONE

EARTH - *Follow the Map*

The earth holds a lot of significance for the soldier. The earth soaks up the blood and sweat of the soldier. The shrubs that sprout from the earth provide cover for the soldier to evade and target the enemy. Bunkers are dug under the earth. All the battles of a soldier are fought on the earth. Most importantly, on the earth lies the path or trail to the enemy.

The final destination of every battle is peace. So when you follow the earth's trail to the enemy's camp, the result after the battle will be peace. However, it would be myopic for the soldier to think that attaining peace *begins* and ends with strategizing, following the coordinates that lead to the enemy's quarters, and employing different weapons of war.

Musashi stated that in his Earth scroll, to know the immense and profound things, we must first understand the small and shallow things. What we see on the battleground—war cries, gunshots, bomb blasts, dead bodies—are the big things. But what escalates into war are the small things that are often neglected by the soldier. And if we lean on the words of Musashi, we can trace the path of peace down to the soldier.

There are two virtues for peace a soldier must possess. These virtues are like map coordinates—following or deviating from them can either restore or remove peace from the world.

Loyalty and Timing: The Soldier's Virtues for Peace Loyalty

In Musashi's days, a samurai is known for carrying two swords—the long sword and the companion sword. The long sword is usually the weapon known as the *katana*[1]. This is the essential sword of the samurai. Asides from being used in combat, the katana sword symbolized the warrior's status and *unwavering loyalty* to his master.[2]

The companion sword, on the other hand, was usually the *wakizashi*[3]. Only samurais were allowed to carry the katana, but the wakizashi could be carried by anyone of the lower class. Because of its use in samurai suicides[4], the wakizashi was also referred to as an "*honor blade*." Samurais were never without their wakizashi. They carried it wherever they went and even hid it under their pillow while they slept. The samurai's wakizashi is likened to the pistol of the modern-day soldier.[5]

The pairing of the wakizashi and the katana is called a daisho, which literally translates to "big little." Daisho is not a weapon in itself but refers to the act of carrying two swords. Samurai warriors discovered that having two swords gave them a competitive edge during battle.[6]

So what does this mean for today's soldier? The katana and the wakizashi—or more aptly put, the daisho—represents loyalty. Beyond knowing how to wield a gun and throw a grenade, the soldier must have the primary virtue for peace: loyalty.

Loyalty is faithfulness or devotion to something or someone. All a loyal person thinks about is what or who they are devoted to. The circumstances around them do not matter so long as they protect the interests of what or who they are devoted to.

Just like the samurai carrying two weapons, loyalty for today's soldier is two-pronged. A soldier must be loyal to *humanity* and *country*. Loyalty to humanity is like carrying a katana, while loyalty to country is like carrying a wakizashi. Both are important, but in times of decision making, one becomes weightier than the other.

Remember, we have established that the soldier's path is one that leads to peace for his country and, ultimately, for humanity. So when he is faced with a tough decision, a soldier should ask himself: *How will this impact my country? How will this impact the human race?* Many disagreements have escalated into wars because people have failed to ask these questions and provide honest answers to them.

The world has experienced wars and crimes against humanity because people—soldiers—are neither loyal to country nor humanity, but to themselves alone. They project their self-centeredness on the rest of the world under the guise of fighting for their nation. But a close examination of the conflict's nuances would reveal that most (if not all) of the wars the earth has experienced would have been avoided if humanity was put first.

For example, World War 1, which lasted between 1914 and 1918, arose because of the competition for imperialist control. Serbia wanted to take over Austria-Hungary's control of the Slavic people of Bosnia and Herzegovina. This strong desire for control led to the assassination of Austria-Hungary's Franz Ferdinand, the Archduke of Austria. The assassination degenerated the conflict between Austria-Hungary and Serbia into a full-blown war that claimed over 17 million lives.[7]

Imperialist nations never clamor for the interests of the countries they want to dominate. The power tussle between Austria-Hungary and Serbia was a contest for increased wealth and dominance, and not for the good of the Slavic people of Bosnia and Herzegovina. When we say "imperialist nations," it is vital to bear in mind that a group of people governs a nation. Therefore, the fight for wealth and dominance was simply a fight for the pockets and pride of people who were ready to sacrifice human lives on the altar of selfishness, people who were only loyal to themselves and not to humanity.

Loyalty to Country: The Wakizashi

You are a soldier because you are defending your nation. Your primary duty is to your nation. Part of the United States Oath of Enlistment reads: ". . . that I will support and defend the Constitution of the United States against all enemies, foreign and domestic; that I will bear true faith and allegiance to the same. . ." So you ought to do what is in the best interest of the nation you serve and represent.

There have been many betrayal cases in military history where people have shown disloyalty to their country, handing it over to its enemies. For example, there was China's Qin Hui. In Chinese history, Qin Hui was a chancellor of the Song dynasty. He was a power-hungry fellow who removed all his political opponents and eventually handed the Song dynasty to the Jurchen dynasty. Another example is power-hungry Emilio Aguinaldo—a man who implored his nation, the Philippines, to surrender to Japanese invaders, with the hopes of getting the Japanese to make him the president of the nation. What about Mir Jafar, who received a bribe from the British East India Company and betrayed India to the British[8]; an action that led to Britain's imperialist rule over India for almost 200 years? The stories of Qin Hui, Emilio Aguinaldo, Mir Jafar, and every traitor in human history boils down to one fact: they were *only* loyal to their personal interests.

Peace is not only the absence of war or violence; it is also the presence of equality, equity, and cooperation. A soldier who shows disloyalty to his nation may not plunge the nation into war but would certainly remove vital aspects of peace like equality and equity. Therefore, as a soldier, you *must* understand that your duty to restore peace doesn't begin at the battlefield—it begins before then. It begins by wearing loyalty around your loins at all times like a wakizashi. When you maintain loyalty to your nation, the need to go into the battlefield may not arise.

Now, there is the question: If the primary duty of a soldier is to his nation, why is loyalty to country likened to the small wakizashi instead of the big katana?

Loyalty to Humanity: The Katana

Loyalty to country is great, but loyalty to humanity is greater. No individual or country exists in a vacuum. We are all connected and interdependent on one another. It is for this reason a soldier must holistically consider how his actions or inactions would impact not just his country, but also the world at large. Barack Obama understood this.

In his address to the nation on September 10, 2013, the then POTUS spoke about the Syrian civil war and the repressive actions of Bashar al-Assad, the president of Syria at the time who had killed over a thousand Syrians with poison gas, sarin. Except for being the world power, the United States actually had no business interfering with the affairs of Syria. As a matter of fact, many Americans either felt that the US had no business interfering, or that interference could escalate into a war, or that interference wasn't worth it. But that night, Obama underscored why the United States needed to attack Syria. His reasons were all founded on the need to respect and protect lives all over the world. He explained that the consequences of America's inaction and indifference could be far-reaching since "other tyrants will have no reason to think twice about acquiring poison gas, and using them."[9] He asked Americans to "reconcile [their] belief in freedom and dignity for all people with those images of children writhing in pain, and going still on a cold hospital floor. *For sometimes, resolutions and statements of condemnation are simply not enough.*"[10]

If we critically examine the Vietnam War, we will realize that the war would have been avoided if the conflicting parties, North Vietnam and South Vietnam (and their allies), put humanity first before their competing ideologies. Both parties wanted a unified Vietnam but wanted to model the country differently. The North wanted communism, the South wanted a country with economic and cultural ties to the Western world.[11] If the belligerents had shoved aside their ideologies and put humanity first, then over 3 million people—of which more than half were Vietnamese civilians—wouldn't have died.[12]

There are times when the interest of humanity trumps the interest of your nation or personal interest. And as a soldier, you have to be rational to understand these times. Samurais did not carry their katana everywhere as they did with the wakizashi. The katana came into play in moments of the battle, in decisive moments. In the same way, you may not consider your loyalty to humanity in every situation.

In most cases, your loyalty to your country comes first. However, in critical moments when the human race is threatened, your decision must favor of humanity. Always bear this in mind, dear soldier.

Timing

Musashi said that there is timing in everything—from music to archery to riding horses. For a merchant, there is a time when his capital rises or falls. The same goes for a warrior; there is a time when he thrives and a time when he declines, a time of harmony and a time of discord. In every skill and ability, there is timing. And Musashi suggests that it is important for the warrior—the soldier—to understand timing.

Nations have successfully attacked other nations that did not understand the power of timing. Timing was all it took for Israel to defeat the United Arab Republic (Jordan, Syria, and Egypt) in what is commonly known as The Six-Day War, which lasted from June 5 to June 10, 1967. After the 1948 Arab-Israeli War, relations between Israel and its Arab neighbors didn't return to normal. Tensions kept mounting until it escalated in May 1967, and both sides started preparing for war.

The United States intelligence predicted that Israel had the capacity to launch a successful attack on the United Arab Republic with little or no warning. However, Israel never confirmed these predictions as the United States never knew the actual timing of the operation. The Israelis were discreet with their plans. They had robust security who did not reveal their plans or preparations. Apart from being discreet, Israel also played a multifaceted game of deception. First, they made Egypt believe that they would attack southern Sinai instead of the north if they were to attack. Second, they put specific measures to give the enemy the impression that an attack was not imminent. Some of these measures included: public statements by the then Defense Minister who told the world that Israel would rather go for dialog and diplomacy than launch an attack; issuance of leave to thousands of Israeli on the 3rd and 4th of June; and announcements that the Israeli government was only concerned with routine matters. The United Arab Republic relaxed. And on June 5, Israel successfully launched a series of airstrikes. What made Israel's attack even more interesting was that it was launched at an hour of the morning when most Egyptian officials were on their way to work and when the Egyptian Air Force chief took his routine daily morning flights.[13]

Reading about The Six-Day War, it is difficult to fathom how the United Arab Republic could be so careless. Who relaxes in time of hostilities? It was easy for Israel to deceive the Arabs because they made light of the time they were in. In a time of war, adequate preparations must be made. Nothing must be left to chance. Israel understood this, prepared, and won. In six days.

A similar scenario had even played out some years earlier during the Second World War. Hitler used a delay tactic to defeat Western Europe, which comprised Holland, Belgium, and France. The Central Intelligence Agency (CIA) noted that these three countries had "ample and repeated warnings," but since Hitler never executed the attack—having delayed for six months[14]—they took the warnings for granted. They even called it a "phony war" as Hitler postponed the attack 29 times, usually at the last minute. Before the actual attack, the countries had received information about it. However, the Dutch and the French didn't heed this warning, dismissing it as another false alarm. Only the Belgians were smart enough to place their forces on general alert.[15]

Just like the United Arab Republic, Western Europe downplayed the importance of timing. They went to sleep in a time of war. No matter how many times Hitler had postponed the attack, they should have been prepared, knowing that it was a time of war. The war had already lasted eight months, and its end was not even in sight, so why were they comfortable?

Israel and Germany had the same tactics: they made their enemy undervalue timing. They "infected" their enemy with a calm spirit, a spirit not prepared to fight. (This is a technique Musashi taught in the Fire scroll, and we will examine it later.)

Musashi rightly noted that there is timing in the whole life of a warrior. Therefore, your actions should be guided according to timing. One does not relax during a time of war; neither does one become hostile in a time of peace unless such a person is an enemy of peace.

As a soldier, every activity is encased in time. Musashi wrote the five scrolls on the basis of timing. But there is something I want you to know: every time should be a time of peace. The timing for peace should not be conditional. Everything should be done towards fostering peace. However, I do not neglect the fact that there would be situations that call for war, but before going to war, make sure it is the only option left.

I say this because many wars have been fought not because they were necessary, but because they were instigated by people who, ironically, "benefit" from the dividends of war. So dear soldier, when faced with a dilemma whether to escalate a conflict, ask yourself: *Is war neces-sary or do I want to fulfill a selfish goal?*

Through *The Five Spheres*, Miyamoto Musashi offered samurais a guide to true swordsmanship. Little did he know that his lessons would be a template for world peace more than three centuries later.

Musashi's Way of Strategy is absolute: kill the adversary. Peace ought to be absolute too, because *only* through peace would we thrive as individuals and collectively as a species. Unfortunately, just like many samurais did not follow the Way in Musashi's time, in today's world, peace in its totality is a mirage.

In teaching his Way, Musashi knew that it was not enough teaching samurais about (his) strategy or timing, he knew that samurais must first possess certain traits which would enable them to become skillful swordsmen who understood timing. Today's soldier must also possess these traits—for if he does, the virtues for peace will come naturally to him. These traits include: honesty, understanding the Way of all professions, distinguishing the pros and cons in every matter, intuitive judgment and understanding for everything, recognizing the unseen, and paying attention to details.

- *Honesty*: This is a fundamental ingredient for loyalty. A dishonest soldier can neither be loyal to his country nor to humanity. He is never on the path of truth. The traitors we saw earlier were dishonest fellows who claimed to be true to their nation but later sold off their countries for selfish gains.

Like Musashi, I am not just telling you to be loyal to your country and/or humanity, I am also letting you know that your loyalty is *dependent* on whether you are honest or not. So be honest with yourself and answer this: *Am I an honest person?*

- *Understanding the Way of all professions*: There are lessons to be learnt from other professions. There are a set of principles that guide every profession. Musashi even noted that asides the Way of the Warrior, there are three other Ways through which men pass through life; they can pass as farmers, merchants or artisans. The farmer understands changes in seasons, the merchant understands how to make profit, and the artisan is proficient in the use of his tools. The importance of understanding the way of other professions is to discover the similarities and differences between our way and that of other professions. Through these similarities and differences, we can pick vital lessons that will help us understand our own way better.

For example, a soldier should understand the way of medicine; the way of the doctor. The doctor is committed to restore health and life to the body. And he does this without considering political affiliations, race or religion. He is committed to only one purpose: saving lives. This leaves a lesson for a soldier, whose commitment should be to restore peace to a broken world and also protect lives.

Understanding the way of others is not limited to professions alone; the soldier should also understand the way, character, or ideologies of other human beings. As seen earlier, the Vietnam War occurred due to conflict in ideologies between the North and South. If the conflicting parties involved had understood that their way is not the only way, that the way of another may be more beneficial, then the war would have been averted.

Dear soldier, perspective is important. Hold on to your perspectives and ideologies because they form the ideals that guide you through life, but also be flexible enough to understand (and sometimes, accept) the perspectives of others. If not for your sake, at least for the sake of world peace.

• *Distinguishing the gains and losses in every matter:* Gains and losses are relative. What constitutes a gain for one person may be a loss for another. In fact, conflicts arise because parties clamor for what will profit them. Sometimes, there are situations that look like they have no gain, but by taking a closer look and looking at the big picture, you would see the benefits hidden like a pearl covered by dust. This brings to mind the story of Desmond Doss, a United States Army corporal.

Doss was the first conscientious objector to receive the Medal of Honor—the highest, most-prestigious personal military decoration awarded to military personnel who had distinguished themselves through their valiance. Why did Doss receive this recognition?

Desmond Doss served in the US Army as a combat medic. What made him an interesting character was his refusal to handle a rifle. His superiors and fellow soldiers, confounded by this decision, decided to persecute him. After several persecutions (including an arrest and a court-martial), Doss was allowed to serve as a combat medic.

In the Battle of Okinawa, Doss was assigned to the 77th infantry Division, which had the task of securing Hacksaw Ridge. In their first attempt to secure the Ridge, the Japanese launched a massive attack which drove the Americans off the Ridge. Now, instead of Doss to escape with his fellow compatriots, he returned to the Ridge to save wounded soldiers. For 12 hours, he single-handedly carried and lowered 75 soldiers from the Ridge. It gets more interesting as he also lowered wounded Japanese soldiers, although none survived at the end.

Logically, Doss's action was unwise. The American army had been overpowered by the Japanese, so there was no need to remain on the Ridge. No gain whatsoever. Staying on the Ridge was foolhardy. But Doss decided to look at the big picture. He knew that these wounded soldiers had families who they had promised a safe return from the war. He knew that the greatest gain is that which values human life. In that moment, as the smoke from explosions and the stench of decaying bodies rent the air, all Doss could think of was saving one more life. Without handling a rifle, Doss was able to restore hope to 75 people—and to everyone around the world that has heard this story. Doss's heroics validate my earlier assertion that a soldier's duty goes beyond strategy, coordinates, and weapons.

* *Intuitive judgment and understanding for everything*: The affairs of life do not exist at the surface. When you encounter a situation, you have to critically examine and understand it before arriving at a definite conclusion. Have a holistic view about everything—factor in the perspectives of others.

Dear soldier, before you pick up your weapon and go to war, carefully evaluate the situation. *Is the war necessary? What are the major causes of the conflict? Can these causes be addressed without escalating the issue into a full-blown war?*

There is a time for war, no doubt, but make sure you understand the situation and *honestly* come to the conclusion that war is the only option left.

- *Recognizing the unseen*: Intuition and understanding everything will help you see things that are not obvious to others. Sometimes, the gains or losses of a venture do not lie on the surface; you have to uncover the nuances to see what others don't see. Just like we saw with Desmond Doss, while others felt the wounded soldiers couldn't be rescued, Doss saw that there was hope for them. It didn't matter to Doss if these soldiers were maimed, all he wanted to do was to save their lives and give them a chance to reunite with their loved ones.

- *Pay attention to details*: This is the only way to recognize the unseen. You cannot afford to be careless as a soldier. Never dismiss anything as unimportant. In his book, *Atomic Habits*, James Clear narrated how the fate of British Cycling changed because they hired a coach who was keen on details. The coach broke down cycling into different processes and started improving on each process. He redesigned bike seats, hired a surgeon to teach the riders how to wash their hands to reduce their chances of catching cold, painted the inside of the team truck white so that specks of dust wouldn't go unnoticed. All these summed up to give British Cycling a well-deserved success.[16]

In a world where conflicts abound, where violence is the default resolution to conflict, it is easy to miss out the details that would birth lasting peace. But this is why you are different, dear soldier. You are a warrior, and you are not just one because of your valiance on the battlefield, you are one because you know the Way to peace. This is a knowledge many do not have. So while others only skim the surface in moments of conflict, you have to dig deeper, scrutinize, and see what others cannot see.

Dear soldier, set these principles to your heart. Master them. Let them guide everything you do. By applying these principles, you will get a broad perspective of issues and know how to handle them as a master of peace. Musashi wrote: *If you constantly pay attention to the Way and develop the culture of hard work, you will not only master your technique but also defeat your opponent.*

Always remember that your opponent is not the next human being, but the systems that keep exploiting conflicts for gain. Contend against these systems. These systems are everywhere—from the racist police officer to the sexist filmmaker, the corrupt governor to the vile drug baron. If you can apply these principles and contend against these systems on a small scale, then you are bound to win on a large scale.

Key Point from Musashi: *In any given path, know how not to lose to others, know how to help yourself, and know how to build a reputation for yourself. This is the Way of the Warrior.*

CHAPTER TWO

WATER - *Soft As Water*

Many often think that a soldier should be one detached from his emotions. He should be stern and feared. He should only focus on war and the power he wields through his gun. Many soldiers have gone on to live according to this narrative, but this narrative is not a true definition of who a soldier should be. A soldier is like water. Water has the tangibility of solid and the fluidity of gas. Similarly, we seldom see soldiers but we know that they are working behind the scenes to keep the peace.

Water is unique. Flexible and assumes the shape of its container. Sometimes calm, sometimes turbulent especially when under the influence of pressure. Refreshing when calm; sweeps clean when turbulent.

In his Water scroll, Musashi, without directly stating it, used some of the attributes of water to guide the swordsmanship of the warrior. He outlined two main prerequisites for swordsmanship: Posture and Gaze. But before explaining these prerequisites, he taught warriors how to prepare their minds, and I have grouped his teachings into three striking points.

1. In the Way of the Warrior, the mind should not be different from the spirit of your daily life. Let your mind be always calm and upright both in your normal life and in moments of battle. Do not change, not even a little. Do not be uptight, yet do not live recklessly. Be focused and keep your mind from wavering.

What Musashi was saying in a nutshell is this: Let the soldier be calm ... just like water. For the one who must bring peace must first be at peace with himself.

2. While relaxing the mind from the environment, make sure the depth of your mind (your inner self) is strong. Do not allow others to influence your mind.

During a storm, the sea experiences sustained winds. Waves come crashing down. There are loud, continuous crackles of thunder. But beneath the ocean there is total calmness. This is what Musashi wants for a warrior. A soldier should be able to maintain calm despite the disturbances he may face. Peace is not only the absence of disturbance, sometimes, it is the ability to remain calm amid the disturbance.

3. Be open-minded. Look at things from a wide perspective, and in this vastness, cultivate wisdom.

Your mind should be as vast as the sea. Stretch out. See the perspectives of others. Understand the way of others. Reflect deeply as you do this. Know that the path to peace sometimes lies in the unseen. So you have to collect different ideas, sift them, and produce what is in the best interest of humanity.

Posture

Musashi outlined guidelines for posture or stance a warrior should take during battle. But what does posture mean for today's soldier? It means how the soldier presents himself to the world. How does the world perceive him? A savior or a villain? Does his uniform instil fear, or is it a symbol of safety? What stance does the soldier take in social issues that plague the world? Is he on the side of truth and humanity, or is he a puppet of destruction?

Musashi's guidelines for posture can be accurately applied to today's world to put the soldier on the path of peace. Here are some of his instructions:

- When you stand, your head should be straight, it should not tilt or droop or look up.

This holds a literal meaning for a protégé of Musashi, but a figurative meaning for today's soldier. Uprightness is a fundamental requirement for the soldier. You must be morally upright. You must also be

35

upright before the law. The fabric of peace is loosened at its seams by people who are not upright. And if you, as a soldier, must restore and keep peace, then you must also not be found wanting.

In the past, many soldiers have been found wanting in uprightness and that is why there is a long list of war crimes today. These crimes were not perpetrated by people or soldiers pressured by war, but by people who were already morally and ethically deficient. Some of the heinous war crimes committed in history[1] include:

- *The T4 Euthanasia Program*: In August 1939, physicians, nurses, and midwives received an order from the Reich Ministry to report infants under the age of three who appeared to suffer from severe mental or physical disabilities. Health workers suggested that parents send their children to certain pediatric clinics in Germany and Austria for treatment. On the surface this looked like a good plan, but the reality was that these children were not to be helped—but killed.

The T4 program, initiated by Adolf Hitler, gave physicians the power to determine which children were deserving of life. The Nazis justified the program saying that the funds used in treating these terminal illnesses could be channeled to "better" the lives of those who had no health condition.

Children were taken to these clinics and put into gas chambers. Their dead bodies were disposed in ovens and their ashes placed in urns, which were sent back to their families alongside a falsified account of their death.

The T4 program ran for two years—from 1939 to 1941—and it was estimated by the U.S. Holocaust Museum that at least 5,000 physically and mentally disable German children were killed.

- *Unit 731*: The details of Unit 731 are even more horrific than those of Hitler's T4 program. Between 1937 and 1945, the Imperial Japanese Army carried out deadly experiments in northeast China. These experiments were carried out on human subjects, mostly Chinese and Russians.

The experiments, started by Lieutenant-General Ishii Shiro, were carried out by a group of 3,000 researchers known as Unit 731. Shiro hoped to use the knowledge of science to make Japan a world power. The aim of these experiments was to develop new treatments for the ailments that plagued the Japanese Army.

Shiro and his team vivisected prisoners without anesthesia; injected diseases such as syphilis, anthrax, and gonorrhea into subjects; and raped female subjects to carry out tests on their fetuses. They didn't stop there: they used prisoners as targets for grenades, burned people alive, and dropped plague-carrying fleas in Chinese villages to study how fast the disease spread. It is recorded that these horrendous experiments claimed between 3,000 and 250,000 lives in a single camp.

What makes the story even more chilling is that these researchers were never tried for war crimes. And here is why: The United States, in a bid to be ahead of the Soviet Union in global weaponry, chose to give these perpetrators immunity in exchange for the information gathered during the course of the experiments.[2]

- *Congo Wars*: Aside mass murders, one significant feature of the war in Congo (which lasted from the early 1990s to 2013) was mass rape. It is reported that the rape was so widespread and routine in Congo that the United Nations decided to class rape as an instrument of war, and not a side effect.

It is recorded that up to 1.8 million women in the Congo have been raped, averaging about 48 women per hour. And what is most shocking is that there is no age limit to the women targeted, as girls as young as 18 months old to women as old as 80 have been victims. In some cases, the genitalia of these women are mutilated, while their families are forced to watch.

In many cases, these women were ganged raped by 2 to 20 soldiers who took turns over and over again.[3]

- *Camp Sumter*: Georgia's Camp Sumter was meant to hold 10,000 prisoners, but Henry Wirz, the Confederate commander of Andersonville crammed 32,000 prisoners of the U. S. civil war into the facility.

Inmates were starved since food was scarce. Sanitation conditions were deplorable as prisoners had to drink the creek water filled with the fecal matter of diseased and dying men. As a result of these, many prisoners came down with scurvy, dysentery, and diarrhea. Prisoners who weren't killed by these diseases were killed by the poorly trained guards who shot inmates indiscriminately without cause. 900 prisoners died each month at the camp, and over 12,000 died between 1861 and 1865.

When Wirz was condemned to death for war crimes, he claimed he only followed orders.

These horrific tales of war crimes show the moral bankruptcy of many soldiers. A person who was not upright before joining the army can never be upright after joining the army. There is no valid reason to waste human lives. Before the horrors of Congo, the U. N. once considered rape a side effect of war, however, it is puzzling to think about why any soldier would want to rape women in the first place. Even without war, rape is already a crime, yet soldiers go ahead to rape innocent women who have already been emotionally and psychologically disturbed by the dynamics of war.

Musashi advised that the warrior's posture must be upright and should not droop, so dear soldier, have sound moral values and stick to them. Do not be influenced by other soldiers or circumstances around you. Henry Wirz, the commander at Camp Sumter claimed he was following the orders of his superiors. And I know this raises the question: *What should a soldier do when he receives orders from a superior?*

I wouldn't ignore the fact that this is a difficult question to answer since one of the golden rules of the military is "Obey before you complain." So should the soldier obey an order that ignores the sanctity of human life? Personally, I don't think so.

The army should not be too rigid in its workflow. Rules such as "obey before you complain" paint an inappropriate image of the army. An image of undue harshness, irrationality, and inability to listen to the voice of reason. When Musashi talked about posture or stance, he wasn't only referring to the posture a warrior should take during a duel, but also to how others—especially the adversary—see the warrior. How others see the warrior depends on how the warrior positions himself. Likewise, how the army, as a body, positions itself based on its rules and regulations, determines how civilians would see them.

The soldier has a license to wield any kind of weapon, but these weapons are not toys to be used anytime the soldier wills; they are actually instruments required to restore order and bring peace to a nation and/or the world. Guns are not more powerful or valuable than human life. So before answering the question, "What should a soldier do when he receives orders from a superior?" we must first understand and accept that rigid rules that seem to enthrone the soldier's will above human life should be done away with. When this is done, the soldier can now a follow some steps towards responding to orders.

I came up with an algorithm that can guide the soldier on what to do when he receives orders from a superior(s). This algorithm may or may not be feasible, but I believe that in a world where the rights and opinions of everyone is respected, these steps would go a long way to stymie gross misconducts and horrendous actions in the military.

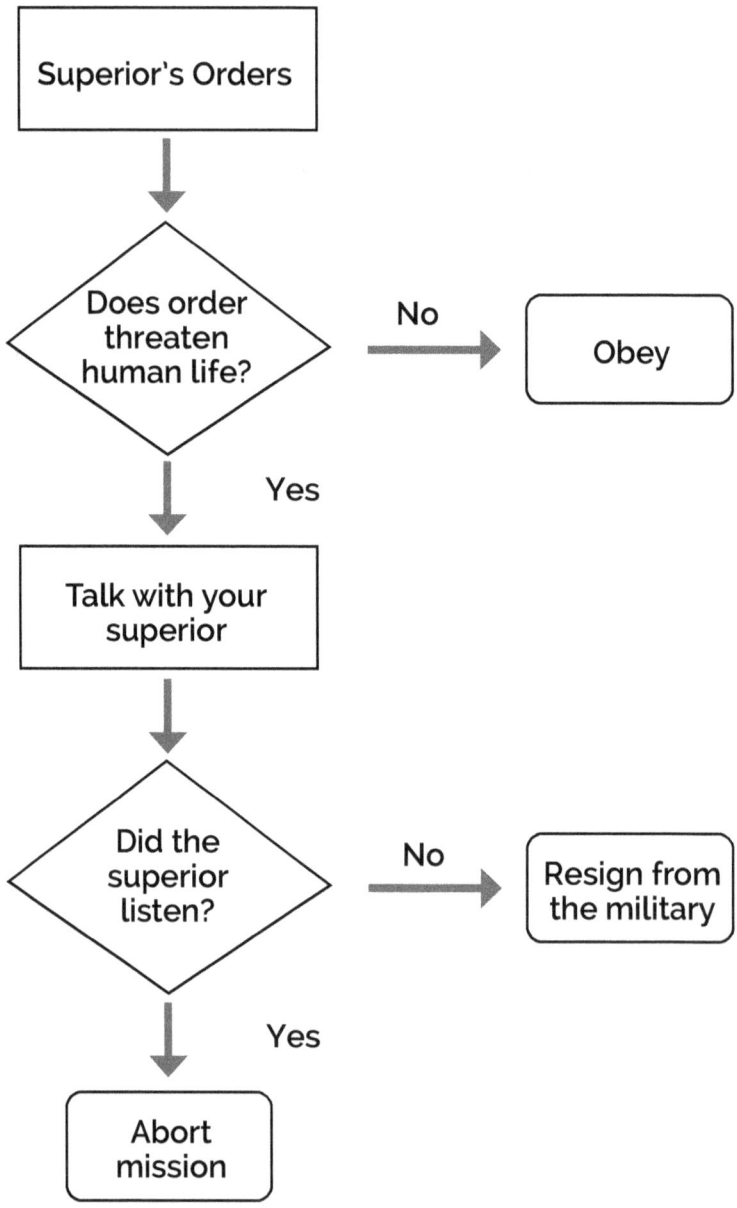

The algorithm above shows the flow of steps a junior officer should take when given an order. The flowchart is self-explanatory, but I want to buttress on some steps. Remember: These steps were developed on the assumption that the "Obey before you complain" rule is not enforced.

When you try to reason with your superior and he still insists on going on with an action that threatens human life, you have two options: either you carry out that action, or you resign from the army.

—You can decide to carry out the order because you don't want to disobey your superior, but would you be able to live with the guilt that you carried out an order that antagonizes the sanctity of human life.

What is even more ironic about obeying these orders is that sometimes, if not most, it is the junior officers that get punished, while the senior officers that gave the order escape without being brought to book. A typical case in point is the story of Henry Wirz of Camp Sumter. He said he was following orders, yet there are no records of his superiors being punished. He faced the music alone.

So dear soldier, would you be able to bear the fact that hundreds, thousands, or even millions of lives were wasted on your account? Think about this. Does the order worth more than human life or the burden of guilt on your conscience? If today's soldier considers these questions and provides honest answers to them, they will be the beacon of light that will guide the soldier through the path of peace.

—Your second option may seem tough and risky, but it is a much better one. You may be labelled a deserter, a traitor, but posterity will always remember you as a soldier who chose the value of life even at the detriment of self. I understand that what I am suggesting is uncomfortable, but sometimes, truth is discomforting. Truth is hard. But we must be on the side of truth at *all* times.

• Do not frown

Have you ever seen a samurai smile? A samurai always wears a serious look; always in a combatant mood. This is understandable, yet Musashi admonished warriors not to frown. While he did not instruct them to smile, the expressions he asked them to have would make their face pleasant to look at. And this also applies to today's soldier.

Dear soldier, you are a human being to be loved and appreciated, not a person to be feared. Being a soldier shouldn't make you lose touch with your emotions. Be friendly. Be cordial.

It was beautiful to see female army officers participate in "Don't Rush" Challenge on Tik Tok. It showed that military personnel can have fun too. And this is what it should be. The public should not perceive you as someone who is unreachable, someone who doesn't have their interest at heart. Let civilians not be gripped by fear when they see you. They are not your enemies.

- The body, from the shoulders down to the toes, is one piece

These words of Musashi apply to the army as a unit. Soldiers should understand that they are representatives of the military. Anything they do or say off the battlefield would affect, either positively or negatively, how people perceive the military.

The core function of the army is to serve the people, defend the nation, and keep the peace. Your actions or inactions as a soldier should not make the people question this purpose. The military is *one* unit, one *body*. So what you do as an individual soldier tells a lot on the entire unit. You have to position yourself rightly at all times.

Gaze

The second prerequisite for swordsmanship outlined by Musashi is gaze. For Musashi, having vision is not enough, the warrior should also know how to use his vision. He instructed warriors that their vision *must* be wide. And this applies to today's soldier too.

Dear soldier, have a holistic view of situations. Let your vision be wide just like an expanse of blue ocean. Do not be myopic. Do not give in to prejudice. When you have a broad view of a situation, you would be able to make sound decisions that would bring glory to your nation.

In chapter one, we saw the story of Desmond Doss. Doss became a lifetime hero because he had a broad view of the situation at Hacksaw Ridge. While other officers, panicky and hopeless, left the wounded to die, Doss *saw* that the wounded could be saved. While other officers thought that the only way to become a soldier is to wield a rifle, Doss proved to them and the world that lives can also be saved without a rifle.

A soldier needs to understand that many issues of life are multifaceted, thus there is no one-size-fits-all approach to solve these issues. To effectively solve these issues, the soldier must factor in all the nuances present and find out the best possible approach that would not be detrimental to humanity.

Musashi divided gaze or vision into two: Perception and Sight. He wrote: *With perception, you look to feel; with sight, you look see. Perception is strong, sight is weak.* And I agree with Musashi.

A lot of people these days have only sight without perception. Hinging on Musashi's definition, I would give two simple equations:

$$Vision + Emotion = Perception$$
$$Vision - Emotion = Sight$$

We are emotional beings and losing touch of our emotions for whatever reason would only reduce us to robotic entities. War crimes are committed by soldiers who only see but don't perceive. Sight is limited, perception is limitless. Soldiers who use the power of the gun to intimidate innocents are myopic. Cold-hearted and emotionless, these soldiers *see* only the present—the quick profit of killing for money, the instant pleasure of rape. They are so insensitive to perceive how their actions would affect their victims, how it would also cause a dent to their image as soldiers.

Dear soldier, your military trainings should toughen your physical body, not harden your heart. Be in touch with your emotions. The world does not revolve around you. Understand that a single action from you is capable of destroying millions of lives. So look at the big picture before acting. Go beyond seeing. Perceive. This is the fundamental step to peace.

Musashi also made another striking point when he wrote: *It is important in strategy that you know your opponent's sword by just looking at it.*

We have likened loyalty to the samurai's sword. So knowing your opponent's sword without looking at it means that you, as a soldier, should be able to detect where the allegiances of the enemy (or even other officers) lie. And the only way to achieve this is through perception. Through perception, you would be able to tell the intentions of the other person through his actions.

An instruction may look good on the surface, but when the soldier goes beyond seeing to perceiving, he would see the flaws and dangers in such an instruction. For instance, one may say that Lieutenant-General Ishii Shiro's objective of making Japan a world power through science was a noble one. Every country aspires to become one of the leading nations of the world, politically, economically, and socially. But a person who doesn't mind using human subjects to carry out deadly experiments does not have the interest of the world at heart.

Sight would tell a Japanese soldier that it is for the good of Japan, but Perception would say that it is not only detrimental to Japan but also to the entire world. Someone may argue that Shiro used human subjects from China and Russia, and so he wouldn't inflict harm on his countrymen. This is a shallow reasoning. A person who does not value life wouldn't hesitate to destroy lives for his selfish gains whether those lives are his countrymen or not. Or didn't Bashar al-Assad of Syria kill fellow Syrians (including children) with sarin gas?

Soldier, perception is a vital quality for you to have. Your ability to perceive the actions of another may be the only step towards saving your country from chaos. Don't be rigid with your ideas. Let your mind be as soft as water, as fluid as a stream unhindered by rocks. Recognize diverse views. Remove the extraneous. Digest them. Then mix them in the melting pot of your heart to produce a single action that would be favorable to all of humanity. After detailing posture and gaze as prerequisites of swordsmanship, Musashi also taught the warrior how to hold his sword. We are going to look at some of the instructions he gave.

• A loose grip on a sword is bad

In chapter one, we established that a sword, whether the katana or the wakizashi, represents loyalty. So here, we would interpret Musashi's words to mean that your loyalty shouldn't be shaken, no matter what. Hold tenaciously to it. Your loyalty to humanity is paramount above any personal principles or superior orders.

Let your loyalty not be bought with money or with the promise of power. A loose grip on loyalty is bad. When people notice that you do not have a firm hold on loyalty, you lose the trust of the good guys and fall into the exploitative trap of the bad guys.

So make your stand clear—that you are always for humanity. And posterity will reward and remember you forever.

- When drawing the sword, think of it only as an object to cut down an opponent. As you cut down your opponent, do not change your grip. Hold the sword in such a way that the hand is not weakened.

Dear soldier, your enemy is not your fellow human being, but the systems that keep stripping peace off the world. And your only goal should be to "cut down" these systems. Yes, in the process you may have to cut down the human beings that promote these systems, but they are not the real enemies.

In cutting down your opponent, hold tenaciously to your sword. Never change your grip. Do not be inconsistent with loyalty. Believe in humanity and be firm with this belief, for this is the only way your "hand would not be weakened."

Desmond Doss never believed in taking human life for whatever (valid) reason, and he held firmly to it. Despite being persecuted, he was resolute, knowing that the rules of the military and the tears of his wife and the pleas of his father do not supersede his belief—his value for life. And this introduces us to Musashi's next lesson: The five approaches for wielding the sword.

The Five Approaches for Wielding the Sword

For me, these five approaches do not only show the warrior where to attack the opponent, but also instructs the warrior on the possible positions where the opponent can launch an attack from. These five approaches are: the first or middle approach, second or up approach, third or down approach, fourth or left approach, and fifth or right approach.

Today's soldier needs to know that the peace he is trying to keep can be threatened through any of these approaches. And to find out how this can happen, we would have to use, again, metaphors.

The middle (first) approach signifies you, the soldier.
The up (second) approach signifies your superiors.
The down (third) approach is the opposing camp.
The left (fourth) approach is your loved ones (family and friends).
The right (fifth) approach signifies your colleagues.
So how can peace be threatened through these different individuals?

You: The Middle Approach

When you enthrone your ideologies or desires above peace, then you are a threat to peace. Although villainous military officers throughout history used their subordinates to carry out their actions, it doesn't take away the fact that these villains did not care about peace or sanctity of life. They were only concerned about their selfish and wicked desires, and because of this, the peace of the world was threatened. There are families who have been scarred for life and races (e.g., the Jews) whose history have never remained the same because of the personal interests of a person or a group of persons.

So dear soldier, understand that sometimes the enemy of peace is not outside, but within. And you can be that enemy. The only way you wouldn't be an enemy is if you always put peace and humanity first. This cannot be emphasized enough.

Superiors: The Up Approach

As we have seen in some stories shared, most of the havoc that have been wreaked on humanity by the military were instigated by senior officers. Think about it: from Adolf Hitler to Saddam Hussein to Idi Amin.

Army officers like the people mentioned above, work their way to the top so that they can have the influence to carry out their nefarious acts. They use the junior officers as pawns to fulfill their desires. Sometimes, they use force and threats to get the junior officers to do their biddings, while at other times, they persuade them through words.

Hitler, for example, was a great orator. He used his oratorical prowess to get Germans to believe that the Jews were a threat to the growth of Germany. As a matter of fact, Hitler wrote in his book, *Mein Kampf:* "I know that men are won over less by the written than by the spoken word, that every great movement on this earth owes it growth to great orators and not to great writers." And through his speeches, he got his countrymen to *hate* the Jews and almost exterminated them.

Dear soldier, threat to peace may come from your superiors. And when this happens, you have to make a decision whether to obey the last order or be on the side of humanity. I have already given you an algorithm.

The Opponent: The Down Approach

We already know that when two or more nations are in a war, they are threatening or tearing down the peace of their nations. This is one way peace can be threatened with the down approach. But another way we often do not take cognizance of is the situation where the opposing nation(s) lure the soldier of the other nation to deliberately sabotage the peace of his nation.

In chapter one, we saw examples of traitors who betrayed their nations to the enemy for fame, power, money, or all three. Soldiers do not just become saboteurs overnight. Saboteurs are individuals who already lack scruples before joining the army. And when the enemy spots them, he uses them to his advantage to carry out his vile plans.

This is the reason you ought to be upright, dear soldier. When you are morally upright, when you understand what is ethical, when you value the sanctity of human life, then you wouldn't be the weak link on the chain that holds peace.

Loved ones: The Left Approach

I used our loved ones to represent the left approach because of this: the heart, which is the center of our emotions, is at the left side of the body. The loved ones of a soldier can cajole him to disrupt the peace of the people.

There are stories of families who go about disturbing others because they feel they are untouchable since they have a family member or friend in the military. Military personnel have been used by their families or friends to intimidate other civilians.

Dear soldier, do not be part of this. Do not allow those you love to use you as a tool to disrupt the mental, physical, or emotional well-being of others. Let them know that you are in the military to serve, not to bully. Your gun is for restoring peace not for instilling fear. Remember that the soldier has to have an upright posture. Let your loved ones understand this.

Colleagues: The Right Approach

Human beings are social animals, and as behavioral science has shown, we pick many of habits from others. It is for this reason that soldiers can be and are influenced by peer pressure. Soldiers learn harmless traits from their colleagues, like drinking, looking good for the opposite sex, and buying things they don't need. Some people have even joined the military because they have friends in the military.

But just like harmless traits are learned, toxic behavior and vile actions can also be learned. If you read novels or watch movies about war, you would see that there are some soldiers who commit crimes like raping and killing innocents, not because it is in their nature to do so, but because they are cajoled by other officers and they don't want to be left out.

Dear soldier, you have to remember again the need to be upright. Through uprightness, you can distinguish right from wrong. Emulate the good. Eschew the bad. Have a firm, independent mind that cannot be pushed into doing wrong. If influence must come into play, let your colleagues be the ones that would be influenced by your (good) actions.

Now that you have seen the different approaches by which peace can be threatened, there is a salient principle Musashi taught: *Position – No Position*.

The Principle of Position No-Position

This principle is like a contradiction of the five approaches because Musashi wrote:

Position – no position means that there is no such thing as sword positions [or approaches]. *No matter the opponent's approach, the terrain, the circumstances, or sword, always have the intention of cutting down the opponent easily.*

While this looks like a contradiction, it actually is not. All Musashi was trying to say is that the warrior shouldn't be focused only on the possible approaches the opponent might use to attack, because if the warrior focuses on them alone, then there is a tendency for his swordsmanship to become rigid and mechanical. Musashi wanted the warrior to flexible—to be able to move in and out of positions, having just one aim in mind: to cut down the enemy. This is why he wrote:

When in the upper position, you can gently lower your sword and adopt the middle posture. Also, when in the middle posture, you can move up a bit and adopt the upper position. In the lower position, you could move up a bit and take up the middle position. Depending on the condition, if you are on the left or right side and you move towards the center, it basically becomes the middle or lower position.

This applies to the soldier too. Don't focus on one approach, thinking that that's the only way peace can be threatened. For instance, you may think that your superiors or opposing nation are the threats to peace, without knowing that the ones close to you are even bigger threats.

So be flexible to read the situation and block every loophole. You can counter one approach with another. Your colleagues can stand with you against the unethical orders from your superior. You, as the middle approach, can educate your loved ones on what it means to serve the nation. You can report erring officers to your superiors for disciplinary action. You can inform your superiors on the plans of the opposing nation. This is the flexibility Musashi recommended. This is position – no position.

———————

Dear soldier, be like water: flexible, yet forceful. Still, yet stretching. Water is an indispensable resource; a requirement for survival for all living things. In the same way, you are an indispensable requirement for the peace of your nation and the world at large. Water comes in diverse forms and you can take up any form: you can be the rain dousing the tensions of the world, or the flowing stream carrying the debris of intimidation and unrest, or the expansive ocean spreading peace all around your nation and the world.

Key Point from Musashi: *Have the spirit of a warrior: Today I will beat who I was yesterday, tomorrow I will defeat the less skilled, and later I will defeat the one that is more skilled.*

CHAPTER THREE

FIRE - *Fierce As Fire*

The fiery side of the soldier is what the world mainly knows. There is a time for the soldier to be fierce. And by fierceness, I don't mean being ruthless to fellow human beings, but being ruthless and resolute to your strategy to restore peace. Have aggressive strategies that would burn off the systems of chaos already planted in the world.

In Musashi's days, other schools of swordsmanship focused on maintaining distance as the best strategy. It was a logical strategy since the warrior has to keep his distance to avoid getting hit, as he looks for an opportunity to strike his adversary. However, Musashi thought and taught differently.

Musashi's strategy was to put the opponent in an awkward position to prevent him from striking. Musashi wrote that the warrior could use some elements to his favor (e.g., the environment). Or he could also make the opponent lose focus by manipulating his psychology.

The Fire scroll in *The Five Spheres* outlines 27 different techniques the warrior could use to apply Musashi's strategy. And we are going to see how today's soldier can also use 20 of these techniques to foster peace.

1. The Topography

Examine the nature of your terrain or environment

This is the first technique Musashi taught the warrior. He instructed the warrior to use his environment to his advantage. And he gave three ways the warrior could achieve this:

- *Sun shouldering*: Musashi wrote that the warrior should stand in such a way that the sun is behind him. But if that isn't possible, then he should position himself in a way that the sun is at his right side. Even if it's an indoor fight, the warrior should ensure that the fire is behind him or at his right side. The reason for this is two-pronged: the warrior would be able to see the opponent clearly, while the opponent wouldn't be able to see.

- *Looking down on the opponent*: Another instruction Musashi gave to the warrior was that he should always ensure that he stands on places that are elevated, so he could "look down on" the opponent.

- *Chasing the opponent to awkward places*: Musashi wanted his students to always chase their opponents into unfavorable terrains like thresholds, lintels, doors, verandas, pillars, and so on. As they chase them to these places, they should not also give them the opportunity to look around and adjust.

So what does this mean for a soldier?

The soldier should study the environment of the nation and/or the world. And by environment, I do not mean physical environment alone, I also mean social, economic and political environment. Systems that threaten the peace use these environments, either singly or in combination, to cause instability and division.

For instance, we saw earlier that the Vietnam War arose as a result of conflicting political ideologies. The French Revolution came as a result of socio-economic issues. The people of France revolted and overthrew the monarchy after being hit by famine, excess taxes, and financial crisis.[1]

Therefore, it is important for the soldier to understand these various elements and how they affect the peace he is trying to restore. Sometimes, restoring peace is not only through force and guns; peace can be restored when the issues affecting these environments are addressed.

So the soldier should ask himself some pertinent questions: *Are the people happy with the political or socioeconomic situation of the nation?*

Who are the actors using the political or socioeconomic conditions of the nation as a tool to disrupt the peace of the nation? How can we outwit these actors? To outwit these actors, we apply Musashi's techniques.

— First, sun shouldering. We can interpret this as blocking the loopholes that can be seen as opportunities by these actors to inject unrest. As a soldier, you can spread political consciousness among the people. Teach them that politics should be for the people and by the people. Teach them to know their rights and stand for their rights. Teach them that political parties or ideologies do not matter so long as the people aspiring into office are focused on promoting the social, economic, physical, and political wellbeing of the people. When you have a politically conscious people who know their rights, the antagonists of peace wouldn't outsmart them to promote their selfish interests. If key players in the Vietnam War had understood and agreed that the value for humanity trumps their differing political ideologies, then the war wouldn't have happened.

Also, actors could come from the angle of poverty. There are countries of the world where the people in government have intentionally made the economic climate harsh so that they can use the frustrations of people as tools for unrest. An individual who is without money, without food, and without hope would take out his frustrations on another human being. Such a person may not mind killing or maiming another under the directives of someone higher just because they've been promised a certain sum of money.

Dear soldier, try to close the economic inequality gap. Teach the people not to depend on their government to create wealth. Tell them that in this digital age, there is no excuse for not having digital skills. Mark Zuckerberg did not wait for his financial liberation from the U.S. government, neither did Jack Ma rely on the Chinese government. They got their wealth through their innovation, consistency, and hard work. Now ask yourself: *Will Mark or Jack attempt to do anything to disrupt the peace of their nation or the world, knowing that if the peace of the world is affected their businesses will also be affected?*

When you show people the need to put their innovation to work, they wouldn't have time to carry out the wicked, selfish interests of others.

— Second, look down on the opponent. At the Democratic National Convention during the campaigns of the 2016 presidential election in the United States, Michelle Obama said, "When they go low, we go high." This catchphrase is the best interpretation for Musashi's "Look down on the opponent."

As a soldier, you have to be a step higher than the enemy at every point in time. Antagonists of peace are bereft of key values that bind the world together. Values such as kindness, respect, loyalty, love, and so on. These values go together with peace, so tearing down peace also translates to tearing down these values.

When they treat you unfairly and show hatred, revenge with kindness and love. When they disrespect you, show respect. When they show disloyalty to the nation, maintain undivided loyalty both to your nation and humanity. This is not only a principle that should be in religious books, it is a principle that should be applied at all times. The world has known pain because warring parties keep fighting at the same level—a level of dirt, impunity, and utter disregard for the rule of law and human life. No one is attempting to go high, to elevate himself from the opponent.

Dear soldier, never go low. Look down on your enemy at all times. I believe that when you always remember that the real enemy is not the other soldier but failed systems, you will always be on the side of peace—the place where you would want nothing but peace even if it costs you your ideologies and desires.

— Third, chase the opponent to awkward places. This is similar to the second point. When you elevate yourself above your opponent, he immediately becomes disadvantaged as he has to stretch himself to get to you. The awkward places for the enemies of peace are the values they have lost. Fighting them with these values will leave them confused, because they wouldn't understand how you fight hatred with love, disloyalty with commitment, disrespect with respect. It is often said that two wrongs cannot make a right. You cannot fight evil with evil. Only good can overcome evil.

Another way of chasing the antagonists of peace to awkward positions is to use tools they don't understand or cannot grasp easily. For instance, recall that I said that some countries deliberately harshen the economy so that they can exploit the poverty of the people. But in this era, one can beat them to their game. How? Through information technology. Take the fight to the internet. Information technology has given people financial liberation. From Mark Zuckerberg to Jack Ma, Bill Gates to Jeff Bezos, Elon Musk to Larry Page, Jack Dorsey to Jerry Yang, Zhang Yiming to Satoshi Nakamoto.

In the internet is a world as real as our physical world. And the beauty of it is that anyone can be anything on the internet. A person does not need to go through the bureaucratic hassles associated with government policies before gaining wealth. So dear soldier, advise people to liberate themselves financially by taking advantage of tools that would be "awkward" for their oppressors.

2. The Three Initiatives

Every battle begins with one of three initiatives. Because an initiative can determine the winner from the beginning, taking an initiative is the most important thing in strategy.

Musashi outlined three initiatives to forestall the enemy:

- *Advance Initiative*: This is when the warrior takes the initiative to attack. Musashi instructed the warrior to be quick and strong outwards, but calm inwards. He advised the warrior to make the most of their mental strength.

- *Postponed Initiative*: This is when the enemy takes the initiative to attack. Musashi instructed the warrior to relax and pretend to be weak when the enemy takes the initiative to attack. Then when he attacks, the warrior can now "explode" and reveal his strength. He advised the warrior to find a loophole in the opponent's rhythm and capitalize on it to win.

- *Simultaneous Initiative:* This is when both the warrior and the enemy attack at the same time. In this initiative, the warrior does the opposite of what the enemy does. Musashi instructed the warrior to approach the opponent calmly but strongly if the enemy approaches him quickly. Then when the enemy gets to him, he can "explode" and attack. If the enemy at any time relaxes, Musashi advised the warrior to strike forcefully and take victory on the spot. If, on the other hand, the enemy approaches the warrior calmly, then the warrior should approach him quickly. Musashi made a striking point when he wrote: *When he approaches, you approach him once to test your sword, then adjust your attack according to his condition and cut violently to win.*

So what do these three initiatives mean to today's soldier?

The battle for peace is a continuous one because we live in a world with degenerated systems. This is why the soldier must first study his environment before knowing the initiative to take.

— First, the soldier can use the advance initiative. This means taking the battle to the antagonists of peace. How does he do this? The primary way to do this is by disrupting the systems that have been established to take away peace from the nation or the world. I have mentioned earlier how the soldier can promote political and socio-economic growth among his people. By doing that, he is launching the attack before the enemy does.

— Second, he can use the postponed initiative. Here, he waits for the antagonists of peace to deal all their cards. He observes them and their actions. This can take months to years. He watches their strategy, how they build their systems. Then when he has gotten all the information he needs, he can now attack.

Now this does not mean that the soldier would fold his arms doing nothing, as he watches the antagonists succeed in taking peace out of the nation—or the world. In a duel, a samurai does not watch and does nothing as he is being attacked; he would definitely defend himself. So, in the same way, as the antagonists attack first, the soldier must defend and/or attack till he wins.

— Third, he can use the simultaneous initiative. And this is the initiative I prefer for the soldier. Personally, I think a lot has gone wrong with the world for the soldier to waste any more time. Therefore, he has attack just as the enemy is attacking too. The antagonists of peace are *continuously* planning on ways to disrupt law and order for their benefit, and unfortunately, they have the economic and political power to do so. This means that the soldier has to be smart in order to outwit them. When they attack strongly, relax so they cannot predict your next move. When they relax thinking you cannot do anything, then you attack. And always remember to adjust your move according to their condition. If the simultaneous initiative is to be summed up in two words, it is this: *be unpredictable.*

3. Pressing Down A Pillow

Don't allow the opponent to lift his head

A samurai should not allow his opponent to lift his head during combat. Musashi noted that it is bad for the warrior to let his opponent move him around and place him on the defensive. It should be the other way round. Musashi also advised the warrior not to get distracted because the opponent would also have the same intention of attack. Musashi wrote: *In strategy, you must stop the opponent before he attacks, strike the opponent before he hits, and pull the opponent out of his strategy before he can strike you back.* When the warrior understands the Way of pressing down the pillow, then he will be able to predict the next move of the opponent—and stop it.

Musashi knew that the opponent may likely want to use the same technique against the warrior, so he instructed the warrior to allow the opponent to do the useless things and not allow him to do anything useful. This is an important element in strategy.

Although pressing down the pillow is a useful technique for the warrior, Musashi noted that using the technique continually puts the warrior on the defensive.

How does this apply to the soldier?

The soldier should be able to predict the moves of the antagonists of peace. In today's world it is even easy to predict what the antagonists would do. Throughout history, we have seen the same systems of oppression, division, impunity, and disregard for human life play out across different countries. So, there is nothing new.

Today's soldier already knows the angle the antagonists can attack from. As we saw earlier, they can either attack from political sentiments, social issues, or economic climate. Knowing this, the soldier can help forestall this attack by nipping these issues in the bud. And I have already stated ways in which this can be done.

But just like Musashi noted, pressing down the pillow continually puts you on the defensive. It is said that attack is best form of defense. This means that when you keep defending you are (indirectly) attacking—and showing the enemy all your moves. In plain words, you are giving them the upper hand. So do not use the technique of pressing down the pillow as your only strategy.

4. Crossing the Ford

When you are striving towards a goal, have the same determination as you are "crossing the ford"

To explain this technique, Musashi likened the warrior to a sailor. Crossing the ford means setting sail even when the sailor's friends choose to remain in the harbor. It means knowing the route, knowing the integrity of the ship, and knowing the wind. When the sailor has understood all these, he can now set sail. And if the wind changes few miles to his destination, he must cover the remaining distance with his oars.

It is the same for the warrior: he must understand his strong points and discern the enemy's capability, then "cross the ford" at an advantageous point. Musashi defined crossing the ford as attacking the enemy's weak point and gaining the advantage.

What does this mean for a soldier?

The most important lesson I want the soldier to get from this is this: *When you are striving towards a goal, have the same determination as you are "crossing the ford."* Determination is the operative word. The fight to restore is peace is a tough one. The enemy is not relenting. And there are times when you'd feel like giving up because you think your efforts are fruitless. But that is not true.

Before setting out on this journey to restore peace, you've already counted the cost. You knew that the orchestrators of chaos are ruthless in their dealings. So never be deterred. Fight their ruthlessness with your fierceness.

Try to get your colleagues or friends or family along in this fight, but if they choose to remain at the harbor, let them be. Don't allow them to discourage you. For love of country, for love of humanity—

this should be your motto. As long as you don't get discouraged, the enemy will definitely get weakened, then you can take your victory.

5. Understanding the Situation

Perceive the enemy's weakness and strength

Musashi wrote that before going to a battle, it is important to understand the intentions of the enemy including his terrain and dispositions. The warrior should also understand the adjustments to the enemy's rhythm and know how to seize the advantage. Then he should use all the information gathered to his advantage to counter all the actions of the enemy. To be able do this effectively, you should have a high intellectual capacity.

Throughout this book, I have emphasized the need for studying all the moves of the enemy. I have also given methods on how this can be done. But in this technique, Musashi made an important point. He stated that the warrior needs to have a high intellectual capacity to be able to understand the situation. And I agree.

Dear soldier, stretch your intellectual capacity through reading. In books lie vital clues for liberation and peace. The antagonists of peace across the world have used similar strategies to carry out their plans. Fortunately, these strategies have been documented in numerous books. And to win the battle, you must read. It is interesting to note that these antagonists know the power of and in books, and they go ahead to try and stop people from reading. For instance, there are countries where history has been scrapped from their academic curriculum. Another example that easily comes to mind is the Nazi book burning of 1933. An event German poet, Henrich Heine saw coming more than hundred years earlier when he wrote in 1821: "Where books are burned, in the end people will be burned."

From May 10, 1933, Nazi-dominated student groups started the public burning of books they tagged "un-German." These books included works from Jewish, liberal, and leftist writers. Over 25,000 volumes were destroyed in the bonfire. Targeted authors included socialists like Bertolt Brecht and August Babel; founder of the concept of communism, Karl Marx; critics like Arthur Schnitzler, an Austrian playwright; and authors they called "corrupting foreign influences" like Ernest Hemingway.[2]

The antagonists of peace know the power in the written word. In a short film by the United States Holocaust Memorial Museum[3], Azar Nafisi, the author of *Reading Lolita in Tehran* said: "Books represent humanity at its best and its worst. [And] The first thing every totalitarian regime does along with confiscation and mutilation of reality, is confiscation of history and confiscation of culture. I think they both happen almost simultaneously."

Ruth Franklin, a literary critic and contributing editor in *The New Republic*, gave a reason why totalitarian regimes do this. She said: "All literature is dangerous to a regime that fears the free flow of ideas because the literature, in its most fundamental way, is meant to forge connections among human beings." And this fear is triggered by the unpredictability of literature, just like author Nafisi rightly noted. ". . . You don't know where it takes you. Knowledge is always unpredictable; there is always a risk. It is like Alice jumping down that hole, running after that white rabbit, not knowing where she goes. And for tyrants, control is the main thing. They don't like this unpredictability, they don't want the citizens to connect to the unknown parts of themselves, of their past, and to connect to the world," she said.

Corroborating Nafisi's words, Franklin added that, ". . . these [totalitarian] regimes are predicated on the idea that the people within them will resign themselves to thinking that this is all there is. And that there aren't any other options."

So dear soldier, you have to defeat the aim of the antagonists of peace. There are other options. War, murders, and the gross undervaluation of human life aren't the only way. There are a lot of options "hidden" within books. In books, you will learn the operations of these antagonists. You will see the world in all its entirety. You will see and piece together the puzzle of humanity. In books, you will see what is meant to be, and what ought not to be.

6. The Collapse

Everything has the tendency to collapse

Musashi wrote: "Everything has the tendency to collapse. A house can collapse, a body can collapse, and an enemy can collapse when the time comes and their rhythm becomes chaotic."

He went further to instruct the warrior to be observant and notice when the enemy falters and begins to collapse. This is the point the warrior can claim victory. If the warrior allows the moment to slip away, the enemy may recover and become defensive thereafter.

In this moment of collapse, Musashi advised the warrior to be direct and vigorous with his attack. "Smash the enemy to pieces so that he cannot recover," he wrote.

What does this mean for the soldier?

Musashi noted that everything has a tendency to collapse. And this is true. However, I would like to add that there are three things that can cause an entity to collapse.

- *Faulty foundation*: A house with a faulty foundation would definitely collapse. A person with a congenital heart condition would collapse.

- *Age*: An old house would likely collapse. People also collapse when they become old.

- *Pressure*: An excavator or a storm can collapse a house. A person can also collapse if they are hit.

Now when it comes to fighting the antagonists the peace, you must understand that their ideologies aren't built on a faulty foundation. This is why it has lasted for decades. So, the soldier cannot hope that these ideologies would collapse because of a faulty foundation. That is impossible.

We cannot also rely on age. The solidity of these ideologies and the consequent indoctrination that follows have made these ideologies to persist for a long time. Thus, the soldier cannot also hope that these ideologies would wane as time goes by.

The only thing left for the soldier is pressure. Attack. The antagonists may be rigid and resolute in their ideologies and actions, but as you attack, as you keep up with the pressure, a time will come when they will falter and begin to collapse. Be observant to recognize this moment and ensure you take victory at this point. Musashi called it "smashing into debris"—breaking the enemy to a point where recovery is impossible.

7. Becoming the Enemy

The one trapped in the house is a pheasant and the one who comes in to cut him down is a hawk

This technique is simple, but Musashi adds to it a layer of depth. He said bandits are often considered powerful when they are trapped in a house during a robbery. But if one puts oneself in the position of a bandit, then one would discover that the bandit is actually weak. Trapped in a house, the bandit feels that the world is against them; he feels desperate and hopeless. At that point he is a pheasant and the one after him, a hawk.

Musashi noted that when the warrior feels that the enemy is strong, he would always find it difficult to attack. But when the warrior thinks of himself as the enemy, he would be able to predict the mental and emotional dispositions of the enemy and discover the most effective point to hit him.

What does this mean for the soldier?

Dear soldier, do what the antagonists failed to do. The world is in this state today because the enemies of peace have never tried to see themselves as the people they were suppressing. They have never asked themselves how their actions or inactions would affect their nation or the world. They have zero empathy. And that is why the world is a torn fabric of chaos.

Soldier, you have to see yourself as the enemy, not to act like them, but to know their weak points. When you put yourself in the position of the enemy, you would realize that they aren't as strong as you feared. You would be able to know their next move, possible mistakes, thought patterns, and expectations. With these information, you can then formulate an effective plan for attack.

8. Releasing Four Hands

If you think there is going to be a deadlock, give up your intention immediately and use some other advantageous tactics to win

A situation may arise during a duel or a battle where both the warrior and his opponent have the same intentions and when this hap-

THE GAME CHANGERS SERIES

pens, the fight becomes a deadlock. This is the spirit of "four hands." In such a situation, Musashi instructed the warrior to give up the intention and try another advantageous tactic. The warrior should not advance at this point, rather he should re-strategize and achieve victory using tactics that the enemy cannot think of.

Dear soldier, in this fight to restore peace, there are times when it would look like you have dealt all your cards yet you are not winning, and the enemy is not winning too. Don't keep trying out the same things over and over again, expecting a different result. Break the deadlock. Analyze the situation and then come back with a better strategy. Don't get attached to one strategy. Be flexible enough to move in and out of strategies depending on the prevailing circumstances. This is the only way you can be ahead of the enemy.

9. Moving the Shade

Reveal the enemy's intentions and you will instantly realize where your advantage lies

There are situations where the warrior wouldn't know the true intentions of the enemy because his sword is either by his side or behind him. This is because the enemy "shades" his intentions. To uncover the intentions of the enemy, Musashi recommended that the warrior "moves the shade." What this means is that the warrior should act as if he wants to launch an attack. This will ruffle the enemy and then his true intentions would be known. When the warrior moves the shade, he not only uncovers the enemy's intention, but also realizes the advantage he, the warrior, has. At this point, the warrior should never let his guard down, else the opportunity would slip away.

How does this apply to a soldier?

I have observed that the antagonists of peace are smart. They seldom reveal their true intentions so that they can make the people believe that they have nothing to worry about. In the short film by the United States Holocaust Memorial Museum, Robert Behr, one of the survivors of the concentration camp, said that there were warning signs, but people like his mother never took them seriously. He said he remembers asking his mother if they should be worried about Hitler but she said to him, "No. We are living in a democracy. We have the protection of the police. Nobody's going to hurt us." But in the end, they were arrested and sent to a concentration camp.[4]

In times when you cannot accurately tell what the plans of the enemy are, feint an attack. If the antagonists of peace have bad intentions, they would retaliate, even in a more brutal manner. But if they have good intentions, they will most likely ask why the attack happened and assure you that they mean no harm.

For a soldier, skepticism is a gift, so you may also think that their call for dialog and explanation is a ploy to get you to relax before they strike. True, that is possible. However, you have to remember that the antagonists do not value life. Surprising them with an attack would definitely ruffle them and they would have no choice but to show what they were planning all along. They would have no time to think about any more strategy. They would also think that one way or another you may have been privy to their plans, so they'd need to launch an attack before it is too late. This moment of unsettlement and destabilization is the right time to launch your real attack and finish them off.

10. The Contagious

To weaken your opponent, infect him…

Musashi wrote that many things are contagious. Drowsiness is contagious, yawning is contagious, even time is contagious. The warrior can get his enemy to a disadvantaged position by transferring his own disposition to him.

For instance, if the warrior notices that the enemy is agitated, the warrior can remain calm, and when the enemy sees this calmness, he would also relax and his will to attack would be dampened. This is the point where the warrior strikes. As a final admonition, Musashi wrote: *To weaken your opponent, infect him with a melancholic feeling, then hopelessness, and lastly weakness.*

So how does a soldier infect the enemies of peace?

The soldier can do this in two ways. It is either he infects the enemy with the true ideology that should govern living, or he infects them with a false strategy.

The first can be done through dialog. The soldier can educate these antagonists on the need for peace. He would teach them the workings of peace and how it is beneficial to all. However, I must admit that infecting the antagonists of peace with this ideology is nearly impossible. They know what peace is, but since they want to profit from chaos, they would rather hinder peace from thriving.

In 2020, there have been demonstrations across continents of the world—from Europe to Asia to Africa. These demonstrations arise because of maladministration and also the deliberate attempt to undermine the value of human life and, consequently, stifle human rights. For example, in Philippines, the anti-terrorism bill was signed into law by the president. Hearing "anti-terrorism," one would think that the law is actually harmless and geared towards protecting Filipinos, but that is not the case. The law stifles the rights of the average Filipino. A part of the law states that suspects could be jailed without charge for weeks. It also classifies terrorism as "engaging in acts intended to endanger a person's life," intended to "damage public property" or "interfere with critical infrastructure," where the purpose is to intimidate the government. With this law, citizens no longer have the right to protest against bad governance. However, the law states that it does not intend to punish advocacy, protest, dissent, industrial action and strikes, so long as they don't create "a serious risk to public safety."[5] But only the government can define what constitutes a risk to public safety and what does not.

Now a government that passes such a law does not have the interest of the people at heart. It is a law that can be taken advantage of to harm even those that promulgated it. It has been noted that the government that signed this law has a "poor human rights record,"[6] so how can such a government understand the language of the peace. Because of situations like this, the best thing to do is to infect the antagonists with a false strategy.

When you know that the enemies of peace are on their toes, draw back and relax. Make them feel like they have succeeded in scaring you away. Make them relax. Make them consider you as weak and insignificant. Make them underestimate you. When they have done this, then you hit them with everything you have got. Their greatest weapon is oppressing and suppressing the people. However, if you can get the people to rise and speak up for themselves, then you would leave the enemies of peace confused. And therein lies Musashi's next technique.

11. The Confused Opponent

There is confusion in everything

According to Musashi, there are three situations where the enemy can become confused: (1) when he senses danger, (2) when he senses failure, and (3) when he is surprised. Musashi advised the warrior to put his opponent in a state of mental turmoil and should not allow him recover from it. He told the warrior to attack when the enemy least expects without giving him time to think or strategize. As the enemy thinks of his next move, the warrior should take advantage of the situation and win.

Dear soldier, spring the element of surprise on the enemies of peace. Let them see that they are failing. Let them also see the danger in their failure. This would get them confused. With confusion comes panic. And when they panic, you can capitalize on their mistakes to gain victory.

12. To Frighten

People are frightened by the things that they never expected to happen

For Musashi, fright is commonplace and the utmost aim of the warrior is to frighten is opponent. The warrior can frighten the opponent with his *body*, *sword*, or *voice*. When the opponent becomes frightened, the warrior can take advantage of the fear and instability.

How does this apply to today's soldier?

Through observation, I have discovered that the enemies of peace keep eroding systems that promote peace because they think the people weak. But when the people would finally arise, the enemies of peace would become frightened. Therefore, just as Musashi said, aim to frighten your enemy.

You can *frighten them with your sword*. In this book we have explained that the sword is a metaphor for loyalty. The enemies of peace are often stereotypical, so they may think that they could easily buy your allegiance. But *never* let this happen. Let them know that your allegiance is on the side of truth, and because of that you are going to employ the two other ways to make them afraid.

Frighten them with your body. Remember earlier, I advised you to liberate the minds of people by educating them on the tenets of peace and why they should demand peace. When you have done that, you would have a large body of people who would never rest until the atmosphere for peace has been created or restored. With this body of people, the last method of making the enemy afraid can now be employed.

Frighten them with your voice. Do not lose your voice for whatever reason. Let your voice be loud. Let it resonate to the ends of the earth. The enemies of peace are always against those who speak the truth. This is why military dictators arrest or even murder journalists, writers, activists, and everyone who is bold enough to speak. But that should not discourage you. As long as your voice remains loud, the enemy would become frightened. Your voice should be heard on the streets, on social media, in newspapers, in media houses. Every platform you have, gives you the opportunity to speak out. Because a loud voice can attract allies, never allow the enemy mute your voice.

13. Soaking in

If you separate yourself from the opponent, you will not win

This is like a situation of "four hands," but instead of withdrawing and re-strategizing, Musashi told the warrior to "soak in" or merge with the enemy. Unlike other techniques where Musashi gave the warrior definite ways to take advantage and win, here, he told the warrior to understand the situation and figure out how to take victory through it.

So, what does this mean for the soldier in his fight for peace?

There are times when the soldier would have to blend in. You would have to do this not because you've been bought over, but because you actually want to know the plans of the enemy. In these times, you would be a Trojan horse. Soak into the enemy. Absorb into their systems. Know how they work. See their strengths and weaknesses. Then use this information to strategize how to create an atmosphere for peace.

14. The Hurting Corners

It is difficult to move strong things by pushing directly, so you have to "hurt the corners"

Here, Musashi recommended that the enemy should be weakened from "the corners." According to him, if the corners are overthrown, the whole body will also be overthrown.

Today's soldier can also apply the same technique. Sometimes, you don't win by hitting directly. You have to be patient to get your ultimate goal. Weakening the corners is like gaining small victories. For instance, your ultimate goal is to achieve peace. However, knowing that the enemy wouldn't grant this easily, you can weaken the corners by establishing other needs like respect for human rights, sound education, and so on. Individually, these are not the ultimate goal, but collectively, they sum up to it. If the enemy starts to respect human rights, it will give people the confidence to demand for changes in the society that affect their peace. In the same vein, a sound education broadens the mind of people to know how they have been exploited, and since knowledge is the first step to freedom, these people would also start clamoring for a change.

So dear soldier, when you cannot hit the enemy directly, chip away the corners of his structure until all of it crumbles.

15. The Three Shouts

Voice is a quality of life

Musashi stated that there are three times a warrior can shout in a fight: *before*, *during*, and *after*. Before the fight, the warrior shouts as loudly as he can. During the fight, his voice is low-pitched. After the fight, he gives a shout of victory. Shouting is important because voice is a quality of life. It shows strength.

In the 12th technique, "To frighten," I have already stated the importance of not being silent as the soldier fights for peace. However, I would like to add a salient point: Many shout when they are not supposed to. The shout of victory should be reserved till the end of the fight. So, what this means in essence dear warrior, is that do not celebrate early. Ensure you have totally defeated the enemy before giving a shout of victory. Giving a shout when the battle is not over may cause your allies to withdraw because they think the battle is over. Do not give a shout a victory when the fight has not even started. Claim your victory, then shout.

16. The Mountain-Sea Transformation

It is bad to repeat an action in the midst of a battle with an enemy

This technique can be summed up into Albert Einstein's words: "The definition of insanity is doing the same thing over and over again and expecting a different result." Musashi told the warrior never to repeat the same move during a battle. Although, there are times when the warrior can repeat a move twice, Musashi noted that it is totally bad to repeat it the third time.

When the warrior launches an attack on the enemy and it fails, then he should try out a different approach. Musashi summarized this technique thus: *When the opponent thinks of the "mountain" then you attack with "sea." But if he thinks of the "sea" then you attack with the "mountain."*

Dear soldier, be strategic in your actions. Don't keep doing the same things that do not work. The absence of peace we experience now in different continents of the world have persisted for centuries. If the world still experiences it, it means that those who had attempted to solve this situation were doing the same things that have never worked.

I think in restoring peace, many have only focused on cutting off the rotting branches instead of uprooting the entire tree. As long as the root is still buried beneath the earth, new branches would still be corrupted. Just as I mentioned in chapter one, the absence of peace is simply a product of the total disregard for the sanctity and value of life. This is the root of the problem. So, all your actions, dear soldier,

69

should be geared towards solving this problem. And this leads to the next technique of Musashi.

17. Pulling the Bottom Out

You have to silence the enemy's spirit by pulling his heart out from below...

All Musashi was saying here is: deal with the root. He advised the warrior to ensure that the enemy is not only defeated at the surface but that his spirit is also defeated, because if the enemy is defeated only at the surface, he may recover. The warrior has to silence the spirit of the enemy for only then can the enemy be *completely* defeated.

I have already discussed dealing with the problem from the root. The antagonists of peace keep transferring their ideology from generation to generation. So, to ensure that this issue does not keep sprouting up from generation to generation, it has to be defeated from the roots. The minds of many need reorientation. People need to be given new perspectives. And dear soldier, this is your duty.

18. To Renew

When there is no resolution, change your perspective

This tactic is similar to "releasing four hands." It is used when the fight between the warrior and his opponent is unresolved. Musashi advised the warrior to step back, think about the situation in a different perspective, then win with a fresh rhythm. *Without changing the circumstance*, the warrior should change his spirit and win through a different technique.

The difference between "renew" and "releasing four hands" is that while the latter requires that the warrior changes his strategy immediately, the former requires that the warrior steps back a bit and think of a new move.

As a soldier, stick to your cause at all times. But when it looks like there is no resolution in sight, step back a bit, look at the situation from a fresh perspective, then launch a new attack. Check what you are doing wrong. Then readjust. The sole aim is to win, so withdrawing for a while to plan and renew your strength is necessary.

19. The Rat Head – Ox Neck

Whenever you become preoccupied with small details, remember that the Way of the Warrior is always a "rat head – ox neck, rat head – ox neck"

This technique is used when the warrior and the opponent focus on minor details and become confused. Musashi noted that when this happens, the warrior should focus on the important details.

Dear soldier, never be distracted. In the fight for peace, there would be issues planted by the enemy to take your attention off the fight. But be smart to understand this. Always redirect your focus to the important matters. Never allow yourself to be distracted.

20. The Body of a Rock

You have the body of a rock when you attain the Way of the Warrior

This is a culmination of all the techniques above. Musashi wrote that when the warrior masters the Way of Strategy, his body becomes like a rock—nothing can touch him, he cannot be moved.

Dear soldier, be steadfast. Be resilient. Never give up this fight. Use all the tactics mentioned above to transform yourself into a rock. The enemies of peace shouldn't win. And this can only happen if you never give up.

Dear soldier, you are a rock, you are light. Be fierce as fire.

Key Point from Musashi: *The true Way in terms of swordsmanship means fighting with the opponent and winning. This is not replaceable.*

CHAPTER FOUR

WIND - *Enigmatic as the Wind*

As the wind blows, it sweeps everything that is not firm away. Sometimes, it has the power to uproot firm things like trees, pillars, and houses. The wind is that powerful. It is also enigmatic because one cannot tell where it is coming from or where it is going to. All we know is that it just blows and moves and signifies the advent of something refreshing: rain.

In Musashi's Wind scroll, he criticized the ways of other schools of swordsmanship. Like the wind, his own Way swept away the doctrines of other schools because they had no solid foundation and did not lead to victory. Musashi's Way did lead to victory. After all, he was undefeated in all his duels, including those he fought with samurais from other schools.

To introduce his Way to the warrior, he needed to first puncture holes in the ways of other schools, not because he just wanted to be a critic, but because he knew that there were flaws in those ways.

This is the same thing you should do as a soldier. Before now, there have been individuals and groups who have sought peace, yet failed because they didn't do it the right way. Therefore, it is not enough for me to present a new way to the soldier without also showing why other paths to peace did not or will not work.

The soldier on *this* path of peace is an enigma. His path is different. It is not a path other have treaded. And in this chapter, based on Musashi's ideas, I am going to show the soldier how this path differs from the previous paths to peace.

1. The Extra-Long Swords of Other Sects

Depending on the length of a sword for victory shows a weakness of spirit

Musashi talked about schools of swordsmanship that had a predilection for extra-long swords. He considered them weak schools who depended on the length of their sword to defeat the enemy from a distance. According to him, their mantra was, "More than an inch gives an advantage." But for Musashi, this mantra showed that they did not understand strategy and were unable to grasp its principles.

So what does an extra-long sword mean when it comes to seeking peace?

Recall that we defined a sword as loyalty. This means that when we talk about an extra-long sword, we are talking about being loyal to other people or groups besides your nation or humanity. There are people who believe that they cannot restore peace if they do not show loyalty or fraternize with certain sacred cows. These people feel that they do not have the resources to fight for peace, thus they need extra hands. They want to pass the bulk of the fight to others while they watch from a distance, waiting to take the glory.

There is nothing wrong in seeking allies as you fight for peace, but make sure your allies are those who are also loyal to the nation or humanity. Make sure they are people who want the same thing you want. Because if they are not *truly* on your side, then they would foil your plans to attain peace.

This is why Musashi raised an important point when he said: *If the enemy is close, like so close that you can grapple him, a long sword would make it difficult for you to cut him. The sword becomes useless. You are restricted by the sword and even worse than a person with a short sword or someone without a weapon.*

Musashi's words mean that if there is a situation where you are close to defeating the enemy, it is possible that the extra allies you have would draw you back if they have an interest different from yours. Your loyalty shouldn't be scattered in different places at the same time. Those you are loyal to may have interests far different from yours, and may only feign support for you for a short time.

Your loyalty is to your nation and to humanity. And that is enough. Being loyal to your nation and humanity should drive all your actions and guide your strategy. Don't ever think that you cannot win alone or with a small group of people who share your ideologies. Even Musashi asked: *Without carrying a* [extra] *long sword, would someone with a short sword lose?* Not at all. It is a matter of strategy, not the sword.

Musashi also noted that an extra-long sword is useless to someone who is physically weak. So if you don't have the mental, emotional and maybe, physical strength to fight for peace, having extra allies won't help you. The duty lies squarely on your shoulder. Don't pass the job to others.

2. The Strong Long Swords of Other Sects

Trying to swing a sword strongly is a bad thing, and it is difficult to win with such a rough technique

Musashi stated that in swordsmanship, there should be no such thing as a "strong sword" or a "weak sword." Swinging a sword forcefully is bad, and when the warrior tries to cut the enemy too hard because he feels he has a "strong sword" then he would likely fail. Musashi also noted that it is wrong to cut forcefully when the warrior is testing his sword.

All the warriors should think about is cutting down the enemy. He shouldn't cut too strongly, neither should he cut too weakly. He should apply only the right force to defeat the opponent. If the warrior strikes too hard, there is a tendency he may shatter his own sword.

So what does this mean on the soldier's path to peace?

What Musashi was saying was that just like the warrior shouldn't depend on the length of his sword for victory, he shouldn't also depend on the strength of his sword. For the soldier, this means that he should not be too overconfident. There are those who had rubbished their efforts in bringing peace because they felt they were so strong. They became hot-headed and unwilling to listen and reason. They felt that their loyalty to the cause superseded that of every other person. At a point, they became unable to separate their personal desires and egos from the fight for peace. And because of this, they never even realized the moments when they should have taken victory.

The soldier shouldn't also consider his loyalty to be weak. If he does this, he automatically loses the fight. Any challenge from the enemy can get him to run away from the fight.

So dear soldier, your victory does not and should not depend on how strong you feel you are. Your ego should not be placed before your fight for peace. The strength of your loyalty does not lie on how rigid you are to what you believe in, but in how discerning you are to recognize what action(s) would foster peace. We have already seen in the Water scroll the importance of being flexible. So let your mind be always on the goal.

3. The Short Sword of Other Sects

The thought of winning using a short sword is not the true Way. Long and short swords have been clearly explained in ancient times. But they do not matter, all that matters is taking advantage of the situation

Just like some schools depend on long swords for victory, Musashi noted that there were other schools that depended on a short sword. Samurais of these schools used the short sword with the aim of jumping in and catching the enemy off guard. However, Musashi stated that aiming for the enemy's unguarded moment is a defensive strategy that cannot be used when the enemy is close or when the warrior is surrounded by many rivals.

There are people who have fought for peace and thought they could handle the fight alone. They sprang up from nowhere trying to catch the enemies of peace off guard. And that is a poor strategy, because these enemies have all the resources to stifle the voice of an opposition.

This is why the soldier must strike a balance. On this path of peace, you don't journey alone, yet you do not journey with everyone. Allies are needed. But ensure that your allies are loyal *solely* to the cause. This is the only way to victory.

4. The Sword Techniques of Other Sects

When it comes to cutting down a person, there is no special way to do that

Musashi had a problem with other sects that invented a lot of techniques and taught them to their students without first teaching the students the true Way of the warrior. By doing this, they turned swordsmanship into a commodity for sale. The students went about feeling they knew all there was to swordsmanship, while in truth, they knew nothing.

For Musashi, victory goes beyond techniques. He noted that there is no special way to cut the opponent down. *Whether someone is knowledgeable or ignorant, whether it is a woman or a child attacking, all it takes is stabbing or cutting... The way to win is to cut first, and not pay attention to small details.*

Just like in Musashi's time, there are people who have developed their own techniques for attaining peace. They transfer these ideologies to people who don't understand what the fight for peace is all about. They just champion a cause because they see others doing so. At other times, they join the movement because of what they think they would benefit. They fail to understand that the fight is to uproot every element that is limiting the peace of the nation or the world.

A perfect example of this is seen in Colum McCann's novel, *Apeirogon*. The book, mostly based on true accounts, explores the conflict in the Middle East between Palestine and Israel as it relates to two fathers: Bassam Aramin; a Palestinian, and Rami Elhanan; an Israeli. Aramin lost his daughter, Abir when she was shot in the head by an Israeli soldier in 2007; while Elhanan lost his daughter, Smadar in 1997 in a suicide bombing attack carried out by Palestinians.

United by a common pain, these men have been touring the world to propagate peace. They have been in many interviews and delivered a lot of speeches and have passed same message all the time: peace. But there is a place where the story of these men relates to what Musashi said about the techniques of other schools.

Elhanan said that many of his countrymen turned against him because he refused to follow their path of retaliation. He said: "I have been called many things, an insect, an Arab lover, a self-hating Jew. They say I am naïve, self-righteous…"[1] Despite this, he remained resolute to what was right. He knew that revenge wouldn't bring the peace Israel needed, the peace he needed. He just wanted the path that led to peace and that's why he said: "If I had found another path, I would have taken it—I don't know, revenge, cynicism, hatred, murder. But I am a Jew. I have great love for my culture and my people and I know that ruling and oppressing and occupying is not Jewish. Being Jewish means that you respect justice and fairness."[2]

Elhanan's words are in line with the principles outlined in this book. The path of peace remains the same, no matter the circumstances. The enemy is not the other human being, but the systems of injustice that have been solidly rooted in the world.

In Musashi's strategy, all it takes for the warrior to win is to make his posture and spirit straight, and also make his opponent weak and fall. In the same way, the soldier should be upright in every way. He should weaken all the actions of the enemy with the deeds of justice, fairness, equality, and value for human life.

5. The Special Sword Positions of Other Sects

The only time to use the "defensive" position is when there is really no opponent

Musashi noted that other schools taught special positions to their students. The positions taught were mainly defensive positions, and Musashi didn't feel it was right. According to him, these positions were drawn from long standing customs and codified into rules, so they had no place in a one-on-one combat. In addition, a defensive stance meant trying to use immobility to one's advantage, and that's not a good trait of a warrior.

The warrior should always take the initiative—he should be proactive. A defensive stance means that the warrior is waiting for others to take the initiative, but this shouldn't be. This was why UAR lost to Israel in 1967, and Western Europe lost to Germany in 1940 just as we saw in chapter one. The UAR and Western Europe allowed the enemy to take the initiative. They were waiting for an attack; they were on the defensive. And by being on the defensive, they gave the enemy the power to control the narrative, to put the odds in their favor. This was the reason Hitler could postpone the attack on Western Europe 29 times in six months. And it is surprising to think that in all those times, Western Europe never thought about launching an attack. They just relaxed, waiting, and dismissing every warning as a false alarm. That is not the true Way of the warrior. A warrior is not careless. A warrior is attentive to details. A warrior understands timing. This is why Musashi told the warrior to: *Do things that the enemy cannot imagine—confuse the enemy, disturb the enemy, or threaten the enemy in order to catch him when his rhythm wavers.*

There are people who claim they want peace, yet they do not take the initiative. They would rather sit still and watch others do the job, then come out to claim the glory. In *Apeirogon*, Rami Elhanan talked about this. He said: "Some people have an interest in keeping the silence. Others have an interest in sowing hatred based on fear. Fear makes money, and it makes laws, and it takes land, and it builds settlements, and fear likes to keep everyone silent . . . We use the word security to silence others. But it's not about that, it's about occupying someone else's life, someone else's land, someone else's head. It's about control. Which is power."[3]

For some people, the path to peace is the path of silence. It is the path of enduring injustice and inequality. It is the path of fear. And fear sets one on edge, it makes one defensive. It makes one skeptical about demanding for the creation of an enabling atmosphere for peace.

But this is not the true way. Dear soldier, you are the wind. They shouldn't see you coming. You are unpredictable. Fear is an emotion that can be predicted. But courage is an element of surprise. Never cower. You know the true path to peace—follow it.

6. Gazing in Other Sects

Once you have trained and grasped the Way of the Warrior, you will also be able to see the distance and speed of any sword.

Musashi observed that other sects teach their students to focus on different things during combat. Some tell their students to focus on the opponent's sword, other teach their students to focus on the opponent's arm or face or feet. Focusing on different things during combat can cause distraction, and Musashi called it "blindness" in strategy.

The warrior should focus on the goal. Musashi exemplified this with a soccer player. A soccer does not have to look at the ball closely before he can perform skills with it. So what is the goal for the warrior? The opponent's mind.

Musashi advised the warrior to not just see, but perceive the opponent's mind. By doing this, he is able to see the strength and weakness of the adversary.

Dear soldier, as you journey towards peace, do not be like others that can be easily distracted. Don't concentrate on the enemy's actions alone; they can be deceptive. The actions of the enemy are minute details; their plans are hidden in their minds. So concentrate on reading the enemy's mind, that way you can predict their next move. Always remember this: If the people of Troy had concentrated on reading the minds of the Greeks, they wouldn't have been carried away by the "gift" of the Trojan horse.

7. Use of the Feet in Other Sects

In our strategy, nothing changes about the footstep

Other schools of swordsmanship during Musashi's day taught their students footwork during combat. Some of the footwork they taught include: floating feet, flying feet, shrugging feet, and so on. According to Musashi, the flying feet made the warrior gallop; the flying feet made him jump and fly; while the shrugging feet made him indecisive.

What Musashi recommended was a firm step. In the Way of Strategy, there is no change to the footstep. The warrior should maintain the same step he uses during his normal walk. He advised the warrior to move according to the rhythm of the opponent. He also should not move too fast so he wouldn't falter, or too slowly because walking slowly may make him miss the opportunity to take victory.

Some people have failed to achieve peace because they were either in a haste or they were indecisive. Hasty—because they felt they have endured injustice and violence for too long. Indecisive—because they knew that the fight for peace is a tough one, thus they were skeptical about whether to go into the fight or remain with the status quo.

Dear soldier, you are different. Your path to peace is a unique one. You know that this path will definitely lead to peace if you are patient and firm to the cause. Be strategic: move according to the rhythm of the enemy, but at every moment you have to remember that the objective is to win.

8. Speed in Other Sects

Speed is not a true Way of the Warrior

Musashi wrote that speed makes a warrior lose coordination and the flow of rhythm. According to him, it is bad to be too fast or too slow in anything. The warrior should see himself as an expert in swordsmanship, and an expert never does anything in a hurry.

Dear soldier, you know the true path of peace. You are the expert. Don't be in a haste. Your decision to restore peace means breaking down deep-rooted systems that have existed for centuries. It wouldn't be a walk in the park. The aim is to win—and winning takes precision, not speed.

There are times when the enemy would want you to be hasty so that you can mistakes. Do not lose your cool. Be calm. Don't let them draw you in. Take charge of the situation.

9. "Interior" and "Surface" in Other Sects

The way to understand is through experience

Other schools of swordsmanship classified their principles of swordsmanship into "interior" or "deep" principles, and "surface" principles. But Musashi disagreed with this. For him, he taught his students the Way of swordsmanship in a manner easy to understand. There was no need for rules or regulations, or classifying the lessons. For principles that were difficult to comprehend, he took time to explain them to his students according to their comprehension ability.

Soldier, you have the duty to educate others on the path of peace. But while you do that, do not hide anything from them. Explain to them why peace is important to the world. Show them the long history of chaos that the world has experienced. Then teach them why they should follow the soldier's path to peace. You are doing this because you know that there has been a lot of distorted information when it comes to the issue of peace. You have to tell a different story and change the narrative. By doing this, you erode the foundations of chaos that have already been built, and gradually enthrone the culture of peace.

Key Point from Musashi: *The sword does not have "depth" or "entrance" nor does it have a "supreme" posture. You only need your mind, and you also need to perfect the attitude of the sword. This is the nature of strategy.*

CHAPTER FIVE

THE VOID - *In the Void*

In Musashi's Scroll of The Void or Emptiness lies the secret for *perpetual* peace. Musashi believed that there is wisdom in believing that one does not know anything no matter how much one knows. When one accepts that they do not know everything, they increase their capacity to learn, to absorb more information. This is a place of nothingness, so there is enough room to be filled up with knowledge.

In this scroll, Musashi left some vital lessons for the warrior. And these lessons are also important for the soldier.

First Lesson: Musashi wanted the warrior to understand that even though he, Musashi, had shown him the true Way of swordsmanship, he should also be willing to learn more. The warrior should understand that learning the art of swordsmanship should not stop at reading *The Five Spheres*. The most interesting thing about the Scroll of the Void is that Musashi advised the warrior to also learn the way of other sects. I believe that Musashi did not give this counsel to the warrior so that the warrior could copy the way of other sects, but because of two reasons: (1) Since the warrior would be fighting samurais from other sects, he wanted him to learn their strategy—to know their strength and exploit their weakness. (2) He wanted the warrior to increase his own knowledge by understanding the way of other sects. After all, Musashi's Way of Strategy was birthed from observing and studying the way of others—and exploiting their weakness.

How does this apply to the soldier?

It is true that I have shown you exhaustively the true path of peace. But you should also understand that we live in a dynamic, ever-changing world. For this reason, you have to step into "nothingness"—the point of believing that you know nothing. This is why one of your qualities as a soldier is to be flexible as water. As you journey on this path to peace, be flexible to accept changes and adjust yourself to them without losing focus.

With the explosion of science and technology, you should know that the methods employed by the antagonists are bound not to stay the same. Just like we saw in the Wind scroll, it is important you move according to their rhythm. It is also important to focus on their mind because that is the only way to predict their actions.

Learn everything that you can learn. Be open to new information. The internet is a vast place to gather information. Read. Listen. Understand. There are times when you would need to read or listen to information that is not line with your goal. But know that you are not consuming this information to be like the enemy, rather you are doing so because you want to get a peek into how the enemy thinks. You want to know their strength, their weaknesses. You want to know what they see as opportunities and what they consider threats.

The place of nothingness is a vast expanse. Do not limit yourself. As long as you keep your eyes on the goal, you are bound to win. Learn from Musashi: He learnt the ways of other schools, yet maintained his own Way of Strategy, and never deviated from it. And because of that he came out victorious, sixty-one times.

Lesson Two: Musashi taught his students in this scroll that they should never allow the true way to be tainted. They had the duty to preserve what they had learnt. In the beginning of *The Five Spheres*, Musashi noted that the true way of strategy had been abandoned. That was the primary reason he wrote *The Five Spheres*. And since he handed down his knowledge to his students, they had the duty to preserve it so that the true Way of Strategy would not fade away again. He wrote to them: *Never let the Way of the Warrior we practice becoming tainted or obscured, not even a little bit. Your mind must never be lost.*

How does this apply to the soldier?

Dear soldier, you have learnt the true path to peace. Do not hoard it to yourself. Remember that the fight for peace is not one you can fight alone. To get other soldiers to join you, you have to educate them. You have to ensure that this path is neither tainted nor obscured. Use every channel possible to propagate this doctrine. Write books. Deliver speeches. Write articles. Tweet. Let this message be heard around the world. Let it reverberate across the nations.

The duty rests on you to successfully transfer this message from generation to generation to generation. This is the only way the peace you fought for can be preserved. If the path of peace be lost, then the protagonists of violence may rise again, and when they do, it would be hard to defeat them again. Why? They have already seen all you've got.

Musashi said that the way of strategy must never be tainted or obscured, *not even a little bit.* I emphasized these five words because only a tiny loophole is needed for the ship of peace to sink. Let those you teach understand this. Let there be a oneness of mind, of knowledge, and of action.

Lesson Three: Musashi told the warrior that unless he understood the true Way, he would always look at human laws through the lens of right and wrong. But the true Way teaches him that human laws are a product of individual prejudices. They are distorted and as such go against the Way of the Warrior. This means that the warrior's swordsmanship cannot be based on human laws because they are already tainted and distorted. In the Way of the Warrior lies emptiness, and in emptiness, lies virtue, intellect, principles, and no evil.

How does this apply to the soldier?

There are human laws guiding human existence. And in most cases, the enemies of peace use these laws to suppress the rights of people. They use these laws to act out their violence, injustice, unfairness, and disregard for human lives. They wield the power to change the law as they see fit.

For instance, the Imperial War Museums recorded that there were "surprising" laws passed in Britain during the First Word War. The most important of these laws was the Defense of the Realm Act (DORA) which was passed to "secure public safety." But the constituents of the law didn't actually secure public safety but infringed on the rights of Britons. The law gave the government the power to prosecute anyone that acted in manner deemed to "jeopardize the success of the operations of His Majesty's forces or to assist the enemy." Some of its measures included: (1) banning whistling for London taxis in case it should be mistaken for an air raid warning, (2) forbidding people to loiter near bridges and tunnels or to light bonfires, (3) instituting the British Summer Time which made clocks go forward so that working hours in the day could be maximized, (4) introducing blackouts in certain towns and cities to protect against air raids, (5) censoring the press which limited the reporting of war news, (6) censoring private correspondence, and (7) restricting the movement of foreign nationals from enemy countries.[1] These laws show the extent the enemies of peace can go to limit the rights of individuals in order to promote their own agenda. In fact, one of the measures of DORA morphed into a restriction of food production which led to the introduction of rationing in 1918.[2]

This example shows the soldier that in many cases human laws do not favor peace. As Musashi rightly noted, these laws are promulgated based on human prejudices. So dear soldier, your only path to peace is the path which you know now. If you want to use human laws to your advantage, then you must find a way to become a lawmaker. And I don't consider this a bad thing. But I am skeptical about that because we have seen over time how power corrupts men and women. However, if you are certain that despite having and being in power, you would *always* follow the path of peace, then it is a good strategy. After all, the path of peace is also a path of nothingness, of flexibility, of applying knowledge geared towards peace.

Key Point from Musashi: *Train the eyes to perceive and see. There are no small clouds. You must understand that when the illusion clouds dissipate, then that is true "emptiness."*

A Practical Lesson From The Duel Between
Miyamoto Musashi and Sasaki Kojiro[3]

The Five Spheres was not just a book of musings for Musashi, it was a documentation of the life he lived as a samurai. One duel that stamped Musashi's reputation as a warrior to be reckoned was his duel with Sasaki Kojiro that took place on the Ganryu Island on the 13th day of April 1612.

Kojiro was considered one of the greatest samurais in Japan. He had *speed* and precision. His sword was a huge no-dachi blade that was *over a meter* in length. The size and weight of the blade made it a brutal weapon, but Kojiro perfected its use like no other samurai had done.[4]

Musashi, on the other hand, was a masterless samurai who was also well known in Japan. As at the time of the duel, Musashi had already sheathed his two katana and was only dueling with a bokken—a wooden practice sword.

On the day of the duel, Musashi arrived at the island three hours late. This infuriated Kojiro, who paced up and down with his hands behind his back. Kojiro was a man with a big ego and he felt Musashi's lateness was an insult to his honor. Three hours earlier, Kojiro was a calm man who even sat in deep mediation as he mentally prepared himself for the combat. It is said that his composure was so remarkable that his retinue of students and servants[5] had no doubt that he would defeat Musashi easily. But every element of composure and calm was lost as Musashi kept him waiting.

He grumbled, cursed and snapped at his servants. One of the officials tried to calm him down by telling him that there was a possibility that Musashi would not arrive because he had developed a weak feet thinking of the prospect of facing him. But Kojiro did not agree with this. He knew Musashi—he had a great reputation as a swordsman and wouldn't flee from a duel. And true to his thoughts, Musashi was just around the corner.

He sat cross-legged in a fishing boat not too far away from the island. As he sat in the boat, he, without haste, carved the boat's spare oar into a bokken with his sharp knife. After he was done, the fisherman rowed Musashi to the island.

When Kojiro saw Musashi, he was even more enraged by Musashi's appearance. Musashi was unshaven. He wore only a simple robe with a sword belt. His feet were bare. Also, he hadn't washed for some time because his robe had many stains and discolored patches. Musashi looked nothing like other samurais of the time. And Kojiro felt insulted by this.

He charged towards Musashi with his sword.[6] Musashi jumped and dodged to the left, and what happened next surprised Kojiro. Musashi did not draw out a sword, but a bokken. A piece of wood.

Kojiro considered the arrogance that would make a samurai approach him with a wooden sword. This moment of consideration which led to further infuriation caused him to falter. He dived towards Musashi with a great sweep of his blade. Musashi ducked in time, with the sword cutting a wisp of his hair. Kojiro brought his sword down to Musashi again, but the latter evaded the blow. Musashi then stepped to the right and hit Kojiro's right side with his bokken. Then he struck another blow to the side of Kojiro's head. As Kojiro staggered, Musashi smashed the bokken into his left side. Kojiro felt his ribs crack, a sharp pain exploded in chest, and he couldn't breathe. The fight had ended as soon as it began. Musashi was victorious.

From this story, we see Musashi apply some of the tactics he later penned down in *The Five Spheres*. He knew that Kojiro had speed, and speed could make a samurai to stumble. Another thing Musashi knew was that Kojiro used an extra-long sword. This meant that although he was a skilled samurai, he depended on the length of his sword for victory—a tactic Musashi considered weak. But what is really striking about this story was Musashi's perception.

He knew Kojiro was a man with a big ego and he decided to use it against him. I believe he had watched Kojiro's duels and knew that Kojiro had great composure. So for him to defeat Kojiro, he had to get him agitated. Recall that Musashi advised warriors to take the opposite disposition of the enemy. If the enemy is calm, then the warrior should agitate him; and if the enemy fights in a hurry, the warrior should remain calm. For Musashi to get Kojiro agitated, he had to exploit his ego. Coming three hours late to the duel was an insult to Kojiro and because of that he lost his cool.

The moment Kojiro lost his temper was the moment Musashi gained victory. This is what Musashi called "Pulling the Bottom Out." He defeated the spirit of his opponent first before defeating him on the surface. Little wonder Musashi said that once a samurai understands the Way, he would remain undefeated. Through the Way—a mind game—Musashi defeated one of the greatest samurais with a wooden sword. Not even a katana. Soldier, when you understand the disposition of your enemy, you would be able to use it to your advantage. Staying focused to the goal should be utmost in your mind. Kojiro was focused at first, but lost his focus because he allowed his ego to override him. As a result, he fought with speed, no precision. That is why Musashi kept evading all his blows. And when the time was right, Musashi who had been *patient* all through, struck him hard and killed him.

PART II

WINNING WARS WITHOUT COMBAT

CHAPTER SIX

An Alternative Approach

The objective of every war is to win. No army engages in a war for fun except in war games. And even during war games, some heightened senses and actions imply that war is a serious affair. Indeed, it is to kill or be killed, and for that reason, most battles and wars are fought to win. After all, victorious war veterans who live to tell war stories are celebrated while very few vanquished soldiers are ever heard of.

But wars are fought for more than just egotistical satisfaction. Of a truth, some conflicts are simply the products of the puppeteering expertise of highly placed politicians acting on their whims or the whims of *their* puppet masters.

Be that as it may, every soldier on the battlefield has one sole objective: to win. It is this objective that Musashi's Gospel is hinged on; defeating the enemy at all costs. Your country depends on it. Your loved ones depend on it. Most importantly, your pride and honor depend on it.

The last chapters you just read took you along the Way of the Warrior. You have been acquainted with the craft and guile of warfare, and you are now more aware of what it means to be a soldier defending the honor and pride of the fatherland. And as a human that has been trained to be a weapon, you are prepared and expected to commit the ultimate sacrifice to ensure that it happens if need be.

If anything, Musashi's Way of the Warrior and his life embody what the ultimate warrior should stand for.

Yet, if you have learned anything from Musashi's treatise on the use of the sword. From the way he draws the elements of Fire, Water,

Wind, and Air into the discourse of the Warrior's Way and his emphasis on entering into that space known as the Void, you should have noticed that there are multiple ways to win a war.

This part of the book will deal with the ability to win a war with minimal (where possible, zero) physical combat.

Could There Be War Without Physical Combat?

Yes, it is possible. Avid students of politics and economics will regale you with never-ending tales of instances where countries and groups of partnering countries have allowed divergent interests to reflect in their international policies. The Cold War of the 1980s comes to mind, and more recently, the US-China trade wars are examples of politico-economic wars that have not escalated into full-blown military wars.

These situations can be mentioned in a discourse of this context because most military wars are products of political and economic aspirations. The soldier on the battlefield is a vehicle or device for realizing these aspirations to all intents and purposes. To borrow a quote from Niccolo Machiavelli's *The Prince*," The acquired kingdoms were conquered by either fortune or the talent displayed by the ruler's army or by a foreign army."

There is a salient question if the soldier must make economic aspirations a reality using blood, sweat, and tears as the currency for achieving said aspirations. This question stems from a conflation of different positions, which are:

1. The need to win wars at all costs using blood, sweat, and tears where possible

2. The soldier's desire to live as long as possible (self-preservation is an inalienable human drive)

If these positions are part of the dynamics of war, then the question arises, "Is it possible to win a war without physical combat? Better put, is it possible to win wars with minimal expenditure of blood, sweat, tears, and everything else in between?

War has been likened to the game of chess. And even in chess games, pawns are sacrificed to protect the queen, the most important chess piece on a player's side of the board. So if pawns are sacrificed to win games (read wars), does it follow that soldiers must always pay the ultimate sacrifice for wars to be won?

These are the questions that this section of the book will explore. Exploring these questions is particularly important given the frightening military might that most of the world's powers boast of.

On The Virtue of Emptiness

To explore an alternative means to winning wars, you'd need to be willing to explore that chthonic space which Musashi describes as the "Void" or "Emptiness."

This concept describes a place that exists beyond human knowledge and understanding. It refers to a realm of ideas where you can create anything because of the flexibility and formlessness that it affords everyone that has access to it.

Embracing the realm of emptiness lends the ultimate warrior the tools required to explore previously unknown options. This capability makes creating an alternative approach to winning wars possible.

How, might you ask?

Well, here is the thing, the ultimate warrior (that's you) must be proficient in using weapons of warfare as he is with his mental faculties. Thus, the soldier who understands the Way of the Warrior understands the importance of a constantly sharpened mind and is willing to master as many strategies as the mind can handle.

To Musashi, the partnership between a sharpened mind and a resolute will offers entry into the realm of the Void, where free yet disciplined thought leads you to a world of immense possibilities for creating the right strategies.

Indeed, you will be walking a path less trodden as you'd be free of the illusions that impair the perception and reasoning of so many a soldier. Illusions can becloud the very senses required to be successful at war.

Yet like clouds, illusions must dissipate at a point. It is at this point of dissipation of the clouds that clarity comes. This is why Musashi likens the Way of the Warrior to the cloud because of the constant transformative process of cloud forming water before falling as rain, only to gather back as a cloud at the appointed time.

Musashi aptly describes the virtue of 'Emptiness' in *The Five Spheres* thus:

In emptiness is virtue, and there is no evil. In emptiness, intellect exists. Principle exists. The Way exists. And the spirit is nothingness.

Once you have grasped the concept of 'Emptiness," enter into a realm of being that predisposes you to take the form required to achieve your immediate goal.

This understanding takes us to the next milestone on your newfound path to victory with minimal physical combat.

Preparation

A mind that has embraced the void of nothingness is open to new things. To walk the less-traveled path known as The Way of the Warrior, you need to prepare your being for a revolutionary approach that takes your enemy by surprise. After all, what is the point of using strategies and ways of warfare that are common knowledge and could be easily countered?

To prepare yourself to achieve your ultimate goal as a warrior, your mind is your ultimate weapon. Indeed, planning and preparation require a reset of your old ways of warfare. We live in a digitalized world. Military equipment has evolved from swords and spears to fully computerized equipment that consists of software that controls the military equipment (hardware).

Think of your mind as software and your physical body as the hardware. Your mind determines what your body does, and when the mind is at its best, the body follows suit. Musashi puts it as clear as day when he notes:

Develop a large mind — a mind like water. Depending on the situation, the mind should be flexible like water. Water can be dark blue. It can be a drop or a vast ocean.

When your mind takes the property of water, it is able to adjust to the situation. And to win a war with minimal combat, you'd need to be flexible enough to adapt to any situation that might arise. He who walks through unchartered areas has to be willing to align his path to the contours that he encounters along the way.

Understanding As A Means of Preparation

Why is it essential for a soldier to understand anything beyond military strategies and perhaps how to make the most of his weapons? The answer to that is this: understanding the nature of warfare is the difference between losing and winning a war. You need to master the "traditional" tenets of war before creating yours.

All the most outstanding scholars and strategists all have one thing in common. They studied the ideas and principles propounded by the great minds before using these ideas as a foundation for theirs. As the ultimate warrior, you'd need to understand the five "determinants" of war as propounded by Sun Wu.

The first of the five is the concept of Righteousness. Sun Wu sees righteousness as the means of making people "willing to join with the king, to make them unite and join forces, to live and die with courage."

We have already established that you are the sword of the king—the vehicle through which his will is realized. Your engagement in battle is born of your conviction that you are doing the right thing. This conviction will come in handy at those points in your where doubt might set in because of the uniqueness of your approach to winning with minimal combat.

The next determinant is the Atmosphere. Sun Wu defines this as "the night or day, hotness or coldness, and change of four seasons." Your battles will have physical locations, all of which are subject to the Atmosphere. Traditional war strategists have a perspective on the seasons and have created tactics based on these seasons. Your ability to perceive the failings and strengths in their tactics will help you formulate an approach that sets you apart.

The terrain is the third determinant, and to Sun Wu, it is the "high or low ground, near or far distance, easy or difficult roads, plains or canyons and the conditions of survival." We will call this the physical location of the battles you will engage in. If you are going to win your opponent with the least physical combat possible, you will need a level of mastery of your terrain. You'd need to understand how the terrain works in your favor or against you. The ideal is to win a war and live to tell the story. Why else would you be looking to win with minimal physical combat? Understanding the terrain is key to coming up with strategies that put your enemies in disadvantaged situations. Afghanistan is a prime example of how physical terrains affect warfare. The relationship between its unique terrain and the fatalities experienced by the Coalition forces, who were unfamiliar with the terrain, is well documented.

The General is the next determinant in Sun Wu's list. Vu believes that he must be "strategic, trustworthy, kind, courageous and strict." These are the characteristics of the ultimate warrior. You can't win the war against your enemies if you haven't won the war against yourself. Having these values puts you in a better situation to make the right decisions that help you achieve your ultimate winning goal.

Martial law is the fifth and last determinant which he who chooses to walk the Way of the Warrior must understand. Martial law in this regard refers to the "organization, management of soldiers and expenditures in the military."

The organization is very important in the military as it provides the structure needed to implement a strategy. For an army to be organized, its soldiers must be well-managed. Managing soldiers also requires the proper handling of the available resources. You must be a "professional" student of martial law, one who is constantly improving on his body of knowledge about keeping his soldiers in the right frame of mind at all times.

Understanding Sun Wu's war determinants prepare you to explore alternative paths to winning wars. Mastery of these factors provides the foundation for building your unique strategies and tactics. To facilitate your understanding of his ideas, Sun Wu listed several situations that you must consider at each point in time:

- Which party has the righteous king?
- Which party has the talented general?
- Which party benefits more from the atmosphere and terrain?
- Which party abides by martial law?
- Which party owns the better, more sophisticated weapons?
- Which party's soldiers train more frequently?
- Which party rewards and punishes more fairly?

The soldier who is prepared for all has the advantage over his counterpart is limited to the traditional ways of warfare. Preparation allows you to make the most of situations as they arise instead of being hedged in the box. Understanding the nature of war is essential to your preparation.

The Nature of War

War takes place on multiple levels, primarily as physical and psychological combat that often involves firepower, troop strength, morale, leadership, courage, effective decision-making, and tactics designed to handle battlefield and non-battlefield situations. Regardless of its form, in the context of this work, war is essentially some form of military combat between two or more parties.

War is strictly distinguished by its scope and goal as typified by the clash of major interests backed by the parties involved. To this end, we would refer to war as sustained (or not) combat between trained soldiers who represent political or economic interests.

It often involved using military forces that attacked enemy soldiers and designated points, appropriated geographical locations, or gathered intelligence. With wars, information, tactics, and strategies are employed to achieve often mutually exclusive goals. Ultimately, an intricate web of interactions must be effectively managed to achieve victory.

One of the most common reasons for war is the enforcer of political will, where clashing political interests quickly degenerate to physical combat. This is the most common form for which a soldier is expected to die for the "honor" of the country. Although there are both defenders and aggressors in this dynamic, both sides of the conflict believe they are in the right, and victory is often seen as a non-negotiable outcome. This approach to warfare leads to sustained effort, expenditure, and mostly irreversible and large-scale destruction.

Indeed, it would seem as if warfare is a primordial aspect of man's existence. Indeed, all of the political states that exist today were created and sustained by wars. Either one state is trying to protect or defend social, religious, or political interests from both internal and external aggressors. History is replete with examples of wars from pre-literate times to the present day.

The Evolution of Warfare

Just as man has experienced physiological, social, and technological evolutions over decades, war has also significantly evolved both in nature and dimension.

The modern age has seen the proliferation of wars between state and non-state actors where guerilla groups with personal and political interests have engaged states within and without state borders. Yet again, the modern age has experienced wars where nuclear weapons capable of destroying multitudes have changed the paradigms of warfare.

Political states now use these weapons and the threat of using them to achieve their goals or prevent bullying from other political states. The pissing contest between the US, China, Iran, and North Korea comes to mind. Of a truth, nuclear weapons have revolutionized warfare in modern times as countries could "easily" obliterate each other with the touch of a button without the need for combat between soldiers.

That said, the proliferation of nuclear weapons appears to be a double-edged sword. One side of the blade is the instant destruction of the earth, while the other side of the blade ensures the nuclear powers exert some restraint.

But modern wars have evolved beyond the weapons used. We are now entering a phase in civilization where technological advancements (namely robotics and artificial intelligence) will soon eliminate the need for armed humans in wars. The United States has already started deploying robots and drones to handle tasks hitherto done by humans: disarming bombs, detecting threats, performing reconnaissance, and firing missiles.

Even military robots and drones are being designed to be deployed in combat areas adjudged to be too dangerous for humans. This is as biological engineers actively seek to eliminate the need for traditional weapons and armies. They have taken their studies to the point where certain human vulnerabilities are being targeted for improvement or replacement. On the flip side, there is talk of bioweapons like a bio-engineered virus being used in place of nuclear weapons in the future—cyber warfare, where the internet and its minions will be used as a weapon of warfare.

To all intent and purpose, man's wars gradually evolve into bloodless combat between non-human actors (read soldiers). Yet again, regardless of its nature or form, war at its simplest is an expression of a conflict of interests.

Understanding Your Place In Contemporary War

Obviously, we are slowly moving towards the kind of warfare that requires little or no physical combat, all thanks to technological advancements. Yet we are not there yet, as contemporary warfare is yet to catch up to the futurist wars captured in many sci-fi movie flicks on Netflix and Amazon Prime.

This is for you who seek to elevate your "warriorhood" to the highest levels possible. You have a lot to learn from the quintessential warrior Miyamoto Musashi who won all the duels he partook in.

Winning that many duels over the years was only made possible by his approach to combat, which was hinged on minimal dependence on physical strength against reliance on technique, strategy, and all the other intangible aspects of warfare. In situations where the surprise was needed, Musashi employed it. When the strategy was the difference-maker, he used it to his advantage. Yet again, the emotional manipulation of his opponents was another tool in his bag of tricks, just as the mastery of his combat skills was another.

Musashi's secret was to go above and beyond the capabilities of his opponents. Where they relied on training, flashy weapons, and battle-tested tactics and techniques, Musashi explored the Void, grasping the power of responding at the moment and adopting a fluid strategy that handled whatever came up.

As you prepare for war, myths, misconceptions, and traditional tactics and strategies must be archived. Because that is where they belong, you'd need a different strategy that is as fluid as water yet as effective as steel. Winning wars does not require a hard and fast formula; instead, the essence is to explore all the possibilities that lie in the realm of the Void. As much as your strategy is vital, it must be creative, fluid, and fitting.

CHAPTER SEVEN

Military Strategy

No one can truly follow the Warriors Way without understanding the way strategy. Miyamoto Musashi won so many duels because he was strategic about everything. From his mastery and use of his sword strokes to how he studied his opponent's emotions and used them to his advantage.

Strategy is critical in conventional warfare. It is doubly critical when you are looking to win your battles and wars with minimal physical combat. To get a grasp of strategy and its place in Musashi's teachings, we'd be looking at how strategy in warfare evolved over the years.

What Is Military Strategy

As the name suggests, military strategy refers to how military campaigns are planned and coordinated to achieve military objectives. Military strategy is reflected in the tactics that an army applies in battle. Let's put things in perspective. Strategy is the way a set of battles are used to win a battle and is often seen in how the troops are used in combat.

The success or loss of any battle or war boils down to the strategy used. We find evidence of this fact in the Greek origin of the word *strategos*, which roughly translates as "the general's art." Every ardent student of war history will observe that despite the influence of technology on military strategy, at its root, military strategy refers to the way military operations are managed to achieve defined objectives.

Military strategy is designed to handle specific issues that often arise in and out of the theatre of war and is often limited by the size,

THE GAME CHANGERS SERIES

training, and morale of forces on the ground. It is also affected by the grade and number of weapons used, the terrain, the weather, and how well trained the enemy forces are. Now that we have established military strategy let's look at how it evolved over centuries.

Military Strategy Over the Years

We could trace the beginning of military strategy to the growth and expansions of political empires worldwide. Some of the notable names in the development include Philip II (382–336 BC), Alexander the Great (356–323 BC), and Hannibal (247–183 BC), all of whom made innovations in their approach to warfare long before Musashi discovered the secret of the Warrior's Way.

Philip II found a way to merge infantry, cavalry, and artillery into a proficient fighting unit that could be easily maneuvered where and when necessary. Alexander the Great is one of history's most accomplished strategists and tacticians. He earned this reputation by being particular about planning, communication, supplies, security, and the element of surprise. Hannibal used flexible attack tactics, unity of command, and an elite cavalry that laid the ground for developing the Roman military strategy that made them some of the most successful armies of all time.

What we know as modern warfare started with the exploits of Gustav II Adolf, king of Sweden (r. 1611-32). Adolf brought back maneuver into military strategy by having a national army structured into small, well-armed, and easily maneuverable fighting units.

Perhaps Frederick II (the Great) of Prussia (r. 1740-86) made the most significant changes in military strategy over the years. To make the most of the challenges he faced at the time, Frederick II used interior lines and a highly disciplined army and horse artillery that he could easily assemble where he wanted to strike his enemies at different points.

Napoleon, I structured his military campaigns so that he could easily maneuver his troops to focus on different battlefields. His battle approach included skirmishing, cannonading, and a great concentration of forces adept at turning and enveloping battlefield maneuvers. It is safe to say that Napoleon heralded the beginning of modern military strategy as his tactics became templates for many army generals that came after him.

By the 19th century, military strategy was again modified by technological changes in the volume, reach, and speed of warfare. Military equipment expanded and improved, so there was a change in the tactics and strategy. Take the U.S. Civil War, for example, where the North and the Confederates fought over political interests. The victory of the North can be linked to a strategy that includes several tactics like the blocking, division, and destruction of the Confederate armies and supplies.

When machine guns and airpower were introduced into war dynamics, the military strategy took another turn. War generals moved from trench warfare to strategic airstrikes on cities and enemy positions. These airstrikes, in particular, greatly changed the face of modern military strategy and warfare. A few well-trained pilots with the latest fighter aircraft could wreak more havoc in less time than even the most advanced ground soldiers could.

Perhaps that is when the first seed of the idea of optimized combat results with minimal physical effort was sown. Because warfare soon moved from fighter jets to nuclear bombs that could obliterate countries with just the push of a button from a remote location. With almost every technologically advanced country owning nuclear weapons, military strategy has further evolved. For one, it engendered some level of responsibility among world leaders who are somehow aware of nuclear weapons' destructive potential. Seeing as none of these leaders value world annihilation over their political interests, military tactics have been forced to adjust to meet the prevailing socio-political conditions.

Warfare is now being executed mainly by small, elite forces that have training in guerrilla war and are equipped with state-of-the-art, light weapons that facilitate speedy deployment and withdrawal to and from enemy lines.

Musashi on Military Strategy

One thing that is clear in our summary of the history of military strategy is the significance of maneuverability to the success of military campaigns. Like we mentioned at the beginning of this chapter, Musashi's unprecedented win ratio in his sword duels is down to his approach to strategy.

In his words, *"when you attain the Way of strategy, there will not be one thing you cannot see."*

If you want to experience as many wins as a soldier in modern warfare, you'd need a great understanding of military strategy. Here are some other insights from Musashi:

"The way to win in a battle according to military science is to know the rhythms of the specific opponents and use rhythms that your opponents do not expect, producing formless rhythms from rhythms of wisdom...Cultivate the power of insights; if strong, the state of affairs in everything will be visible to you."

Musashi's book is a bestselling eclectic treatise that is currently a source of instruction in several fields of thought because the majority of the chapters in the book focus on how you can gain leverage over your enemies. Coming from a place of experience(what with so many wins), Musashi's firsthand experience with strategy is evident in how he tries to show soldiers how to win as many wars as possible using the correct strategic principles.

One of such principle is the need to learn as much as possible, even if it is one's enemy that one has to learn from. The reason is even the most loathsome enemy is not without strengths. To Musashi, learning from such an enemy is a great strategy.

For one, studying your enemies' habits, strengths, and rhythms enables you to arrive at unexpected winning strategies that put you in a favorable position to win your battles. It is a lot easier these days with all the technological advancements that we currently enjoy.

The idea is to mine as many insights as possible from your study of your enemy. The higher the quality of the insights, the better you arrive at a really great strategy because you get to see the battle from their perspective. Once you understand your enemy's view on a battle, you are better positioned to arrive at countermeasures and counter-tactics that give all the advantages that you need.

As counterintuitive as it is to study your enemy, it is an effective approach that you don't want to write off because it gives you one of the most critical advantages that you could ever take advantage of timing:

"Strike fast when you realize the opportunity. Do not flinch your attention at the point, and your opponent will not be able to react. Mow him right down without even giving him time to blink his eyes."

Timing is of the essence in most things in life, especially combat situations. It is a vital cog in any military strategy as knowing when to strike or retreat is key and is the difference between a successful and failed military campaign. Many major battles have been lost because one of the parties missed their opportunity to strike.

But studying your enemy is not as easy as it seems. Mushasi believes that:

"When opponents come at you, appear weak at first, then overcome him... The important thing in strategy is to suppress the enemy's useful actions but allow his useless actions."

You'd need to master some subterfuge when dealing with your enemy. As a master strategist, you must be steps ahead of your enemies. And to do that, you must be willing to adjust your tactics to match the demands of the environment or any pressing situation. Disinformation might be a necessary tactic when you discover the need to throw your opponent off their position of power. For instance, you might need to respond to attacks by feigning weakness, after which you attack at the right time.

Another instance of disinformation is trying to convince the enemy that you will be doing one when you will do another. This tactic could be deployed by calculatingly letting out information so that the enemy believes that the source of information is authentic and that they got a "scoop." The thing with this tactic is that it could lead the enemy to waste resources on "useless actions" when deployed correctly. One real-life illustration is in the third world war.

At a point in the war when they needed to launch their D-day invasion, the Allied forces had to use deception to mask the launch of their major offensive. As part of the ruse, General Patton was given command of a landing force comprised of airfields, dummy tanks, landing craft, oil storage depots, and airfields. All of these things were done in full view of the German spies and military command.

The Allies then proceeded to bomb the Calais region when the Normandy area was the real target of their attack. They used their double agents to relay the wrong information while fabricating radio traffic that sold the illusion that a large invasion force was being assembled in the southeastern region of England. The Allies executed these measures so well that the Germans could not deploy their troops effectively to counter the Allies' attacks.

Why Is Strategy Important To You?

The focus of this part of the book is winning wars with minimal physical effort. To this end, having a clear and focused strategy goes a long way in the success of this approach to conflict. For one, you'd be taking an uncharted path, and so the pitfall to be experienced are more, and the potential for failure is higher. Without a well-thought military strategy, you are almost likely to fail.

On the flip side, you have everything to gain if you find a way to create a strategy that prepares for all the eventualities that might arise at each point. To Musashi, *"The principle of strategy is having one thing, to know ten thousand things because it is important to see distant things as if they were close and to take a detached view of close things."*

But all that mastery and understanding of things outside come to nothing without self-mastery. That is why self-mastery is the first step to effective military strategy. Musashi succinctly describes it thus *"Study strategy over the years and achieve the spirit of the warrior. Today is victory over yourself of yesterday; tomorrow is your victory over lesser men."*

Why Use Strategy

"…a skillful leader does not need to use the battlefield to subdue the enemy. He captures the enemy's city without having to attack. He destroys enemy countries without putting his troops in great risk. All is to preserve the

force by making use of strategy. Therefore, there is no wear and tear, and still, there is great benefit. This is the strategy of offensive art..." -Sun Vu.

(The Law of War: The Art of Competition Benefits in War, Business and Life)

You could simultaneously fight a war on two levels: the psychological and the physical. Psychological warfare is targeted at the will of an army, while physical warfare tends to affect the capabilities of your foes. When applied correctly, numerical and weaponry advantages are removed, and the war is won at less human and material costs.

Any military leader worth their onions will incorporate attack levels in their strategy because both the physical and psychological work is in tandem for a soldier to function optimally. A fitting analogy would be to see the psychological side as software that powers a hardware component (the physical side)

For the rest of this section of the book, we will use the word "will" interchangeably with the psyche while "capability will refer to the physical. Now that that's out of the way, let's look at physical-based and psycho-centric strategies that could be used to win a war.

Physical-Based Strategies

These are strategies targeted at the physical or tangible aspects of warfare.

Executing Physical Damage

One of the targets of war is to inflict as much physical damage as possible on the enemy. It often involves physical violence as a means of annihilating the enemy. The sustained annihilation of one's colleagues at arms has a debilitating effect on the capability of even the most motivated soldier.

Granted, inflicting physical damage on an army has led to many wins, but the context of this treatise is to seek alternative means of winning a war with minimal body bags being flown home.

If inflicting damage is a surefire means of winning a war, then a difficult question arises 'What is the number of soldiers an enemy has to lose before they concede defeat? In some instances, soldiers on a battlefield lay down their weapons and either flee or surrender when they conclude that a battle has been lost.

One might be tricked into labeling such soldiers cowardly and disloyal in discharging their duty to defend and protect. However, the number of dead soldiers and the rate at which they are killed will disorient many soldiers and cause them to save their lives first.

Thankfully, the destruction of an army does not have to come from the death of soldiers. Most modern armies are greatly enhanced by the quality and caliber of their weaponry, so a lot of modern military strategy is often based on these weapons.

Naturally, it follows that getting rid of these weapons will greatly affect the enemy's tactics and strategy and give you the upper hand. There is ample evidence of wars that have been won using this strategy, right from the Boer Wars in South Africa through the Arab-Israeli Wars to the Taliban's deft maneuvering in Afghanistan a few months back. The destruction of enemy weaponry and structure has always been a viable tactic for winning wars with minimal human casualties.

Effecting Disruption

This is yet another military tactic that works like a charm when used right. Every army is based on the efficiency of its structure, where different parts function as a whole. The disruption of a military organization renders the organization ineffective even when there is no physical loss or death of the organization's members. The attack is targeted at the structure and not the humans involved in running the organization.

Disruption can occur in an army's organization by surprising them or executing one's operations faster than they expect. Taking action before the enemy will affect how effective their response to any attack is, and this could lead to complete paralysis of the enemy army's organizational structure. A thoroughly startled army will not implement any tactics properly, nor will it defend its positions well.

The element of surprise can be a great ally once you are ready to decide and implement your actions as soon as possible. However, you would need to avoid hastiness in your bid to execute your actions faster than your enemy. You must be prepared and sure of your actions, or you will lose the element of surprise when initiating action.

Evasive Tactics

Another tactic is using evasive tactics, where you carry out military operations so that the enemy can't put the finger on your tactics or strategy. The principle behind this strategy is that it is difficult to defend and attack every position effectively. Therefore, when you attack the enemy through positions that they are not prepared for, they are forced to scuttle any plans they have, which could disrupt their tactics.

You might also choose to attack the enemy in areas where they do not have the manpower to defend effectively or counter your attack. The principle behind the evasive strategy is to scuttle whatever formation or tactics that the rival army might have. When done properly, the enemy's forces will be disrupted, and you could be a step closer to victory over them. A prime example is the hit-and-run tactics.

Guerilla warfare is a prime example of evasive tactics, and it has been effectively used to destroy powerful armies throughout history.

This strategy is hinged on short, unexpected attacks and a lot of maneuvering that allows the attackers to withdraw and avoid engaging the enemy. It has been used to expose and weaken enemy defenses before the enemy can respond in force.

Attacks by Special Forces units and terrorists are some of the more recent examples, although this tactic finds expression in the Lusitanian War, the Battle of Manzikert, the Battle of Ain Jalut, the Turkish War of Independence, the French and Indian Wars, the Vietnam War, the Soviet-Afghan War and America's recently abandoned military campaign in Afghanistan. All of these wars saw smaller armies forcing their larger enemies into tactical disadvantages using guerilla warfare.

Breaking Communication and Logistic Lines

This is a strategy where you target the communication system of the enemy army. We have already established that an army needs a fully functional and cohesive structure to operate. This structure is built and maintained via open lines of communication.

One of the best ways to break up an army's structure is to cut its lines of communication. When reports and commands along the army's hierarchy are not fully communicated, it becomes difficult to arrive at a clear picture of the situation. Consequently, it becomes difficult to formulate a strategy or even the tactics needed to attack or defend.

It becomes easy for you to isolate and attack your enemy positions because they cannot call for support since you have severed lines of communication. This strategy is often effected by jamming radio frequencies, cutting wires or capturing messengers. You could also achieve the same result by deliberately dis-informing the enemy by feeding them inaccurate information that will negatively affect the reports and the orders issued so that things are tilted in your favor. Another angle of disinformation is to cause resentment within the rank and file of the enemy's army via wrong information that puts the sender(s) and the recipient(s) at loggerheads.

Once you can break up the lines of communication, you increase the chances of disruption and ultimately a loss of cohesion and effectiveness in the army.

You could also opt to severe the transportation lines that link different divisions/units of a military campaign. The transportation routes are just as important as communication lines because they provide support, reinforcements, and supplies to each unit.

There are always points/areas between these units that make them vulnerable to attack. Once you can block the communication and logistic lines between these units, you limit the movement of supplies and reinforcements, which are essential to the success of any military campaign.

This strategy has always played out in military conflicts for a while now. During World War II, cargo ships containing much-needed supplies were targeted and sunk. The German Navy couldn't sink as many ships as the Allied Forces, and so Britain was able to keep a supply chain on the Mediterranean Sea. Consequently, this allowed the Nazis to be attacked from North Africa, and it significantly affected the outcome of the war.

In the Battle of Ilomantsi, the Finnish forces were outgunned and outmanned by the Soviets. However, their successful attacks on Soviet supply lines forced the Soviets to retreat, leaving valuable military equipment in the process.

Eliminating a Key Player/Component

An army is an organization with multiple components working cohesively. Yet a key player or component keeps the structure functioning optimally. This concept is not limited to a human factor, but it includes any part of the military campaign vital to its success.

The key player in the human context could be the general in charge of the military campaign, some of his trusted lieutenants, the elite forces, or even the head of state. You could also target key equipment and infrastructure significant to the military campaign, like destroying airfields and key military bases, nullifying vital codes, or blowing up train tracks or key roads.

Psycho-Centric Strategies

"In doing battle . . . you achieve victory by irregular means. So if you are good at irregular warfare, you will be as inexhaustible as the sky and the earth."-Sun Wu.

If the enemy's capability is the hardware and his mind is the software, you could affect the software so that the hardware no longer functions. The mind is more potent than most military strategists acknowledge, and so you'd be entering uncharted territory when you opt to explore ways of affecting your enemy's psyche.

Psycho-centric strategies are designed to break the enemy's will to fight and oftentimes win him over to your side. Like most military strategies, it has its roots in pre-modern warfare.

Genghis Khan is one of the most popular of that era. He was exceptionally skilled at instilling fear in the hearts of his enemies by spreading rumors about the vicious Mongol horsemen in his army. He was known to have his soldiers carry three lit torches at night to suggest numerical strength. He also had a reputation for catapulting severed human heads over the walls of enemy settlements as a shock tactic.

During WWI, armies used planes to drop flyers and non-lethal artillery rounds behind enemy lines as a means of spreading propaganda. The German and Allied Forces had units that specialized in psychological warfare, which they used in WWII. Both sides also used radio broadcasts to their advantage. The Nazis and their allies, the Japanese, used radio broadcasts like "Axis Sally" and "Tokyo Rose" to spread false information about their victories to demoralize the Allied Forces. The Americans were able to one-up them with their play at "leaking" false orders that deceived the German high command into preparing for an Allied invasion at the wrong location.

ISIS (one of the more recent terrorist organizations)employs social media and other online platforms to implement psychological campaigns calculated at currying support and recruiting fighters from all over the world.

 Let's look at some techniques that strategists have designed to reduce the enemy's will and help you win the war with fewer body bags.

Causing the Enemy To Lose Confidence in Themselves

Constantly failing at something has a dampening effect on anyone's psyche. Soldiers at the battlefront have to go through very dehumanizing, mind-altering situations which task the mind even after retirement. It is one thing to win a battle after going through those brutal conditions after achieving the goal.

It can be devastating when an army has to go through these harsh conditions and still lose battle after battle. After a while, the soldiers start to lose confidence in their abilities, no matter how well trained or equipped. Once the soldiers' morale is low, they no longer have the will or zeal to fight.

Ever heard the saying, "It's not the size of the dog in the fight but the size of the fight in the dog ?" Roughly translated, this means that the will to fight is the critical factor in winning any fight, battle, or war.

The power of the will is the singular reason why wars are won and lost.

It is also the secret behind rag-tag armies and guerillas holding their own against fully trained, well-organized armies. Find ways to cause losses to the enemy's military campaign, even if it is as small as an attack on their communication and transport lines or supplies. As long as you inflict the losses inflicted strategically, it will start to tell on their psyche after a while. Sometimes you could even strategically use disinformation to create an appearance of defeat to achieve a loss of confidence in the enemy's need for the military campaign. Most military forces take the time to compute the cost of resources expended and their casualties. And even when such information is on a need-to-know basis, word always gets out, and in those instances where the information is less than great, it will dampen the soldiers' morale. You could opt for this technique to sow the wrong ideas in the enemy.

Effecting a Loss of Confidence in the Military Campaign

A loss of confidence in one's ability as a soldier will degenerate into a loss of interest in the military campaign. The reason for this is simple. After sustained losses, soldiers tend to lack motivation and ultimately see the military campaign as needless and wasteful exercise, especially when they feel that the losses are a high cost to pay for whatever interests the way might be pursuing.

Most military commanders understand this fact. That is why they are constantly looking for ways to improve the soldiers' morale before, during, and after battles. The aim of attacking the enemy's mind is to get them to review the losses that have been inflicted on them in terms of the results. In situations where the losses do not seem to match the promised results, there will be a loss of confidence in the need for the war.

Soldiers are programmed to die for something: defending their homeland or protecting it from external aggression. For example, look at the furor that the loss of American soldiers in Somalia, Iraq, and Afghanistan caused and see how it affected those military campaigns. A military strategist who can manipulate the enemy's mind to lose motivation and doubt the validation of a military campaign has won half of the war.

How?

Most times, this loss of interest in the war often goes beyond some disgruntled murmurs in trenches and at gatherings of soldiers. The loss of interest can degenerate into large-scale desertion of soldiers or even full-scale mutiny that could threaten the lives of the commanding officers. An army's military might depend on discipline and organization. Once that is lost, the soldiers are nothing more than a group of armed men with little or no direction or purpose. These minute things deteriorate to the stage where you could easily pick them off. Or even co-opt them into your military campaign, which is a win–win situation by all means.

Which Approach Is The Best?

It all depends on your approach to the war. Are you looking to achieve a hard and fast destruction of the enemy's military equipment? If yes, then that would require specific, concentrated, and concerted efforts to get things done as soon as possible. It is essentially an all-or-nothing approach to warfare.

Physical-based strategies target the speedy destruction of the enemy or its equipment and all. It is based on the principle that the swift destruction of the enemy's military strength is the fastest way to end the war with minimal damage. Military strategists who subscribe to this approach to warfare believe that eliminating the enemy's strengths will cause a collapse of the enemy's forces and lead to surrender or defeat. Sadly, many physical-based strategies do not always work if the advantage of military might is not there. You'd be in a suicidal situation if you opted to go all out against an enemy that has more soldiers and more military hardware than you. The sheer difference in numbers will defeat your aim of winning the war with minimal casualties.

Psycho-centric strategies apply a progressive approach to winning away. Attacking the enemy's will to fight is a gradual process that takes time. It is based on the principle that attacking the enemy's will to fight can lead to a surrender of enemy forces with minimal losses for the protagonist. Now, while there are fewer casualties with this approach, it takes time and is just as complex.

The reason for this complexity is that it often depends on the situation and the key players' ability to execute the plans as effectively as possible. Another downside is that an enemy that is the wiser to your antics can outmaneuver you and use your tactics against you.

So which approach works best for a military strategist who intends to win the war with as few casualties as possible? This question recognizes the fact warfare is dynamic, and the results of a well-planned war are often light-years apart from the projections on the drawing board.

The best approach is to blend both systems to arrive at what we would term as the 'Ultimate Strategy".

The Ultimate Strategy

Mushasi captures the need for an ultimate strategy when he submits that:

"In strategy, it is important to see distant things as if they were close and to take a distanced view of close things."

A distanced view of close things involves an objective approach to handling issues. Here is where you step out of the immediate situation to get a better view of the state of things. Call it thinking out of the box, if you will but what Musashi is trying to say is that your approach to strategy should be different from most and, by extension, unpredictable. Hence "…see distant things as if they were close and to take a distanced view of close things."

Taking such an approach to strategy makes you flexible and difficult to anticipate. Your enemy does not know what strategy you might deploy and if you can alternate your moves mid-campaign. For instance, destroying the enemy's manpower and equipment might cause a defeat or a surrender if properly executed, and certain situations work in your favor. But in some cases, with the right amount of destruction of the enemy's forces or sustained disruption of its military operations, you could achieve the same effect.

In such an instance, there is a blend of physical-based strategy and the psycho-centric strategy. The sustained destruction of the enemy forces and their equipment was an example of a physical-based attack on an army's physical capabilities. At the same time, the disruption of their military operations via sabotaging their preparations and lines of communication and supplies and destroying vital components is an aspect of the psycho-centric strategy.

The psycho-centric approach aims to convince the enemy that a loss is inevitable based on past and current experiences. If he wins by some odd twist of fate, it would be a pyrrhic victory that he'd be hard-pressed to justify.

For Sun Wu, achieving a flawless victory in a military campaign is inseparable from great strategy:

"Military strategy is like flowing water. The characteristic of water is to avoid high places but drain into low places. So, victory in the war is due to avoiding strong enemy positions attacking weak enemy positions. Water depends on the terrain to adapt. Combat depends on the enemy's situation to arrange. So there is nothing certain in war as the water never holds a certain form." - *The Law of War: The Art of Competition Benefits in War, Business and Life*

However, Sun Wu only recommends the destruction of the enemy's army after attacks on the opponent's strategy and diplomacy to destroy its alliances have failed.

His ideas are further reinforced by the thoughts of Niccolo Machiavelli thus:

"…you must know that there are two kinds of combat: one with laws, the other with force. The first proper to man, the second to beasts, but because the first is often not enough, one must have recourse to the second. Therefore, it is necessary for a prince to know well how to use the beast and the man. Thus, since a prince is compelled of necessity to know well how to use the beast, he should pick the fox and the lion because the lion does not defend itself from snares, and the fox does not defend itself from wolves. So one needs to be a fox to recognize snares and a lion to frighten wolves." — *The Prince: Chapter XVIII*

In sum, these great minds believe that you have to deploy a balanced strategy that is flexible enough to adapt to situations yet powerful enough to achieve the desired result. Military commanders have had to change the way they operate in the field. But to do that, you need to be in a state of calm amid the chaos around you.

The Power of a Calm Mind

Military combat has an ugly aspect to it. Such is the horror of this violent yet primordial facet of human reality that our consciousness is affected whenever we are involved in violence. It doesn't matter if we dispense or receive it; the outcome is the same; some measure of stress is generated.

Now stress wreaks havoc on the brain. Humans (and indeed all animals) are wired by nature to protect themselves in the face of danger. It is an unconscious and automatic reflex. So whenever we are in dangerous situations, our bodies secrete stress hormones like cortisol and adrenaline. Once these hormones get into the system, they put us in a state where we either fight or run from danger.

That wouldn't be so bad if it were not for the physiological reactions that come with these biochemical reactions. Some of these reactions include a faster heart rate, a trembling solar plexus, sweaty palms, a constricted throat, a rigid jawline, a tightening of the back of the neck, and shallow breathing, and we breathe in more oxygen. Many combatants have experienced this set of reactions at one point. The best of them are those who have mastered the ability to calm their minds even when their bodies are stressed.

For most people, even soldiers, it becomes difficult to make complex decisions, which can be dangerous for soldiers at war. All that is important is how to deal with the imminent danger. Interestingly this response to stress is meant to be a short-lived one.

The reason is that all that cortisol that is pumped into the body starts to take a toll. And so, after a while, one's health starts to deteriorate. But most importantly for soldiers, stress affects decision-making, which is vital in creating and executing an effective military strategy.

The reason is that stress narrows the focus to oneself and possible survival and prevents you from seeing the big picture. You can easily observe more in a less stressful situation, and you find it easier to communicate better. When you are in a calmer state, you manage your energy better, your mind is clearer, and you focus better. You are ultimately more productive, creative and you are more innovative.

Most military organizations focused on hardening the bodies of their soldiers and improving their proficiency in the use of weapons and the execution of tactics. Drawing from the analogy we used earlier in this book; the focus has been on making the hardware better.

Thankfully that is changing. There is now a focus on the mind and its ability to be trained like a muscle. There is a trend in modern military training that sees training the mind as a means of improving soldiers' performances on and off theatres of war. The new catchword is "mindfulness": a crucial part of modern military training.

Mastering the Art of Mindfulness

"If you correct your mind, the rest of your life will fall into place" -Lao Tzu.

Mindfulness is known to offer a range of benefits, including enhanced mood, immune function, attention, and pain tolerance, among others. It is also known to decrease stress while heightening cognitive functioning. Interestingly, the practice of mindfulness has been introduced into military training. This is due to the recognition of its potential to enhance soldiers' performance on and off theaters of war. Interestingly, the concept of mindfulness is central to belief systems that promote peace and oppose conflict. Yet soldiers are using mindfulness practices as tools to help them manage the stress and attendant trauma that is part and parcel of warfare.

So what exactly is mindfulness?

Well, simply put, the idea of mindfulness training refers to practices that train the brain to remain in the present. Folks who have mastered the art of mindfulness can relax, lower their blood pressure, enjoy better sleep, become more focused and alert, optimize their motor functions and improve their relationships.

Why Is Mindfulness Important For Soldiers

For soldiers, in particular, mindfulness training improves their abilities to perform at their best when off-duty, during drills, and in a theater of combat. It is also used to decrease pain, stress, and trauma that is associated with post-deployment and post-traumatic stress disorder (PTSD). Soldiers also use it to enhance their impulse control.

Mindfulness training makes it easier to enhance one's ability to pay attention to the present moment while acknowledging your current emotions, thoughts, and sensations evenly and without bias. It efficiently eliminates issues like mind-wandering, worrying, and trying to appraise the past. With mindfulness, you have tunnel vision that is focused on the present so that you don't get distracted from current events. You simply accept your current reality without any judgment.

The good thing about mindfulness is that it is a skill, and like all other skills, it is transferable and can easily be acquired. Better still, you get better at it the more you practice you put into it. Once you can find the time to practice mindfulness regularly, you will get better at reducing your impulse to get triggered by stressful situations. At the same time, you get better at maximizing your awareness, concentration, and decision-making. That way, you make better decisions; you are more proactive and less reactive.

During drills, soldiers who practice mindfulness find it easier to be safe when trying out new drills. Their memories are sharper, so they can remember even the most challenging tests and qualifications like shooting drills and other important training exercises. These drills are designed to put them in real-life situations and help develop the ability to eliminate distractions while handling their mind-body management of performance anxiety is crucial to their ability to perform in theatres of combat efficiently.

Mindfulness also helps improve situational awareness, which is vital in combat situations. For example, a soldier who is given to a mind-wandering will not be aware of his environment or the particular situation he finds himself in. In addition, appraising situations with bias or judgment will generate the kind of stimuli that affects your ability to optimize the resources you need to execute tasks, prevent disaster, or promptly and effectively respond to crisis situations.

Soldiers will be less lethal and less resourceful during combat situations if their minds keep wandering and they find it difficult to focus on a situation fully. With practical mindfulness training (no matter how short) for even relatively short periods (for example, 8 hours over eight weeks), soldiers will have better focus and improved situational awareness. They will also be better equipped to tolerate the different combat environments (Volatile, Uncertain, Complex, and Ambiguous) that they might encounter during a military campaign. So with well-honed skills, they can respond to stimuli appropriately. Such soldiers will also have a higher pain threshold than others outside the mindfulness training.

But mindfulness practices are not all about dealing with combat situations. There will be "dwell times" when soldiers are off duty. This is when soldiers create bonds, and friendships are cultivated. A soldier who cannot handle the stress and trauma of warfare will have poor interpersonal relations and will often be isolated even in battle because they lack the right connection with other soldiers.

On the flip side, clients who take mindfulness training will be able to build and maintain productive relationships with colleagues and loved ones. They also find it easier to relax and de-stress themselves.

Mindfulness training is particularly important during intensive training periods before deployment. This is a crucial period because soldiers are being physically and psychologically prepared for getting into stress-prone and potentially dangerous situations. In addition, mindfulness training imbibes the training better and makes them better soldiers in real-time combat situations.

Several studies (notably at the University of Miami and the University of California, San Diego School of Medicine, and Naval Health Research Center) have carried out mindfulness studies on American soldiers. For example, the study at the University of Miami revealed that mindfulness training facilitated the attention span of soldiers, prevented mind-wandering, and could improve cognitive abilities.

The study at the University of California revealed that soldiers who practiced mindfulness techniques could cope with the demands of combat situations a whole lot better than those who didn't.

Why Mindfulness is Crucial For The Ultimate Warrior

Musashi is believed to have never lost any of the 72 duels he fought in his lifetime. Besides being a master of martial arts, he was a master of his mind. He was an unalloyed proponent of meditation, and he is known to have used his knowledge in his fights.

Musashi's mastery of mind and matter should be the blueprint for the modern-day soldier looking to walk the Way of the Warrior. Let's put things in perspective for a minute. How was it possible for Musashi to defeat tens of warriors, some of whom were younger, stronger, faster, and more skilled than him?

Baring the use of magic (black or white), such a feat could only have been possible if he knew when his opponents would move before they did. That would mean that he had a strategy that was flexible, efficient, and, most importantly, challenging to counter. Creating and executing such a strategy would require some mastery of the mind, and we would be safe to assume that he practiced some form of mindfulness or the other. His thoughts on the "Void" lend credence to our assumption.

"Your mind must never be lost...Polish the twofold spirit of your mind and your will."

These are words on marble for every modern warrior. You need to step out of the box that has led most soldiers to believe that they only need hard bodies and quick fingers to stay alive during the war. Step into Musashi's void and let this mental space provide the clarity of thought and purpose you need to avoid being one of the body bags on the next flight home.

As a commander of men responsible for the success of combat missions and the lives of the men under you, mindfulness is non-negotiable for you. There are times when things will never go as planned, no matter how many consultations and plans are made on the drawing board. There will also be times when the success of a mission and low casualties will become mutually exclusive. Tons of other distractions would threaten your decision-making at crucial points during a military campaign.

It would be best if you stayed calm in the face of conflict. Your life and the lives of your men depend on that. Being in control of your mind long enough to see things for what they are without an iota of bias or judgment is the difference between an effective military strategy and a botched one that leads to casualties.

Being mindful is key to your strategy as the Ultimate Warrior. In Musashi's words:

"Think accurately and clearly. Think big. Develop the "empty" nature in your strategy."

The Warrior and the Ethics of Warfare

War takes a toll on even the most emotionally detached warrior with iron-clad self-mastery. After seeing enough bloodshed for a while, you start to wonder if it is all worth it after all. You might even begin to question the rationale behind large-scale bloodletting. Is war obligatory? If yes, how then should it be staged?

The thrust of this treatise is winning a war with minimal casualties on your side while inflicting maximum casualties on the enemy. One begins to wonder at the means to achieve that goal. Are drones and long-range missiles considered ethical means for achieving these goals? What about distinguishing between enemy combatants and non-combatants. More so, is death the only signifier of defeat?

Miyamoto Musashi is famed for winning about 60 life-or-death duels by the time he was 29. Yet it is believed that at a point, he stopped killing his opponents as he entered the duels with a wooden staff with which he attacked until the opponent tapped out. Moreover, he did this even when his opponents intended to kill him or cause grievous bodily harm, at the very least.

One can deduce that Miyamoto's change of "tools" (for want of a better term) signaled his change in perspective about the goal of combat. Of course, one can argue that he was tired of the bloodletting that often comes with such duels, but even that in itself shows that he saw combat differently at that point. Indeed, the bulk of his writings was about winning with the least loss possible and for that perception to materialize in the choice of a wooden staff in armed combat suggests one thing: the application of ethics to combat.

According to Musashi, the warrior's path is paved by discipline, focus, restraint, and honor and is maintained by moral and ethical codes. One could draw parallels in his philosophy to the Just War Theory advanced by St. Augustine in the 5th Century and St. Thomas in the 13th Century.

Two of the more popular concepts in this theory," Jus ad Bellum" and "Jus in Bello," which mean "the reasons for going to war" and "the conduct of war", respectively, describe wars as ethical or unethical. Based on the Just War theory, a war was deemed ethical when it was waged by a legitimate authority that fought for a just cause and with the right intentions. Such a war was often the last resort and should be deemed as a last resort when every attempt at dialogue fails. It is also expected that in an ethical war, there had to be discrimination between combatants and non-combatants.

In reality, modern warfare straddles this description because there are a lot of wars that have been waged using unethical means like drones, landmines, torture, and chemicals. There is also a plethora of instances where both enemy combatants and non-combatants have been killed in a war, especially when the use of military force was deemed "disproportional" to the scope of the war.

Machiavelli advanced the opinion that princes gained and kept power by waging wars and going by the growing tensions between Russia and the rest of the EU, wars might not end anytime soon. However, we might yet see a situation where both sides of a war attempt to achieve a bloodless victory.

Does Just War Theory Count in Post Modern Warfare

There is an aspect of Just War theory that deals with the corpus of rules or agreements like the Geneva and Hague conventions structured to delimit the kinds of warfare that were deemed "acceptable." Interestingly, these agreements are subject to religious beliefs, race, and language differences. When both sides of a war see each other as subhuman because of these differences, ethics of war rarely apply. Just War theory will rarely apply in the genocidal wars that have been waged across continents. Yet warfare has always been influenced by rules of engagement. At the time, several codes of warfare prevented attacks on non-combatants like children and women. In addition, there was some sense of "honor" that made it "unsoldierly" to participate in certain acts of war. That is not to say that these codes were always subscribed to giving the accounts of the activities of the Teutonic Barbarians, Vikings, Huns, and the Mongols(of the Gengis Khan era), among others.

Because

"You must know that there are two kinds of combat: one with laws, the other with force. The first is proper to man, the second to beasts, but because the first is often not enough, one must have recourse to the second." -Niccolo Machiavelli, *The Prince*

Indeed, the current narrative of the efficacy of the Just War theory in promoting the codes of warfare is an interesting one. On the one hand, there is an increased awareness of the need to get soldiers to imbibe the tenets of Just War theory. On the other hand, interestingly, more military academies create courses around the justification of war and its application.

Sadly, that has not put an end to war crimes as genocidal campaigns are still on the rise, just as extremist attacks have become the new normal in some parts of the world.

So does Just War Theory matter in postmodern warfare? To answer that question, we'd need to take a look at the theory and the concepts upon which it is built.

The Concept of Jus Ad Bellum and Post-Modern Warfare

Jus Ad Bellum is built on the idea that a just war must be fought for a just cause; it must be a last resort and be instigated by a legitimate authority. It must also be informed by the right intention and be most likely to be successful using proportional means. Now, these tenets might be definite, but it affords some level of flexibility to their application as all of the tenets are relative and could be interpreted based on the context of the situation.

The Idea of Just Cause

What could be considered a just cause in a war between opposing parties? Each side of a war that is the recipient of an act of aggression would term retaliatory attacks just, seeing as the right to self-defense is an inalienable human right. To this end, it is difficult to define what "just cause" means in the event of a physical and mental injury, trade embargoes, perceived slights, and the appropriation of a state's boundaries.

Let's take, for example, the conflict between Russia and the EU over Ukraine's decision to become a member of NATO. Clearly, both sides of the conflict have legitimate arguments. Ukraine has the right of association, while the Russians might have adopted their stance because of the economic and political implications of such a move by Ukraine. If both sides perceive the achievements of their interests to be of utmost priority, it would be difficult to argue that neither of them is acting unjustly.

So going by Russia's relatively unprovoked bombing of Ukraine, Ukraine will be morally justified to launch its attacks. And going by the prescriptions of Just War theory, *both* sides will be justified to pursue such a campaign. Defensive reaction to physical force (anticipated and implemented) can be justified to all intents and purposes as long as the acts of war are implemented to prevent or retaliate against aggression from external aggressors.

This leads us to the question, "Is it justified to launch the first attack to prevent a war. Again, in the illustration of the Russia/Ukraine imbroglio, is it justifiable for any of the parties to launch an attack in the belief that it could forestall a full-blown war?

Will any of both sides be justified if they borrow a leaf from this submission:

"There is no avoiding war, it can only be postponed to the advantage of your enemy." - Niccolò Machiavelli.

This submission leads us to the next tenet:

War as the Last Resort

Wars have ripple effects that often takes a while to correct. And so, war should only be used when other options are off the table.

Proper Authority

The concept of proper authority revolves around the belief in the state's sovereign power. Yet, arriving at such a position is problematic because not all declarations of war that are seemingly accountable and legitimate really are. Certain military policies and campaigns pursued by these countries might not be justifiable. Indeed, more modern societies have developed the ability to walk that space that is influenced by the political forces of sovereignty, accountability, and necessity.

Right Intention

The tenet of right intentions is hinged on the belief that wars should be waged to pursue just causes and not because of selfish interests. So, in a sense, a pursuit of a national interest via war might be termed unjust.

This might be a bit problematic in itself. Earlier in this book, we established that most wars are extensions of political interests that are often mutually exclusive. In this context, such wars will be termed selfish and unjust. Consequently, gauging the right intentions is tricky because intentions are relative, and what might be right in one content might be wrong in another. So, what one person sees as the right intentions might be the wrong intention to the person on the other side of the war. For example, both sides of the Russia/Ukraine crisis can claim to be pursuing the standoff because they both have the right intentions.

Reasonable Success

This is yet another problematic tenet in Just War theory. It suggests that a war should not be waged until it is absolutely clear that the possibility of winning is high. So in such an instance, the pros and cons of a military campaign need to be ascertained before such a campaign can be launched. Going by this submission, the US military campaigns in Vietnam, Iraq, and Afghanistan can be deemed unjust.

However, while this tenet and approach to warfare might be deemed practical and even realistic, there are existentialist issues that it does not cater to: "Would it be right to refuse to defend one's territory because the chances of success are low" "Would it also be right to refuse to seize the opportunity to obliterate an enemy when the opportunity presents itself."

Proportional Means

This tenet straddles the ethical aspects of warfare. It deals with how wars should be waged and states that a war is just when the means used to win a war are proportional. More like don't bring a gun to a knife fight or a tank to a gunfight. To understand this tenet, let's put things in perspective first. Let us say that Russia invades Ukraine with tanks and soldiers. Now, if/when Ukraine decides to counter-attack, it must never embark on its campaign using nuclear weapons. The idea is to even out the attacks on both sides. If Ukraine hypothetically attacks with a nuclear weapon and Russia survives, there will be yet another round of attacks. But if Ukraine were to respond with proportionate weapons, Russia won't feel that they have been one-upped, and the conflict could reach a logical end.

The Case Against *Jus Ad Belum*

The principles of *Jus ad Bellum* we just described provide pointers towards revisiting military ethics. There are quite some problematic issues in the principles largely because of their open-ended nature that supports multiple interpretations. Given that war is a complex and relative affair, the Jus Ad Belum concept might not completely cover all the angles of the discourse on military ethics. However, it provides a foundation for our understanding of what it means to apply ethics to military warfare.

However, the brutal character and devastating scope of postmodern warfare of war despite the codes of warfare, the prominence of Just War theory across different fields, and its impartation in military academies are telling. History is replete with examples of the brutality of modern warfare, from the bombing of civilian centers in Germany and Japan through the dropping of nuclear bombs on Hiroshima and Nagasaki to the bombing of Ukraine by Russia in the first quarter of 2022.

It would seem like ethics and war might be unmixable because they represent two ends of a stick that could never meet. However, from our description of the principles of the *Jus Ad Belum*, it is clear that nine times out of ten, existential realities (manifested as political interests and military necessities) would always displace the issues of ethics in warfare. Heck, the very nature of warfare makes the discussion of ethics and morals a needless exercise.

That said, the warrior looking to walk the Path and make his own path within that Path must understand the balance that an understanding of the ethics of warfare lends him. And to get a better understanding of the ideas contained in Just War theory, we will be looking at the *Jus In Bello* concept and its relationship with post-modern warfare.

Jus In Bello and Post-Modern Warfare

With the *Jus in Bello* concept, which deals with "just" conduct in warfare, there are three tenets upon which this concept is built: Discrimination, Proportionality, and Responsibility. The tenet of discrimination assumes that there are legitimate targets of warfare, while the tenet proportionality deals with the amount of military force considered ethically appropriate. Finally, the tenet of responsibility focuses on where the responsibilities of the warring parties lie in warfare.

The Principle of Discrimination

Going by the *Jus in Bello* concept, indiscriminate attacks are considered unjust because the non-combatants are not considered legitimate participants in the war and are expected to be excluded from the theatre of war. This is based on the assumption that these parties, by virtue of their existence and activities, are not active in the business of war which is essentially the killing of combatant soldiers.

A perfect analogy for this situation is boxing. It is a crime to throw a punch at someone going about their business of life. Yet anyone who steps into a boxing ring is by virtue of that space assumed to be in a situation where it is legitimately acceptable to throw and receive punches.

Combatants in war are in the same situation. Based on their training, dressing code, and their bearing of arms, they are in a space where it is acceptable by the codes of warfare to kill or be killed: whether their duties are combative or not. On the other hand, it is assumed that non-combatants do not have this status. As such, waging war on unarmed and untrained persons is considered by the principle of discrimination to be an illegitimate activity. This also extends to surrendered soldiers or soldiers turned civilians who have laid down their arms and are no longer active in warfare.

The Principle of Proportionality

"Do not fight but subdue the people." - Lao Tzu *The Book of Ethics*

This principle assumes that combat-related action must be proportional to the objective of the action. It is similar to the same tenet of *Jus Ad Belum* except that for *Jus In Bello*, the extent and violence of warfare is modified to minimize destruction and casualties. It essentially seeks to reduce overall while doing the right thing regarding the level of force that is appropriate in a war.

Of a truth, there will be the possibility of the wrong kind of military force being used against combatants in a war. Military history is replete have been instances where combatants have been killed even after they have surrendered, just as there are instances where non-combatants have been killed in the course of a war.

Does the proportionality principle raise questions about the concept of highly selective killing or assassination? The idea behind such killing is that such specific killing of key threats to peace and stability and war crime criminals as long as such targets are legitimate.

To a large extent, it would make a lot of sense if a legitimate target is killed to avoid further bloodshed or further the objectives of a military campaign. The tendency of such a form of attack generates a chain of retaliatory attacks of the same nature, just as it could be applied in other spheres of human interactions.

The Principle Of Responsibility

The *Jus in Bello* concept advances that soldiers in a war should be held accountable for their actions. It is morally permission for combatants to kill their counterparts to a large extent. However, it becomes an act of irresponsibility when a combatant knowingly opens fire on non-combatants or pursues fleeing soldiers for the thrill of it. Such acts will lose the legitimacy of warfare and enter the realm of war crimes.

The tenet of responsibility is linked to the tenets of the *Jus* ad Bellum and *Jus in Bello* because some measure of responsibility informs the nature of wartime activities. There have always been instances of soldiers going against orders from higher-ups because obeying such orders went against their sense of responsibility.

While this might be a drop in an ocean of barbaric attacks executed in the name of war, it serves as a model for the modern warrior who seeks his path on the Way of the Warrior.

Such a warrior is guided by an internal compass built from the highest values. That is the only way to prevent being consumed by the deepest depravity that is often kindled by acts of war.

The Case Against *Jus In Bello*

"Do not fight but subdue the people." - Lao Tzu *The Book of Ethics*

That would be the right path to follow in an ideal world. But a soldier on the war front has little or no time remembering the principles of discrimination, proportionality, and responsibility with the combination of the cacophony of gunshots, the surge of adrenaline, and the overwhelming drive to stay alive. Now that is the scenario of symmetrical warfare where it is soldier versus soldier. Applying Musashi's admonitions of keeping it mind over matter both in and out of the theatre of combat becomes extremely difficult.

It is even more difficult when fighting in less regular situations where one has direct interactions with a civilian population of supposed non-combatants that provide cover for the enemy. For example, American soldiers in Vietnam, Iran, Iraq, and Afghanistan have often had situations where they were done in by a civilian population that appeared may not have borne arms but were actively in support of the enemy.

The concept of *Jus In Bello* is further challenged by modern weaponry and the change in military strategies that have been occasioned by the asymmetrical warfare that has become the order of the day.

Jus Postbellum

> *Where the soldiers stomped, the thorns grew there.*
> *After winning big battle, there must be a crop failure.*
> Lao Tzu *The Book of Ethics*

At the end of every war, one of three things happens: the army is either defeated, victorious, or has agreed to a truce. Regardless of the outcome, things are never the same before the war. That is where the last and least popular concept of the Just War theory (*Jus Post Bellum*) comes to play.

Jus Post Bellum is pertinent to any scenarios that play out in the aftermath of a war. It is expected to show some amount of graciousness to the vanquished. Non-combatants should not be punished even as their rights or traditions should not be trampled on. It is also worth considering the rehabilitation of the vanquished.

It is important to treat the aftermath of a war delicate because

"It is important to remember that there is nothing more difficult to solve and more dangerous than the adventure of creating a new regime." - Niccolo Machiavelli *The Prince*

One never has to be soft or hard, or you risk making more dangerous enemies than you started with. Therefore, it is important to avoid exploiting the conquered politically or economically. Now, although the thesis of Jus Post Bellum is the ethical handling of a vanquished side regardless of its enemy status before the war, it bears repetition to note that you must tread carefully at this point because rehabilitating the vanquished side might lead to unwitting humiliation and the provocation of a burning desire to revenge.

Yet, a ruthless approach to the situation might generate the same results.

Ethics and the Concept of Bloodless Wars
Conducting a war has a saying:
One does not dare to be a master
But just want to be a guest
One does not dare to advance one inch
But just wants to take a foot back
That is advancing without contest
Set a battle without having to raise your arm
Capture the enemy without having to use a weapon
Lao Tzu *The Book of Ethics*

There is so much technological advancement that it would take a lot to implement the concept of a bloodless war truly. For example, there are so many remote, precision weapons that might ensure the safety of an army's ground forces. But what happens when the army has the same military might and can easily launch effective remote attacks. For instance, let's say both armies have access to the latest toys on the market: drones.

Drones have become the latest addition to the "bloodless" philosophy of modern warfare. They are believed to be affordable, and they eliminate the possibility of a drone-wielding army losing a lot of its soldiers. Drones are remotely controlled by pilots who don't have to see combat firsthand, so the war might be "bloodless" for them, but what about the victims of the drone strikes?

In the recent war between Armenia and Azerbaijan, many of the victims of drone warfare were non-combatant civilians. This raises moral and ethical issues regarding the incidence of war and its consequences. If the idea of a bloodless war is to minimize heavy military casualties, what is the rationale for killing non-actors in the armed conflict? However, in wars fought between standard armies and insurgents without high-tech weapons, some insurgents often evade or launch attacks using the local civilian population.

There is so much technological advancement that it would take a lot to truly implement the concept of bloodless war. For example, there are so many remote, precision weapons that might ensure the safety of an army's ground forces. But what happens when the army has the same military might and can easily launch effective remote attacks. On the flip side, there are bound to be casualties on the other side.

Except there is a move in the military space to replace human soldiers with robots. That might be the level of warfare where we have bloodless wars. Until we get to that point, we will still have to find ways to marry the ideal of bloodless wars with our current realities, if that is ever possible.

To achieve a semblance of that union, the human factor will have to come into play. Essentially, we will need a stronger application of a universal code by which armies across the world conduct war.

The Need for a Code

Regardless of the changing face of warfare, one constant is that humans play vital roles in and out of it. Technology and equipment aside, war is essentially the attempt at using any form of violence to get another party to submit to your will. It is one of the most selfish endeavors because while it aims at getting another to submit, you are simultaneously trying to maintain and possibly, improve your sovereignty.

The current realities of war as we know it is constantly shape-shifting, hence the need to keep one other constant: codes. There are both written and unwritten codes for combat that have guided combat over the years. But all of those are universal external codes that are only effective to the point at which the individual practices them. It is different with a different set of codes and personal convictions that, after all, is said and done, drive the individual's thoughts, words, and ultimately actions in and out of combat theatres.

We emphasize the importance of personal convictions because, as popular as the Chivalric codes of the time, there were many casualties during the Medieval era. And a significant number of these casualties were non-combatants. Moreover, over the years, there were changes in these codes (ostensibly for the better)to match the changes in technology and consciousness.

Yet, what we know as war crimes persist (they may not have been seen as that during man's darker, bestial days), howbeit on a different scale.

Be that as it may, to Musashi, the modern warrior exists for one reason:

"The only reason a warrior is alive is to fight, and the only reason a warrior fights is to win. Otherwise, why be a warrior? It is easier to count beads."

So as long as there are legitimate sovereign states with often mutually exclusive interests, there will always be soldiers like you to protect and preserve those interests. And where there are soldiers, wars are inevitable. Yet to Lao Tzu:

"Weapon is an ominous tool. Gentlemen don't use it. Only used for reluctance."

This takes us back to Musashi's position about mastery over the mind as the ultimate weapon. Knowing when and how to use your military training is the essence of a soldier who seeks the way. If you are in a war to win, then the best path would be to take actions subject to moral conditions. After all, if war is to be waged as a last resort meant to prevent a worse outcome, why be reckless with the power that you wield?

As a soldier in the current military space, you'd need a clearer understanding of the power of your mind to be able to win wars with minimal casualties. When you get to the level where you can pick your fights on your terms with the right strategy, the war is half won.

Being able to control and apply your mind, which happens to be your greatest weapon, makes the difference between if you become a casualty of the war or if you live to tell war stories as a war veteran in your senior years. The key lies in the codes that you live by.

We are in one of the most technologically advanced epochs of our time. We have reached heights that most folks could only have been dreamed about a few decades back. However, our advancements have proven to be a double-edged sword that has also caused us harm concerning the devastating character of the global military space. We have reached the crossroads where we realize that there has to be a paradigm shift as far as our wars go. Or else we risk global self-annihilation.

Thankfully, the thoughts and teachings of great minds like Niccolo Machiavelli, Lao Tzu, and Miyamoto Musashi provide a Way out for the modern warrior. But knowing about the path is one thing; staying dedicated to that path is another. With constant re-evaluation and restrategizing, it is possible to win wars with minimal casualties. It will only require a dedication to master oneself and to make that persistent mastery over self a religion:

"Today is victory over yourself of yesterday; tomorrow is your victory over lesser men." - Miyamoto Musashi

CONCLUSION

There is an interesting twist to the duel between Musashi and Kojiro. Although Musashi was victorious, tears dropped from his eyes as the fisherman rowed him away from the island. He had just defeated—destroyed—one of the greatest samurais in the land, and he didn't see the purpose in doing that.

For Musashi, he didn't gain anything from the victory, but the land had lost a great warrior because of him. Musashi believed that Kojiro had a lot to offer to swordsmanship because his skill as a swordsman had been honed from years of experience. And all that was gone because he, Musashi, had killed him in a pointless duel.

Musashi continued to study and teach swordsmanship, but he never killed an opponent in a duel again.

Dear soldier, I have written the concluding part of Musashi-Kojiro's duel as the concluding part of this book because I want to let you know that restoring peace has a purpose. Unlike Musashi who took out a great samurai from Japan, you are adding something great, something valuable to the world by restoring peace.

This is the point where there is a little contrast between you and Musashi. Musashi cried because he regretted his victory, but you would rejoice when you gain victory. It is said that when Kojiro died, his retinue of servants, students, friends, and officials rushed towards Musashi to attack him but he was gone before they could get him. Yours would be different: On the day you win this fight for peace, many would rush towards you, not to attack you, but to praise you and thank you for bringing to them what they have desired all along.

When this happens, know that it is your chance to share the knowledge you have gained. Know that it is your chance to ensure that the path of peace is not tainted or obscured. Seize the opportunity to propagate everything you know. Teach them to always follow the map. To be soft as water. To be fierce as fire. To be enigmatic as the wind. And to step into the void.

THE ENTREPRENEUR'S BATTLE PLAN

Winning Strategies For Business

INTRODUCTION

I t is not a new fact that money sits at the center of everything we do. It may not be mentioned as one of life's necessities like food, shelter, and clothing, but the truth remains that we can only get these necessities through money. Even important intangibles like love and health need money to thrive. It is for this reason that there is an unending quest for financial freedom.

Seeking freedom means that one is held captive by something or someone. And to be free, one either has to be given freedom or fight for freedom. Financial freedom cannot be given. Life does not throw a briefcase of euros on your laps. Life is not that generous. So, you *need* to fight to be financially free.

The first step to financial freedom is making your money work for you. There are several ways to do this, like having a business—in other words, entrepreneurship—tops the list.

Entrepreneurship offers independence in key aspects of one's life-time, money, creativity. This independence heightens its allure. But here is the hard truth: The business world is a highly competitive space that is out to swallow your vision and crush you to the ground. It is a battleground. As a businessperson, you'd face stiff opposition from existing businesses that already have a large portion of the market share. You'd face opposition from new businesses who are trying to stamp their presence in the market. You'd face opposition from economic policies and the global economic climate. And ultimately, you'd face opposition from yourself—from that little voice in your head telling you to give up, telling you that it is impossible to surmount the challenges.

Considering the many enemies within and without, you have two choices: back out of the fight, or forge ahead till you gain victory. If you are still reading to this point, it means that you've chosen the latter. Well done. Because you have done this, I will present to you, through this book, working strategies to conquer the business battlefield.

These strategies are based on Sun Vu's *The Law of War*—a book that has guided military strategies and warfare for thousands of years. It is recorded that during his lifetime as a military strategist and general, Vu never lost a battle. He didn't achieve this feat because he had the strongest of soldiers, but because he understood that every battle is unique and, as such, should be approached differently.

Sun Vu and Miyamoto Musashi (whose ideas on military strategy formed the basis for my book, *On The Soldier's Path*) had similar ideologies on warfare. Both men believed that warfare went beyond weapons, so they never followed the conventional paths to warfare. They understood that battles are as mental as they are physical. And for this reason, they developed their own strategies.

A military general in Sun Vu's time would have interpreted battle readiness to mean taking up arms and marching to the battlefield, but for Vu, battle readiness meant having the perfect strategy for each situation. It meant being enigmatic, unpredictable. It was a principle that led to countless victories, not just for him but for generals after him that depended on his principle.

Dear reader, see yourself as a soldier, only that you are fighting a financial war—a fight for your freedom. And here is an exciting fact: you will win this war because you have this book in your hands.

The Entrepreneur's Battle Plan is a step-by-step guide for navigating the rigorous terrain of the business world. It is a journey that begins from you getting it right at The Drawing Board (Chapter One) and terminates at how to use spies to win in the business battlefield (Chapter Ten). Between the start and endpoint lie several tactics (e.g., unpredictable maneuvering), resources (e.g., having a winning team), and qualities (e.g., resilience) you must possess to come out victorious. Each chapter of this book is summed up with words of affirmation. These words of affirmation will inspire you to take action. It is not enough to furnish you with strategies for business; it is important you take action. Taking action begins with getting your mind ready and unburdened from any limitation or doubt. And this is what each chapter will help you do.

The victor or vanquished is never known before a battle. But by having this book in your hands, you know you are coming out of the Business Battlefield a victor. Sun Vu's strategies worked for him and those after him. And it is on this knowledge that you should build your trust, knowing that you will win. With this in mind, let's march to the battlefield.

CHAPTER ONE

The Drawing Board

"Give me six hours to chop down a tree, and I will spend the first four sharpening the ax." — Abraham Lincoln

Many have an unintentional approach to business. For them, business is more of an escape route than it is about offering value and solving a need. By a stroke of luck, some have been successful with this approach, but for others, it has backfired. A lot of people go into business as a last resort. They are unemployed; they start a business. The economy is bad; they start a business. They hear that a particular industry is booming; they start a business. In countries in Africa, for instance, youths are advised to go into business as a way of being gainfully employed since their governments have failed them. While this may be a logical reason for starting a business, it has made many jump the gun and venture into businesses that at their worst, lack a solid foundation, or at their best, subsistent.

The first step towards starting a business is to have a plan. Every step in your business should be mapped. This is not to say you must get everything figured out at once. Plans and visions are bound to evolve, but before they do, you must have them first.

Sun Vu stated that there are five determinants that a soldier must plan towards during a war. They are Righteousness, Atmosphere, Terrain, General, and Martial Law.

Righteousness

About righteousness, Sun Vu wrote: *Righteousness is a way of making people willing to join with the king, to make them unite and join forces, to live and die with courage.*

The popular mantra is that the customer is king. Others even say that cash is king. These positions are understandable, but the ultimate truth is that in business, you—the entrepreneur—is king. You navigate the ship of the business. Your failure to navigate the ship as you ought to would lead to its capsize.

Now that you know you are king, the question you should ask is: *Why should people join forces with me?* These forces can be categorized into two: your team and your customers. The bulk of the work starts with getting the right team. If you can get the right team that buys into your vision, getting the customers would be easy.

Your Team

One thing you should know is that your vision is so big for you to fulfill alone. Think about behemoth companies—Microsoft, Apple, Amazon, Facebook, Alphabet, Tencent, Walmart, etc. Do you think they would have been global brands if their owners had decided to build alone? That would have been impossible.

Human resources are the greatest resource on earth. Although it is a resource that is difficult to control, it plays a vital role in any business. Your team does not only consist of your employees, but it also includes your investors and partners as well; it includes anyone who plays a role in your business. Your business, even if it is a startup, is a chain. And a chain is only as strong as its weakest link.

Know this: Humans are soils. Humans can take in your vision, nourish it, and make it grow. Before you make people willing to join you, you must first understand that just like there are different soil types for farming, humans can also be categorized by soil types. There are sandy humans and loamy humans. You should know the features of each category so that you can spot them and know which to utilize and which to avoid. Everyone shouldn't be on your team. Selecting the wrong soil as part of your team may be the beginning of the end of your business.

The Sandy Humans

Sandy soil is light, warm, acidic, and low in nutrients. Drains water easily. Nutrients are easily washed away by rain.[1]

Sandy humans have all the qualities of sandy soil.

1. Light: In terms of soil texture, heavy soil has a high proportion of clay, while light soil has more sand than clay.[2] Heavy soil, although hard to till because of the *stickiness* of clay, is more fertile than light soil.[3]

Sandy humans are not fertile. They can easily kill a vision. They do not have the patience or the capacity to *stick* with you till your vision starts to yield fruit. In this case, clay is a symbol of loyalty, faithfulness, and dedication to you and your cause. Sandy humans lack these qualities. They are light; they have no substance. The essence of building a team is to have people who can enhance and spread your vision. Sandy humans cannot do this. They contribute nothing to the growth of your vision.

2. Warm and drains water easily: Water is life. It is needed for the growth and sustenance of every living thing. Therefore, a soil must have a good moisture-retention capacity. The moisture content in a soil also helps reduce its temperature. Unless it is in a plant's nature to thrive in high temperatures, all plants will die if the soil's temperature is high.

Here, water is a metaphor for passion. Every business needs passion for success. Passion pushes you to become better, to never give up. But sandy humans lack this vital quality. They lack drive. They easily lose their passion and enthusiasm for the vision.

Asides passion, water also represents encouragement, the voice of reason. Running a business can be overwhelming, especially in the business's budding phase. This is why it is necessary to have people who wouldn't add to the heat of running the business, people who will encourage you to strive harder, people who will soothe you in times of distress, people who will be your voice of reason in times when you think giving up is the best and only option. Sandy humans aren't these people. They lose passion easily, so they can't encourage you to keep up with a vision they do not believe in. Sandy humans add to the heat of running your business. Your business cannot thrive with their presence.

3. <u>Acidic</u>: Acids are toxic. They corrode whatever they come in contact with. They stunt the growth of plants. Sandy humans are usually toxic. They possess qualities (e.g., rudeness, carelessness, greed) that are unhealthy for a business. Many business owners underestimate the value of character when recruiting employees. They focus on skill and experience, relegating character to the background. But skill and experience are not enough to maintain consistent patronage.

Human beings are emotional species. They have a sense of worth. No one will continuously patronize a business where they are disrespected or where their rights are trampled on. Sandy humans have toxic traits and attitudes that are capable of sending your customers away. Thus, you need to know the kind of people you bring to be part of your vision. As the business owner, you may have all the traits required to keep the customer happy, but you cannot attend to every customer at every time. For this reason, you need the *right* people to attend to the customers just as you would have. And sandy humans are not the right hands for the job.

4. <u>Nutrients are easily washed by rain</u>: Recall that sandy soils have low amounts of clay, so they cannot retain or hold moisture and nutrients. Sandy soils are loose soils, and the little nutrients that can be found in them are easily washed off by rain.

Sandy humans lack resilience. They lack staying capacity. You may think that they love and want to be part of your vision all the way, but when the rains come, they lose their integrity and loyalty. When the storms of the business world hit (e.g., economic recession, unfavorable policies, inflation, stiff competition), sandy humans will be revealed for who they are—people without substance.

Nutrients are also a metaphor for ideas. You can only expand your vision as an entrepreneur through ideas. Your team, apart from being employees and investors, should be your think-tank. They have seen and imbibed your vision. Thus, it is only rational that they come up with key ideas that would grow the vision. Sandy humans lack ideas, and in cases where they do have ideas, their ideas do not stand the test of time. Why? They do not think in the long term.

By their nature, sandy humans are impatient and are only interested in quick gains. As mentioned earlier, they lack resilience and staying capacity. So, their suggestions for your company would only be focused on what can bring quick, small gains today, and not what will bring huge profits tomorrow, albeit slowly.

If you make the mistake of implementing their idea, you will discover that it won't stand the test of time. If you are unlucky, it may destroy all you've built.

The Loamy Humans

Loamy soil is rich in nutrients. It has high water-retention capacity because it contains a significant proportion of clay. It can also drain water easily. It is easy to till.[4]

So, who are loamy humans?

1. They are heavy with nutrients: They are resourceful people. They are a hotbed of ideas. They understand and accept your vision. They have ideas to push and expand your vision. Just tell it to them, and they run along with it as if the vision is their personal project. They contain clay—they are loyal and dedicated. They have staying capacity. They are there through the thick and thin of your business.

Plant your vision in their hearts and watch it grow.

2. Retains water: Their passion never dies. They are committed to your cause. All they desire is to watch your vision expand. They are there to calm you down when the going gets tough.

3. Easy to till: These people understand that you are in the driving seat, so they are willing to follow your lead at all times. They are independent and smart enough not to be micromanaged, yet loyal enough to flow in your direction. Some people would want to take over your business because they feel they are indispensable.

You would encounter challenges when you have such people in your team. Loamy humans do not think they are indispensable. They do not put you in a position where you would have to choose between working with them and saving your business. They treat your vision as theirs and wouldn't do anything to jeopardize it.

Your business would thrive in the presence of loamy humans.

Now that you know the qualities of sandy and loamy humans, the next step would be to know how to spot these people.

Spotting sandy or loamy humans may be quite difficult because it takes time for an individual's true character to be revealed. However, I believe that the best way to know a person's character or value is to listen to what they say when they are not under duress. Listen to their comments on social, financial, or business issues, then you would be able to tell their character.

In the next chapter, I will outline the steps to follow to spot sandy or loamy before selecting your team.

To expand your business, you must be able to plant your vision in the hearts of others. It is an important step. Once you can do this correctly, then it would be easy to move on to the next determinant—atmosphere.

Atmosphere

Sun Vu wrote: *Atmosphere is night or day, hotness and coldness, and change of four seasons.*

As an entrepreneur, you have to be discerning of seasons. A business is built to evolve and those who will profit from it are those who understand seasons. Many companies are fettered by mediocrity because they cannot comprehend seasons and/or tailor their activities according to seasons.

The Four Business Seasons

Just like the earth has four seasons, there are four seasons in business: spring, summer, autumn, and winter. Peter Brodie, a member of Forbes Council, described the four seasons thus: "In spring, you build business plans, create new services and products, and design new marketing materials. In summer, everything is in full swing. You're busy supporting existing clients, and you continue to promote your services to attract a growing list of new ones. In autumn, the pace of work slows. You still have a core list of clients, but your services and promotional materials grow tired and jaded. Then, in winter, the cold settles in, with no growth or new clients in sight. You're dependent on what you've stored away in preparation for this bleak time."[5]

What you do at each season of your business determines how successful you would become. These four seasons are important and they all have their use—including the autumn and winter seasons.

As a new entrepreneur, the first season you enter is the spring season. Here, you are bubbling with ideas and passion. You make plans, draft strategies, and implement these strategies. You create. You build. You grow. If you get the spring season right, then you would have an exciting summer.

In summer, you watch everything you've planted yield fruits. You consolidate your work with more promotions, more investments, and more innovations. But this phase is not meant to last forever because autumn is just by the corner.

In autumn, there seems to be a tapering of success. It may seem as though you are fastened to a spot. There is no enthusiasm from your clients. Business slows down. The numbers aren't as high as they were before. And just when you are trying to overcome autumn, it starts to snow. Winter has come.

Winter comes with a pause. A biting cold. A depressing phase. No new clients. No innovation. No development. No increase in the numbers. And there is nothing you can do about it.

You must understand these seasons so you wouldn't channel your energy to the wrong activity. The spring season is not a time to rest; it is a period to sow. A season of implementation. A season of action. It is the season where you make the right connections. It is the season to get people into your team. Create and test new products. Improve your customer service. It is not a time to relax. Usually, the spring season is exciting—you are exhausted by all the work, yet you are thrilled by what you are building.

The result of your hard work during the spring season will be revealed in summer. Mind you, not every seed that was sown would germinate and yield fruits. This is why the summer season is important. It is a time to assess yourself. What did you get right? What did you do wrongly? How do you improve and scale up what you did right? What approach would you use to correct your mistakes? Summer is not just a time to enjoy the bubbles of success, it is also a time to reflect on how to consolidate this success. It is easy to get carried away with the warmth of summer and not notice when autumn begins to creep in.

With conventional weather, autumn marks the transition from summer to winter. Nature knows that it would be too sudden to switch between two temperature extremes with no warning, so autumn is that season that prepares us for winter. Similarly, the autumn season of business is meant to prepare you for what lies ahead in winter. Once the decline starts happening, once you stop seeing the bubbles, it means it is time to prepare yourself mentally and financially for winter. Don't allow yourself to be caught unawares.

Winter may be a cold and depressing period, but it is a time of evaluation. Don't lose track of your vision because you feel things are not the way they should be. The winter season is the time to brainstorm and think out new ideas. It is a time to relax with your team and evaluate the next step to take. The ideas you birth during winter are the ideas that you would implement during spring.

Every season is important. And in the world of business, the winter season of one businessperson may be the summer season of another. Peter Brodie put it rightly when he pointed out that there are neither winners nor losers in the business world; there are only seasons to be enjoyed.[6] The business world is an interplay of individual seasons. The period where you are winning and recording huge success is the same period another is at a consistent loss. There is no way to eradicate autumn and winter, leaving only spring and summer. Brodie stated that "most service professionals would like to make the warm, busy days of summer last forever. But too much sun and heat—too much work—will dry things up and create cracks. Both you and your business need periods of rest. You must give way to autumn to recover from the summer frenzy."

These seasons do not have definite lengths. But as an entrepreneur, your goal should be to have longer summers and shorter winters. "The duration is determined by the quality of work you invest into the business during spring. If you take the time to plant and propagate healthy seeds, you'll have long summers and short winters."[7]

Trends

Another aspect of atmosphere you must be able to discern as a businessperson is trends. Sometimes the seasons of your business are determined by the general trends of the market. Just as your business is bound to evolve, the market or industry is also bound to evolve. I have categorized business trends into five types: Uptrend, Downtrend, Sideways, Fads, and Disruption. Every market or industry reflects one or more of these trends from time to time.

Uptrend

This is the period in the market or industry where the value of products is consistently rising due to the high demand for the products. During this period, vendors make huge revenues. The upward trend coincides with the summer season of many entrepreneurs.

For instance, the online education industry experienced a boom during the heat of the coronavirus pandemic. There was massive adoption of online education during the lockdown. Many schools and individuals had to fully adopt online learning to keep up with their curriculum. For instance, when the Chinese government instructed 250 million full-time students to resume their studies through online learning, it resulted in what was dubbed the largest "online movement" in the history of online education as about 730,000 (that is, 81 percent of K-12) students attended classes online through the Tencent K-12 Online School in Wuhan.[8]

The World Economic Forum states that even before the coronavirus pandemic, there has been a massive adoption of online education worldwide. Global edtech investments reached 18.66 billion USD in 2019, and the overall market for online education was projected to reach 350 billion USD by 2025.[9]

With reports like this, entrepreneurs in the industry can accurately position themselves to have a significant market share before the uptrend stops. Other industries that experienced an upward trend due to the coronavirus pandemic include lifestyle of health and sustainability and wellness, delivery/logistics services, remote work, and entertainment industries.[10]

Downtrend

As you already know, this is the opposite of an upward trend. During a downtrend, an industry experiences a steady decline in value. Due to some political or economic factors, the interest of people towards an industry may dwindle. The downward trend coincides with the winter of many entrepreneurs.

An example of an industry that has experienced a downward trend is the global airline industry. Although the industry witnesses a rise in passenger and cargo traffic, it has been steadily declining because of volatile fuel prices and steady competition in the last five years. Between 2019 and 2020, it had revenue growth of -12.8 percent. This decline worsened with the coronavirus pandemic.[11] Richard Branson's Virgin Atlantic had to file for bankruptcy protection four months after Virgin Australia went into administration, owing 6.8 billion USD to over 12,000 creditors.[12]

A downtrend does not always translate to a total collapse of an industry. It is often a temporary setback—a pullback—so that the industry can regenerate itself. Some entrepreneurs and investors see downtrends as the perfect opportunity to make more investments. For instance, when many investors were trying to protect their investments because of the pandemic (I write of the pandemic because it is the most significant factor that impacted every industry around the world), the Oracle of Omaha, Warren Buffett invested 6 billion USD in five of Japan's biggest trading companies.[13]

Sideways

This is a term popular in finance industries like the stock market, forex, and cryptocurrency. But it can apply to other industries or sectors. In a sideways trend, the market neither moves up or down. Supply and demand for products in the industry are equal. Sideways trend precedes an uptrend or a downtrend. It is also known as consolidation because investors hold on to their assets since they don't know the direction the market would take.[14]

It suffices to say that a sideways trend that precedes an uptrend will coincide with the entrepreneur's spring season, while a sideways trend that precedes a downtrend will coincide with autumn.

Fads

We can describe a fad as a short-lived trend. A fad storms a market or industry, creates a buzz, and fades away as quickly as it came. Most times, fads are not genuine. For instance, between 2016 and 2017, the cryptocurrency industry was agog with the fake currency called OneCoin. It was dubbed "The Bitcoin Killer." Ruja Ignatova, the lady behind the project, called herself the Crypto queen and persuaded people to invest in her crypto project which would rival Bitcoin. But it was only a Ponzi scheme. The so-called digital asset was not on the blockchain—the technology that backs cryptocurrency assets. Dr. Ignatova made $4 billion selling a fake cryptocurrency to the world, then disappeared without a trace.[15] And the fad ended.

At other times, fads may be genuine but lack the tenacity to remain and compete in the market for a long time. An example of a genuine fad is Pokemon Go—a gaming app that made waves in 2016. Although it is reported that the gaming app had a record year in 2019, raking about $900 million through in-app purchases,[16] its 2016 buzz was gone.

It is difficult to predict what is a fad and what is not. Some products have been classed as fads and they ended up being staple products. An example is Twitter. Between 2009 and 2010, many questioned if the microblogging app had perpetuity or if it was another fad.[17,18] In 2013, a blogger even described the app as an internet force—"a force. . . for 140 characters worth of banal nonsense."[19] But can those words still be used to describe the app with a current market capitalization of over $37 billion?

The greatest innovation ever known to humankind was also classified as a fad. In 1995, Clifford Stoll, a technologist author and columnist for Newsweek claimed that the internet would never work and would die after 1996.[20] I don't need to write about the outcome of that prediction. The internet was never a fad; it was a disruption.

Disruption

Merriam-Webster Dictionary defines disruption as a break or interruption in the normal course or continuation of some activity, process, etc.[21] Therefore, a disruption is more than a trend or a fad; it is a new way of life.

In his insightful *Forbes* article, Caroline Howard stated that disruption uproots and changes how we think, behave, do business, learn and go about our day-to-day life. Quoting Clayton Christensen, a Harvard Business School professor, Howard explained that a disruption "displaces an existing market, industry, or technology and produces something new and more efficient and worthwhile. It is at once destructive and creative."[22]

Every disruption begins as a new trend, and sometimes, they get labeled as fads. We saw earlier how there was a prediction that the internet wouldn't survive, but more than two decades later, it has become the fulcrum for our every activity. The internet disrupted and replaced analog methods of doing things. Some people have missed huge financial opportunities because they were unable to spot and take advantage of disruptions. In 2010, a young man attempted to auction off 10,000 bitcoins for $50. No one knew if he succeeded or if he had a rethink and retained the digital asset. If we assume he sold off all his bitcoins, that means he auctioned off his opportunity to become about 180 million dollars richer ten years later. The blockchain and cryptocurrency industry is disrupting and revolutionizing global financial systems as we know them. With cryptocurrency, people can now actually have money as a store of value. Although the industry has been in existence for 10-11 years, it is still a budding industry when compared to the stock market and Forex. The New York Stock Exchange (NYSE) had a market capitalization of $25 trillion as of April 2020.[23] Forex has a market capitalization of around $5.1 trillion.[24] However, the cryptocurrency market is just a little over $758 billion as at 2020.[25] Smart entrepreneurs and investors are getting on this disruptive train before becoming saturated in the nearest future.

Jeff Bezos was a man who recognized a disruption and took advantage of it. He decided to take advantage of the web after reading, in 1994, that the web had grown 2300 percent in one year. He made a list of 20 products he could sell online and settled for books. The information on the internet then was less than 1 percent of the wealth of information available today. Yet, Bezos believed in the future of the internet. He left the hedge fund company, D. E. Shaw, where he had risen to vice-president to start his company: Amazon.[26] That singular belief in the internet—a disruption—has made Jeff Bezos the richest man in the world today.

Your ability as an entrepreneur to recognize and understand the atmosphere (seasons and trends) you are in would determine how well you would navigate your terrain. It is just like a physical journey. A road may be rough or the sky may be bumpy with clouds, but the journey becomes even more difficult and hazardous if the atmosphere is unfavorable.

Terrain

Geographically, terrain has to do with an area of land and its physical features. Nayturr.com defined terrain as the earth's horizontal and vertical surfaces. By identifying the different types of terrain, we can determine the most suitable habitats for humankind. The site listed 14 types of terrain, namely: canyon, desert, forest, glacier, hill, marsh, mountain, oasis, ocean, open, river, swamp, tundra, and valley.[27]

Just like identifying terrains can help us determine the suitable habitat for humankind, identifying business terrains can help you determine where and how to pitch your business. In this book, I will use some geographical terrains as allegories for business terrains. Thus, there are three types of terrains in business: canyon/valley, desert/oasis, and forest.

Forest

A forest is an area of land completely covered with vegetation—grasses and trees. Forest trees are perennial and survive for a long time. New trees would have to go through the process of growing as tall as the old trees. And to do this, they would need to compete for resources with the old trees. It would take a resilient tree to survive and grow as it should.

What does this mean in business?

In business, the forest is the commonest terrain. It is a terrain where there are multiple businesses, a terrain of stiff competition. An entrepreneur in this terrain would have to strive hard to stand tall above other trees or, at least, be on the same level with them. Except there is an innovative side to your business, it is unprofitable to be in this terrain because it is often saturated.

Desert/Oasis

A desert is a large, often hot, and dry piece of land with little or no vegetation due to factors like lack of water, bad soil, or salt poisoning. Most often than not, there is no water source in a desert. However, there are cases where there is an isolated area in a desert surrounded by a water source such as a spring, pond, or small lake. Such an area is known as an oasis.

Your business can be an oasis in a desert. You can venture into areas that others see as dry and unfavorable. The desert/oasis is often the toughest terrain, but its returns are huge *if* it eventually pays off. This was the story of Elon Musk's Tesla and SpaceX, especially the latter. A lot of people believed that it is ridiculous to venture into rockets. For them, rockets were the exclusive preserve of huge government organizations.[28] Yet, it was in this supposed desert that Musk decided to be an oasis. Today, he is the second richest man in the world.

Being an oasis in the desert requires taking calculated risks. It requires playing in a field where others have not played before. Thus you need to count the cost before venturing into the business. Elon Musk's idea almost crashed. SpaceX had three launch failures. If the fourth launch had failed, then that would have been it for the company. Yet, Musk believed in his idea and was funding it from his personal money. At a point, he had to sell his car.[29]

If you believe in the validity of your vision, you can aim to be an oasis in the desert.

Canyon/Valley

A canyon is a big gorge in the ground found between escarpments or cliffs *due to erosion from a river or other weather conditions.* A canyon is similar to a valley—a low area between mountains or hills with a river flowing through it. By geographical definition, canyons are formed due to erosion. This means that they were not hitherto present but were created over time due to atmospheric conditions.

What does this mean for an entrepreneur?

Some businesses or industries spring up or expand due to a drastic change in the economic climate. For instance, after 9/11, experts and researchers began investigating methods for improved surveillance technology. Technologies considered include remote-controlled airliners, bio-monitors, remote video monitoring, light guns, super thin flexible body armor, and missile disrupters.[30]

Another example is the explosion of certain industries due to the coronavirus pandemic. Telemedicine, pharmaceutical, online education, e-commerce, online payment, and delivery industries all recorded massive growth due to the pandemic. Just like erosion or adverse weather conditions create a canyon, the pandemic created canyons of businesses.

What this tells us is that entrepreneurs should always seek the positives within adversities. Seeking the positives in adversities is an indicator of a high adversity quotient. In adversity lies a lot of business opportunities. Adversities often reveal new problems; these problems would require solutions. And that's where you come in as a businessperson. Ask yourself: How can I offer value amid these challenges? What solution can I provide? How can I be a canyon?

General

As mentioned earlier, you are king, you are the leader. You are the magnet that attracts every other person to your vision. You are the commander. The general. Because of this, there are qualities you must possess. You must be strategic, trustworthy, kind, courageous, and strict/firm. Your team should possess these qualities too, but they can only do so if you show them the way. When your business expands, you'd have team leads who would oversee different aspects of your company. They can only carry out their leadership function if they see and act as generals. But first, they must learn and imitate the chief general: you.

Strategic

Entrepreneurs have to understand the atmosphere and terrain so that they can be strategic. No general goes to war without a battle plan, a strategy. Going to war without a strategy is suicide. While there are things you'd still have to learn through experience, a business without a clearly defined plan would fail. There is no guesswork in business. Every action taken must be a product of purposeful thought and a documented plan.

Members of your team should know your strategy and the roles they have to play. Divide your vision into short-term, mid-term, and long-term goals. The accumulation and attainment of these goals will lead to the overall success of your vision.

Have the right strategy for you cannot go wrong with one.

Trustworthy

One factor that limits new brands from competing favorably with established brands is trust. Over the years, big brands have created value and gotten their customers to *trust* that they would always deliver. For this reason, a new Samsung phone or iPhone or Play-Station 5 can get sold out within hours to days of release. People are ready to be among the first buyers because they trust the company launching the product.

Before people can trust your product, you need to be trustworthy first. Many businesses do not survive because they were started and maintained by cutting corners. They offer substandard products, claiming that their products are the best. Customers buy the products, use them, and discover they've been scammed. Since no one gets a second chance to create a first impression, the business begins to die.

Trust is a vital attribute needed for the success of a business. Neil Patel stated that trust is the foundation of strong business relationships, and entrepreneurs with a high level of trust are more successful at retaining employees.[31] This means that one fundamental way to have the right team is to be trustworthy. Patel further stated that to build trust, an entrepreneur must first see it as a priority.

Kind

Your products or services aren't offered to machines but human beings. Thus, you have to be kind when dealing with people—both employees and customers. Many entrepreneurs are so focused on their business that they have lost every sense of empathy and kindness. The only language they understand is money. This is a wrong approach to business. It is one of the dangerous drawbacks that can destroy a business. We will see this later.

Do not lose your humanity because you are an entrepreneur. Running a business can indeed be daunting, but you must not miss the opportunity of forging and sustaining human connections. Recognize the worth of humans and make sure you do not diminish their worth.

It is important to note that being kind does not translate to turning your business into a charity organization. Being a people pleaser is another dangerous drawback to a business. You have to maintain your business's image and worth without losing the qualities that make you human. Use your discretion to strike a balance.

Courageous

By starting a business, you have already displayed immense courage. Never lose this courage. The business world is a den of hungry lions ready to devour you as soon as you step into it. One needs to be courageous to be able to maneuver the challenges and come out strong. Without courage, you would be unable to apply the strategies you've mapped out. The lack of courage is a syndrome that can cripple a business. Four signs accompany lack of courage: doubt, fear, discouragement, and quitting. These signs follow an order and creep up as questions. Once you don't nip them in the bud early enough, your transition from doubt to quitting would be swift.

- Doubt: Am I sure this strategy would work?
- Fear: Am I sure nothing will go wrong if I apply this strategy?
- Discouragement: Am I sure I can compete with the top players in the industry?
- Quitting: Am I sure this is what I should be doing?

As an entrepreneur, these questions would pop in your mind once in a while, but "no" should never be your answer. Always say, "yes." Be positive. Let your positivity refuel your courage. Let it remind you why you are on the journey in the first place. Let it remind you that you can win.

Strict/Firm

Sun Vu required the general to be strict, but I think "firmness" should be a better word. Being strict is being a wood—rigid, unyielding, unwilling to adapt to change, losing touch with one's emotion. On the other hand, being firm is being a metal—strong, stable, resolute, malleable.

As a businessperson, you have to be firm, else you'll be taken for granted. Your team and customers should know and understand your place as the boss, the custodian of the vision. Let them know that you are open to ideas provided that these ideas are in line with the company's culture and vision. Never lose your humanity but draw the line between business and pleasure.

This is one of the challenges people who have remote workers face. Remote workers often feel that working remotely means eating your cake and having it. That is, they get paid monthly for a job while they live like they are on vacation. An entrepreneur that faces such a challenge should be firm and let the workers know that order *must* be maintained at *all* times.

People are most likely to disregard the order of a leader who is not firm in running an organization. Firmness is one true way of gaining respect. The people know that you respect and value their human worth, but you are not ready to sacrifice your company's success on the altar of laxity.

Martial Law

Sun Vu wrote that martial law refers to the organization and management of soldiers and military expenditure.

Organization and management are the principal duty of an entrepreneur. This is why many entrepreneurs bear the title "Chief Executive Officer" or "Managing Director." Even though the company has different experts handling a company's technical and financial aspects, the entrepreneur still has to oversee, organize, and manage them.

You don't need to be a techie or financial guru before you can oversee the financial aspects of your company. Brian Chesky, the co-founder and CEO of Airbnb, oversees an tech company, yet he has no tech background. He created Airbnb by hiring those who could handle the tech aspects of the company. Not being a tech guru didn't mean he would cede the company's organizational and managerial control to the tech experts. As long as Airbnb is concerned, Brian Chesky (alongside the other two co-founders) is the brain behind its success. He had a vision, knew what he wanted, and found people who could bring that vision to life. Even if he steps down as CEO, the new CEO would run the company using the template Brian had put in place.

The entrepreneur has the job of overseeing every aspect of the company, whether they are knowledgeable in the field or not. This is why Vu said that in martial law, a general not only manages soldiers, but also the *expenditure* of the military. A general is a man of war and strategy, yet he has the duty to manage the military finances. This does not mean he would take up an accountant's job, it only means that he has the prerogative of stating how funds would be disbursed.

This is the same for the entrepreneur. See yourself as a soccer coach. Not all soccer coaches know how to play soccer. Their forte is team management and tactics. You are just like them. So get a team. Hire accountants, tech gurus, marketing personnel, graphic designers, social media experts, and so on. But always remember that how these different professionals carry out their duties depends largely on your directives.

Pledge to Action

I affirm that:

I believe in the validity of my vision.

I believe I can meet a need in the world with it.

As a result, I will attract the right people to me.

I will attract people that will stick with me and grow with me.

I will navigate the harsh seasons and tough terrains.

I understand that tough seasons do not last.

So, I know I will enjoy the blissful moments of summer.

I have the eyes of an eagle to spot uptrends and disruptions.

I am ready to take advantage of these trends and win.

I will be the general who is strategic, trustworthy, kind, courageous, and firm.

I let go off fear, doubt, discouragement, and quitting.

I am ready to launch my vision.

So here I am at the drawing board.

CHAPTER TWO

The Attack

"Without a plan, there's no attack. Without attack, no victory."

— Curtis Armstrong

The planning phase is the most important phase in starting a business, but if you fail to launch, your plan becomes only a dormant, documented dream. The dictionary defines attack as "to set *work* upon a task or problem." The attacking phase is the work phase. Sun Vu called it the combat phase. At this phase, you test the strength of your vision, the viability of your ideas.

Sun Vu stated that during combat, the general recruits his soldiers and makes provision for expenses such as food, weapons, repairs, etc. During combat, you breathe life to everything you had documented in your plan. By attacking, you will be giving flesh to the five determinants—Righteousness, Atmosphere, Terrain, General, and Martial Law—you considered at the drawing board.

I have already explained how to attack three of the five determinants namely: Terrain, General, and Martial Law. So in this chapter, we will be focusing on the first two determinants—Righteousness and Atmosphere.

Righteousness

According to Sun Vu, righteousness is all about inspiring others to believe in your vision and join hands with you to bring it to fruition. In the previous chapter, we saw that human beings are soils, and just like there are different soils on the earth, there are different human soils. Now that you know the characteristics of sandy and loamy humans, the next step is how to recruit the best soil for your business.

Sun Vu noted that a general who knows how to use soldiers would not have to recruit soldiers twice. In business, continuous recruitment is necessary to fill in gaps and meet company needs, however, when you manage your team effectively, you will have people who will stick with you for the long haul. So how do you select your team as a budding entrepreneur?

Steps to follow for team selection (How to spot human soil types)

- Do not rush into recruitment immediately. By recruitment, I mean conducting interviews and employing staff to begin their duty immediately. I know this contradicts what is currently obtainable because if you don't recruit, how do you get people to work with you? The answer lies in the next step.

- Get a group of people and present your vision to them. These people may be your family, friends, colleagues, and so on. Gather them together and share what you have in mind with them. Do not attach any reward to your vision. Do not entice people into working with you. Only present to them your roadmap and allow them make their choice.

As a startup, you have the opportunity of interacting with people and telling them about what you have in mind. Ask them if they would want to come on board. You would be at peace knowing that someone is working with you because they believe in what you do and not because they expect to be paid.

Don't get me wrong—payment is necessary. Money is motivation. But many people want to receive payment without offering value. And the only way to offer value is by understanding the vision of a business and aligning every action to this vision.

- After you have gathered these people, observe them. The sandy or loamy traits of individuals are often revealed with time. Thus, you have to pay attention to the little things and the big things your team members do. You can know sandy or loamy people through the questions they ask. Sandy people ask questions or say things like:

- What will I benefit from this?
- Why is it taking so long to see results?
- Are you sure we aren't wasting time with this vision?
- I am not sure I can handle this; you'd have to go through this alone.
- Let's take what we can get now. We don't know tomorrow.

The last point may seem logical, but if the founders of Silicon Valley companies had taken only what they could get at the beginning of their business where would they have been now?

Loamy people think long term and ask questions or say things like:

- » How will this benefit the company in the long term?
- » Does the action align with the vision of the company?
- » I know it is tough, but we have to keep pushing on.
- » Let's appreciate the little wins of today because they are pointers to what tomorrow holds for us.

- Spotting loamy individuals does not automatically mean they would be part of your team. There is a vital quality you must look out for in them: passion. You may ask: "If loamy humans are not passionate, how come they ask questions or make statements like the ones outlined above?" Indeed, those statements or questions spell passion, but are the individuals passionate about *your* business. A person can have all the characteristics of a loamy soil, yet they may not be passionate about your vision. Your prospective team members reserve the prerogative to choose or determine where they would flourish in their personal, career, and financial development.

If a person feels that your vision or business would limit their growth, they may not be passionate about it. For instance, a person who has a flair for fashion may not devote to your real estate company. Put them in your company and they would only be forced to work. It is not that they do not believe in your vision or its viability; they just have an interest in a different vision.

Steve Jobs understood how important passion is, that's why it was the fundamental requirement he looked out for when recruiting. He searches for passion was spurred by an experience he had. In the early days of Apple, Jobs had hired two managers to be part of his journey to building a successful company. It was a wrong move. Jobs had to fire them. He called them bozos who knew how to manage but didn't know how to do anything. After that experience, Jobs went for people who knew their opinions and had the passion to flow with the company's vision. He said that he "wanted people that were insanely great at what they did, but were not necessarily those seasoned professionals, but who had at the tips of their fingers and in their passion the latest understanding of where technology was and what they could do with that technology."[1]

Passion, most times, trumps qualifications. A passionate worker will strive to imbibe any skill that will make him an asset to himself, to you, and to your company. But a skillful worker bereft of passion is useless to you. In fact, such a person becomes a liability—slowing you down, drawing you back to levels you should have superseded. It was this for reason, Jobs did not care about the resume of his employees; all he wanted were passionate problem solvers. He found one in Debi Coleman, an inexperienced 32-year-old lady who had a degree in English Literature. Jobs used her to replace the managers he had fired. She worked as Apple's manufacturing chief, and in three years, she became the company's CFO.[2]

A passionate employee doesn't need to be managed. He or she knows what the company is all about and takes initiative that will fulfil the company's goals and objectives. For Jobs, great employees should not be managed. He explained that so long as the employees are *passionate*, smart, and motivated, they would manage themselves. Jobs didn't hire people who he would teach their jobs, he hired those whom he could share his vision and they would work towards the same goal. Apple had a litmus test for spotting such people: they would show the interviewee the Macintosh prototype. If the interviewee's eyes did not light up, if they were not excited, then they didn't belong with Apple.[3]

- When you have successfully spotted and separated the sandy and the loamy team members, and found the ones passionate about your vision, then you can now proceed on your entrepreneurial journey.

The need to have the right team cannot be overemphasized. Bill Gates stated that the ability to build a team is one of his superpowers. Building a team is a skill Gates developed over time as he built Microsoft. He said that it usually took five to six years to assemble *teams* of engineers, alongside understanding what works and what does not. For Gates, it was a game of patience. That skill he developed more than forty years ago has come in handy in these times. In his quest to eradicate global issues like malnutrition and poverty, and diseases like malaria and HIV/AIDS, Gates and his wife, Melinda have had to build and oversee teams of researchers, strategists, and other partners. Gates Foundation has about 1,500 employees around the world.[4] It is with these teams that he had saved the lives of 122 million children by accelerating vaccines getting to children to prevent diseases like pneumococcus and rotavirus[5]; it is with these teams that he had reduced malaria cases and mortality by 40% and 60% respectively[6]; and it is with these teams that he aimed to prevent more than 11 million deaths, 3.9 million disabilities, and 264 million illnesses by 2020[7].

It is not just about having a team but having the right team. In an article for American Express, Donna Fenn shared two stories that buttress the importance of having the right people in your team.

First is the story of the founders of the popular ice-cream company, CoolHaus. The co-founder of CoolHaus, Freya Estreller and her partner, Natasha Case, believed that a particular angel investor was a great fit for their budding company. This investor had earlier invested in a cookie company that was a co-packer of CoolHaus, so Estreller believed working with the investor would be strategic. But contrary to what they had thought, the partnership did not go as planned. The investor was concerned with the company's day-to-day running and didn't allow any room for mistakes. Such close supervision could be suffocating and unhealthy for a startup. Fortunately for CoolHaus, the investor agreed to convert his equity to debt.

CoolHaus would go on to land $1 million in funding from Bobby Margolis, a former CEO of Cherokee Group. Margolis was a perfect contrast to the first investor. He looked at the bigger picture and was not interested in the daily operations of the company. All he was interested in was to make the company grow into an international brand. Sharing what the experience with the first investor taught her, Estreller said, "We mistook common interests for common vision." She advised businesses to "be clear about the value, beyond money, that your investor adds to your business." In 2014, the company raked in about $6 million in revenue.[7] *Forbes* recorded that in 2018, they had gross revenues of $11 million.[8] This was possible because they corrected their mistake and worked with the right kind of person.

The second story is of Deepti Sharma Kapur, owner of FoodtoEat, an online ordering service where customers get access to restaurants, food trucks, and caterers. Kapur, desperately needing a team to build her customer base, made a big mistake: she hired too quickly, and in the process, hired salespeople who neither understood the company nor its vision. They were only looking for jobs. At a point, she had to let some of them go. The experience taught her to rely on references from people in her industry. Kapur said that the first question she asks when she wants to recruit is, "What do you know about the industry and our company?" This new approach gave her company a boost. As of 2014 when Donna Fenn shared this story, the company was working with more than 900 food vendors and served corporate clients like Tumblr. In 2013, the company grossed a revenue of $500,000.[9]

Atmosphere

Like a meteorologist, the entrepreneur must be able to study the business atmosphere and use his study to make informed decisions. Meteorologists are not psychics, so they cannot accurately tell what the weather will look like tomorrow, next week, next month, or next year. They only make *educated* guesses, which may be right or wrong. But right, most times. Likewise, you should be able to study your atmosphere and make educated predictions of the future using past and present events. So how do you do this? The answer is simple: research.

Your level of knowledge cannot go beyond the level of information you have. You cannot predict economic or market trends if your knowledge about the economy or market is shallow. There are three forms of knowledge for making educated guesses or forecasts about the industry or market. They are qualitative knowledge, quantitative knowledge, and knowledge of causal relationships.

Qualitative knowledge

This is subjective knowledge. It is knowledge obtained through market research and interactions with industry experts. Here, you ask the question: *What knowledge can I gain from my studies, interactions, and experiences?* It analyzes present events, although interviewed experts may relate these present events to past ones. *Investopedia* stated that it deals with "intangible, inexact concerns that belong to the social and experiential realm rather than the mathematical one."[10] Here, you would rely on observation, insights, and industry experience. There are several methods of obtaining qualitative knowledge. Smallbusiness.chron.com outlines four of these methods: Delphi Method, Jury of Executive Opinion, Grassroots Forecasting, and Market Research.[11]

- *Delphi Method*: This is a consensus approach where experts gather to air their views and deliberate on *an* event or issue. The convening of experts in such a situation may become an ego contest, a display of hubris spurred by knowledge and, maybe, wealth. An expert with a strong personality may want to overshadow the opinions of others. To solve this problem, the Delphi approach requires that experts fill out questionnaires and surveys independently, instead of meeting face to face. An analysis team reviews the answers, making changes where necessary to the review material. The team repeats this process until a consensus emerges.

- *Jury of Executive Opinion*: Here, you rely on the opinions of high-level managers. For instance, you may gather department managers or advisory board members, present them with company or industry statistical data, request their opinion, and arrive at a consensus.[12]

- *Grassroots Forecasting*: With this method, you obtain knowledge from those closest to the end user. You ask them about consumer perception and consumer expectation. The responses obtained would help you make informed decisions regarding your product or service—and how to make it *fit* for the end user.

- *Market research*: This is a level ahead of grassroots forecasting. Here, you meet with the end users directly. You obtain subjective, qualitative data through consumer survey, interviews, and/ or panels, then use these data to make "accurate predictions about the size, scope, demographics, and buying habits"[13] of your market.

There is an important point to note about qualitative knowledge. Same way you, the entrepreneur, tries to gather knowledge about the market, is the same way the market gathers information or knowledge about you and your company. You want to gain knowledge about the market so that you can fashion your products and services to meet the market, but how do you know the market would be willing to patronize you? For this reason, you need to position yourself so that when the market carries out its own research on you, you would be found worthy.

A lot of companies fail to do this and then wonder why they record poor sales even when they have done their homework. Customers also do their homework, and a minor flaw can turn a customer off. Tim Smith pointed out that customers are more crucial to a company's success than the management and employees since customers are the source of revenue.[14]

Customers are the direct recipient of a company's actions, whether good or bad. This is why Smith advised that an investor looking to invest in a company should try being a customer first. In an example, Smith said that if an investor was considering investing in an airline with excellent financial performance, such an investor should try being a customer. Suppose on trying to use the airline, the investor finds a bug-ridden website, cranky customer reps, petty extra fees, and resentful passengers, it becomes obvious that the company does not prioritize its customers.[15]

Qualitative knowledge is subjective and may be tainted by bias. But an entrepreneur who allows his bias or emotions to becloud his business sense and objectivity is not yet mature to lead. Business, most times, is about doing what is best, not what you *feel* is best. Cognitive bias has been shown to be one of the reasons business leaders make poor decisions. Norman Marks, a global thought leader and internal auditor, revealed that he had been affected by cognitive bias while making business decisions. He trusted people because of their charm instead of challenging their knowledge of the subject. He hired individuals with perfect resumes and certifications instead of others who probably were more creative and curious. He respected those in authority to the point that he ignored the fact that they could default on their commitments.[16]

As an entrepreneur, study the market and take decisions according to market conditions.

Quantitative knowledge

This is knowledge obtained through historical market data. Here, you predict the future of the market using past trends. You ask yourself: *What information can I get from market trends and patterns?* You collect and analyze measurable and verifiable data such as revenues and market share in order to understand the activity and performance of a business or industry.[17] With quantitative knowledge, you do not have to rely on your instincts or experience to make business decisions. Everything you need lies in the trends and patterns in the market.

There is one fundamental fact every entrepreneur should know: there is nothing new in the world. Everything we see has happened before. So, when you get into an industry to start a business, it is important you analyze what has happened and position yourself to get a sizable share of the industry.

One mistake many entrepreneurs often make is that they focus so much on their desire to be innovative that they forget that innovation is not only about creating something *entirely* new. Innovation also means improving on what is existing. Ross Simmonds, a digital strategist and marketer, stated that innovation happens from imitation.[18] This is what you should gun for when analyzing market data.

Your aim should be to spot trends and patterns, and build your business according to these trends and patterns. Check what has existed before and replicate an improved version.

Instagram copied the Stories feature from Snapchat. Sega took a cue from Nintendo's *Super Mario* to create the game, *Sonic the Hedgehog*. Xiaomi's user interface is remarkably similar to Apple's. These companies have used the imitation game to gain a sizable portion of the market. Although Facebook does not release the revenue numbers of Instagram, it was predicted that in 2016, Instagram had a revenue of about $2 billion, towering far above Snapchat's $463.1 million. With the release of *Sonic the Hedgehog*, Sega took 55 percent of the market, displacing Nintendo which once accounted for 90% of America's video game industry in 1990. Xiaomi may not have ousted Apple from its top position in the smartphone market, but by imitating Apple, the company made a revenue of about $14.5 billion in 2017.[19] These companies were able to record breakthroughs because they worked with past trends and patterns and positioned themselves in the market.

There is a confluence point where quantitative knowledge and qualitative knowledge meet. Qualitative knowledge gathers information from the market, interactions with business players, and entrepreneurial experience. Removing the layers from qualitative knowledge, we would discover that it is a knowledge most times backed by quantitative aspects of the market. Qualitative information or knowledge is simply the surface outlook or the finished form of quantitative information. Kimberlee Leonard puts it better when she stated that quantitative data tells us what is happening, while qualitative data seeks to develop underlying reasons for the data.[20]

A simple case study to understand this confluence is what goes on in the stock or cryptocurrency markets. The candlesticks show the trends and patterns of the market within a certain time frame. This is quantitative data. Technical analysts study these candlesticks and predict what is going on in the market—at what price level is there a concentration of demand, at what price level is there a concentration of supply, what is the market sentiment? An investor who studies these charts would be able to determine the right time and price to enter and exit the market.

For you as an entrepreneur, the data you get from the Delphi method, Jury of Executive Opinion, and so on are birthed not only from experience and instinct, but also from quantitative data. Use this data to position yourself favorably in the market. Do not allow your emotions or sentiments becloud your decisions. Now, this is not to say that there is no place for instinct in business. There is. But following instinct is discretionary. There is no formula to tell how to make use of your instinct. If your instinct has always led you down the right path, then trust it. But also trust the numbers too. Numbers don't lie.

Knowledge of causal relationships

You obtain this knowledge by marrying cause and effect. You predict the outcome of one event based on the functioning of another. The question asked here is: *If that happens, what happens to this?* As an entrepreneur, you should not trivialize certain situations or events, because even the most minor event can impact your business. A macroeconomic variable as basic as the GDP of a nation can affect an entire product database.[21]

There are mathematical and statistical variables used to study causal relationships. This is not a mathematics or statistics text, so I wouldn't bore and bug you with such information. However, I came up with certain variables which you need to watch out for as an entrepreneur. I divided these variables into two groups: external variables and internal variables.

The external variables are factors outside your control which could have a positive or negative impact on your business. There are six variables in this group and are popularly referred to as PESTLE factors or variables. They are politics & policies, economic, social, technological, legal, and environmental factors.

The internal variables are factors within your control; factors within your organization. They are purely human factors: you—the entrepreneur, and your team—employees and investors. We have discussed the internal variables in chapter one and we will also see them in other chapters. For this reason, this chapter will only focus on the external variables.

- **Politics & policies.** An entrepreneur should not neglect politics. This is not to say that you must dabble into politics and governance. But as an entrepreneur, you should know that politics and governance birth policies that can impact your business for the better or the worse. This is why top business moguls anticipate elections of their home countries and even other countries—like the US, UK, Russia, and China—that control the global economy. We have seen cases of governments imposing tax laws or trade tariffs that affect businesses. As a matter of fact, it was the tax laws of certain governments that gave rise to illegal structures like tax havens, and legal ones like tax inversion.

Modern-day innovations like robotics and blockchain technology are focused on building decentralized systems that cannot be regulated by the government. This is because over time, we have witnessed the overregulation by the government stifle the growth and innovation of businesses. Businesses have left certain countries or moved their headquarters to other countries because of stringent laws. In 2014, Burger King left the United States for Canada. With that move, the company saved about $275 million in taxes.[22]

The politics of your home country and that where your business is domiciled should concern you. For instance, New Zealand has been ranked the *best* place for doing business according to 2018 report by the *Wall Street Journal*.[23] The country still ranked number 1 in 2019 according to the World Bank.[24] It is a country not just with a free economy, but one with a stable democracy. The government encourages businesses to invest and create jobs. The country favors foreign direct investment and encourages entrepreneurs to expand into New Zealand. Manufacturing businesses easily thrive in the country because of its robust infrastructure, good transportation network, logistics services, and energy production. The country allows foreign entrepreneurs to apply for loans and funding. It is also a country fraught with startup accelerators, venture capitalists, and local business investors.[25]

Based on simple causal relationships, we can easily deduce that a business set up in New Zealand has every chance to be successful. Your knowledge of causal relationships between the political atmosphere and the business world in such a country enables you to take sound decisions for your business. This is not to say that a country like New Zealand does not pose a challenge to businesses, especially foreign companies. For example, the Prime Minister of New Zealand, Jacinda Arden had made statements antagonizing immigration and foreign investments. In 2018, the parliament passed a law preventing non-resident foreigners from acquiring property in the country.[26] Say you had a desire to expand in New Zealand even though it is neither your country of origin or residence, such antagonism from its leader and the law passed by the parliament already suggest that expanding into that country may be impossible—at worst, and tough—at best.

This brings me to my next point: study leaders. It is important you study the lives of leaders—study their beliefs, their culture, and their ideologies. By doing this, you would know what to expect when they come into power. There are leaders whose entry into power determines if your business would thrive or die. A leader that understands entrepreneurship would most likely make laws that favor businesses. Indonesia's president, Joko Widodo is a good example.

Widodo, the seventh president of Indonesia has a business background. He is the first president of Indonesia with a business background. Before taking the mantle of leadership, Joko Widodo owned a small furniture business. His vice, Jusuf Kalla was also a business mogul (built the Kalla business empire from his home province) before getting into politics. The Joko-Kalla duo used their business knowledge to cut red tapes which slowed down businesses. The duo also improved the country's World Bank's Ease of Doing Business index from 104th to 73rd position.[27]

Now, there have been debates stating that laws became favorable for businesses in Widodo's tenure not because the government wanted to favor business owners, but because principal actors in government own businesses.[28] While this may be the case, it does not rule out the causal relationship between Widodo's leadership and Indonesia's entrepreneurial climate. A foresighted entrepreneur who has studied the life of Widodo would have positioned their company to benefit from the new policies.

Have foresight. Be knowledgeable. Predict likely events that may occur with a change in power or policy, then position yourself to benefit from it—if it would be a positive change or avoid it—if it would be negative.

- **Economic Factors.** As an entrepreneur, you may choose not to bother about how national and international politics impact your business, but you *must* be concerned about the economy. The economy revolves around wealth, money. And what sustains your business is money. So, if the economy is affected, your business would also be affected. It is the most direct causal relationship of all the factors. A small shift in the economic balance could cause a large change in your business.

BBC UK noted that the economic climate can impact a business in four major ways: unemployment, changing levels of consumer income, interest rates, and tax rates.[29] So how do these sub-variables affect your business?

For BBC UK, unemployment is not just a state where people are out of jobs; it is a situation where the economy is not fully utilizing the workers available.[30] When this happens, households have less income and reduced purchasing power. And this has a direct impact on businesses. There would be lower sales and, consequently, lower revenue. Lower revenue means that the company may be unable to pay salaries. Inability to pay salaries would lead to laying off workers. And the cycle continues.

However, unemployment may become beneficial to certain businesses. As a result of poor purchasing power, consumers seek cheaper alternatives, which are often less-quality goods and services. The owners of these alternatives experience a boost in sales, thus directly benefiting from unemployment.[31] As an entrepreneur, you can decide which result of unemployment you would want to ride on. Would unemployment affect your business negatively, or is there a way to use it to your advantage? Amazon did the latter, as we would see later in this chapter.

Unemployment can also impact the level of consumer income. It is expected that in a country where unemployment is at its peak, citizens would have lower income and reduced purchasing power. But in a case where the economy thrives and citizens enjoy a high, steady income, then there is a propensity for higher spending.

There is this thing that money does to a person. When you are broke, you live by a scale of preference. You know that you cannot meet all your needs at the same time. So, when you are at the grocery store or a clothing store, you go for only what is necessary and affordable. But this changes as soon as money comes. Maybe you won a lottery or got a raise—your purchasing will and power become heightened. There is a propensity for you to even spend on what you do not need.

Now, the wise entrepreneur can take advantage of this trend. When there is economic prosperity, your thoughts as an entrepreneur should be channeled into making products or services that attract customers. The truth is many have money, but they do not know where or how to spend their money. The onus lies on you to be creative with your products and services. Give people what they need in a way they've never seen before—and their money becomes yours.

Variables like interest rates and taxes are also important. They impact the overall cost of your business. This is why news about behemoth companies avoiding taxes never gets old. The discourse on corporate tax is a complex one. It is not just a financial discourse, but a moral one.

On the one hand, companies *should* pay taxes to countries where they have a presence. These taxes are for the benefit of the citizens. But on the other hand, there is a situation where the governments of these countries do not use these taxes for the socioeconomic development of the country and its people. Companies know this, so they avoid paying. It becomes a story of the fight between two elephants and the grasses being collateral damage.

During the Covid-19 pandemic, giant tech companies like Facebook, Google, and Microsoft avoided tax in developing nations to the tune of almost $3 billion. ActionAid, an international NGO committed to working against poverty and injustice, pointed out that that sum "could pay for 729,010 nurses, 770,649 midwives or 879,899 primary school teachers annually in 20 countries across Africa, Asia and South America."[32]

While interest rates and taxes directly impact the cost of your business, you have to strike a balance between taking the financially smart option or the morally unethical option. I understand that when it comes to these issues, there are a lot of grey areas. To do the right thing, there should be interplay of your business sense and moral codes.

- **Social Factors.** The social climate of a place shapes the behavior of the people and what they buy. Social variables are vast. They range from lifestyle and education to religion and social classes. This is another aspect of your PESTLE analysis where you need to strike a balance. You are an entrepreneur. You are human—a social being, not a robot.

You have your beliefs, values, sexuality, principles, religion, habits, and every other quality that makes you human. And your business is serving different people with diverse social characteristics. Thus, you are bound to experience social conflicts in your entrepreneurial journey. It will be unwise to allow these conflicts interfere with your business. This is a mistake you should *never* make.

Your brand, products, and services should not discriminate or stereotype individuals or communities no matter your religious, sexual, ethnic, or racial inclinations. Drop your inclinations at the door and embrace humanity. Some popular companies did this after the death of George Floyd and the subsequent outrage that followed. PepsiCo scrapped its 130-year-old breakfast brand, Aunt Jemima after admitting that the image of the black woman originated from a racial stereotype. Colgate stated that it would rebrand its top-selling Chinese toothpaste, Darlie whose original name was Darkie, meaning "black person toothpaste." Dixie Beer asked the public to help them pick a new name because it wanted to change its name which has connotations of slavery.[33]

Being a socially aware brand can do a lot of good to your business. As humans, we are social beings. This is why social topics are sensitive issues. They affect our emotions and sense of value. People do not want to be associated with brands that do not consider their emotional wellbeing and sense of value. In recent years, we have seen our societies morph into places with high energy and a strong desire for freedom. We are no longer in a world where people cower in silence to the dictates of superior individuals or corporate bodies. People speak out. Social media has made the average person a media house, a loud voice. And speaking out plus the cancel culture we now see, can leave a *permanent* dent to your brand and company.

Many entrepreneurs and business managers neglect the impact social issues can have on their business. Recall, we are talking about causal relationships. As an entrepreneur, you have to understand the social climate of the world. In this current world, anything you say or do may be used against you in the court of social media. There is a mob online waiting to lynch you without giving you a fair trial. Michael Hogan wrote that there is "a barrage of judgement waiting to be unleashed at the smallest provocation." He went further to state that "every nook and cranny of an organization is subject to scrutiny. What used to be relatively simple is now anything but, and organizations are left damned if they do and if they don't."[34] This may be complicated and exhausting, but it is important you bear it in mind so as to take actions that wouldn't put your business at risk.

Social issues are too weighty to ignore that the outrage can even start from your employees. Jack Kelly, a senior contributor for *Forbes*, pointed out that in the past, employees followed company orders without question. But that has changed. He wrote that there is a wave of employees given to activism who intentionally seek employment in companies who share their social and ethical beliefs. If they happen to be in a company that derails from any of their core beliefs, these employees protest immediately.[35] This was the case with online home goods and furniture company, Wayfair.

In 2019, the company had sold bedroom furniture worth about $200,000 to a government contractor who operated immigration detention centers on the US-Mexico border. Hundreds of Wayfair employees were displeased with this—they didn't want their company to profit off children being in concentration camps. They expressed their displeasure to management, asking for the sales to be canceled. When the CEO refused to comply with the demands, the workers staged a walkout.[36]

It was a complicated case, which started a two-sided debate. Those on the side of management argued that if those beds weren't sold, then the children in those camps would have slept on cold, hard floors. But pro-employees countered this argument by stating that if the company were interested in the children, they would have donated the beds instead of profiting from it.[37] The company ended up donating the profit made from the sales to the Red Cross.[38]

The story of Wayfair underscores how significant the effects of social conflicts could be to a company. Jack Kelly went ahead to paint a picture of other negative results that could have played out depending on how the public reacted to the protest. Kelly stated that the protests could have backfired on the employees (and the company) in several ways. One: Amazon is one of Wayfair's biggest competitors. If consumers had decided to support employees and trigger the cancel culture, they would have boycotted Wayfair's products. This would have meant lesser sales and revenue. The company would have had to lay off employees to cut cost. Two: If a staff who had protested was fired, the staff might perceive it as a penalty for participating in the protests. Such staff may go ahead to sue the company. Three: Staff who are not promoted or given salary raises or bonuses may also perceive that they are being punished for taking part in the protests, especially if staff who didn't participate in the protests get promoted or a salary raise or bonus. These three scenarios could culminate into a toxic work environment.[39]

- **Technological factors.** Business demands a lot of you—production, distribution, marketing, sales, etc. Thus, it is only wise that you adopt up-to-date techniques for running your business. Irrespective of what your business entails, it is necessary to use technologies to facilitate business processes.

Although we are moving towards an era of utmost dependence on machines, technology does not downplay the importance of human resources—they only help improve business operations and guarantee absolute productivity.

The development of technology has played a significant role in business development, especially in automating processes. Automated processes *directly* influence and increase productivity and reach. Kweilin Ellingrud pointed out that automation can handle 45 percent of repetitive tasks—and give workers time for higher-value tasks like problem-solving and creating new ideas.[40] In the end, there is smooth production and distribution of goods and services, healthy customer relationships, and a flexible working environment.

Furthermore, technology helps maintain healthy business relationships. Internet technology like Skype helps you to connect with your workers. And social media platforms like Facebook, Instagram, and Twitter enable you to access your customers directly without the need for a physical meeting. This means that at any time, you can maintain human connections—a vital ingredient for any business to thrive.

In chapter one, we saw an exposition on fads and disruptions. In this era, every fad or disruption will come as new technology. So, have foresight. Be knowledgeable enough to spot disruptions when they appear. Remember, companies that took advantage of the internet in its early days are big winners today. I know you would want to remind me of the internet bubble of the 2000s. But know this: markets crash from time to time, but a market or industry with resilience is one you should be in. More than two decades after the crash, the internet is here.

- **Legal factors.** Every business is subject to the law of the land in which it operates. The corporate laws of the nation where your business operates govern, to a large extent, the mode of operations of your business. Legal factors are closely related to the first variable in the PESTLE analysis: politics. And we have seen how politics and policies can positively or negatively affect a business. However, we will turn our focus on how legal factors can affect your business independent of politics.

Legal experts, Samuel D. Brickley and Brian M. Gottesman, stated that the essence of laws is to create standards, resolve disputes, maintain order and protect the rights of citizens.[41] As a business owner, you would not be comfortable with every law. However, you must be aware of these laws and their relationship with your business.

Legal factors that could impact your business include laws on taxation, organizational law, consumer laws, employment regulations, securities and immigration, contract laws, intellectual properties law, etc. Let's see some of them.

Organizational Law

This is probably the fundamental legal factor that has a significant stronghold on businesses. From a business name to the type of entity selected before registration, this law determines the scope of activities of a business. Organizational law also manages the creation, operation, and termination of a business. The legal status of a company (e.g., limited liability company or a limited liability partnership) determines its taxation, employee, and customs regulations.

Employment Law

Chapter one looked at selecting your team. Besides being guided by personal principles, there is also a legal side to choosing your team, your employees especially. Employment law focuses on the welfare of employees, including mode of payment, work ethics, etc. This law gives employees the right to report any form of misconduct exhibited by their employers to the authorities. In other words, it ensures that the employer and employees maintain a healthy relationship without any form of discrimination based on gender, color, religion, or race. When you align this with the social variables and the real-life cases we saw earlier, you would understand why employees can take drastic decisions such as a protest against management.

Consumer law

Consumer laws are designed to facilitate legal relationships between consumers and business owners and protect consumers from fraudulent companies. You may wonder how this affects your business if it's all about the customer. It affects you because these laws ensure that you do not make the customer uncomfortable during patronage and after patronage as they use your product. For example, business owners are expected to disclose a reasonable amount of information about their policies, products, and services to the public. So irrespective of what you do, your customers have the right to know basic details about your products.

Intellectual properties law

This law is designed to protect products or services such as books, machines, music, or paintings created via a human mind, ensuring that no one takes credit for them without the owner's permission. It gives a person or business the right to sole ownership. However, someone else can use the property if the owner permits. And the rights of such a person are also protected under the law. Chapter five will show how some top companies used this law as their "indirect army" to stay on top of their industry.

Products and services law

The products and services you provide as a businessperson must be checked and tested to ensure that they are suitable for consumption by the target market. The standard of a product or service is checked based on the ingredients used, manufacturing process, environment, the professional status of producers, and quality. However, product laws vary depending on business location.

Taxation

Just like organizational law, the growth of a business depends on the tax regulations in a state. Some states/countries are more tax-friendly than others. That is why businesses in some states flourish more than others in other states. Business owners are strongly advised to first observe and understand the tax policies in a given state before rolling out products and services. As stated earlier, taxation is an important factor that it has led to practices like tax evasion and tax inversion.

Antitrust law

This law is particularly for businesses with a similar target audience or similar market structure. Due to unhealthy competitions and rivalries that could spring up between two or more businesses, this law ensures equal and healthy competitions by regulating business activities, such as price-fixing, bid-rigging, and unfair monopoly. But if competitors understand that they could collaborate, maybe this law would not have existed.

Other examples of legal factors that affect businesses include health and safety law, import and export law, and fraud law.

While these laws appear cumbersome, they determine the growth of any business in a geographical area and are mostly not negotiable.

- **Environmental Factors.** They determine the nature of a product or service and consumers' reactions to them. For example, no one will readily purchase a heater in an already hot environment. This means that if you must record reasonable growth in business, your product—depending on your industry—must align with the weather conditions of your business environment.

Although no business, small and large, has control over these factors, marketing strategies could be developed around these environmental factors to have an accurate picture of market trends and how your business can thrive in a particular area.

There are various environmental factors affecting business development, such as climate change, green agenda, environmental policies, pollution, natural resources, pandemics, recycling, waste disposal, etc.

Environmental policy

The major environmental factor affecting businesses is environmental policy. Environmental policy is the commitment of a business to government regulations and other policy mechanisms that revolve around environmental issues. No business progresses without adhering to environmental policies, as the law compels organizations to change their operational routine to meet stipulated standards.

These environment policies also vary depending on the type of business and the natural features peculiar to that environment. For example, the environmental policies for a company that deals with the production of food items are different from the policies guiding a skincare company. But these policies ensure there is a conducive environment for all to grow simultaneously.

Climate change

Another environmental factor that determines the success of a business is climate change. Climate change can be a threat to businesses if not taken into proper consideration. With the increasing issue of global warming and hostile weather conditions in recent years, it is difficult for organizations to operate equally in every weather condition. Agricultural-based businesses that directly depend on an adequate water supply to grow will be affected if climatic changes result in reduced rainfalls. Although erecting an irrigation system could be an option in such cases, it is expensive and might only be plausible for large-scale businesses.

As a business owner, you must have first-hand knowledge of your business, understand that it is susceptible to climatic changes, and identify favorable areas. Are your products and services suitable for all weather types? Interestingly, consumers are also becoming aware of this factor and are most likely to patronize brands that align with their environment, as they seek both satisfaction and convenience.

Green Agenda

Business-related activities affect the environment as much as the environment affects the growth of businesses. Every business owner must understand the need to have environmental-friendly policies to achieve desired business goals. The Green Agenda is an example of a friendly environmental policy that helps organizations manage their operations to ensure minimal impact on the local and global environment.

To be environmentally accountable, you need to develop operational plans which are beneficial to both the company and the physical environment. These plans must highlight the mode of production and operation, waste management system, and general work ethics.

Pollution

Environmental pollution is not a new phenomenon, but it is one of the greatest problems facing humanity. Both developed and underdeveloped regions have a fair share of this burden. Pollution is also one of the primary environmental factors that affect business strategies. It can cause some major environmental events, resulting in the disruption of supply chains or a relative increase in the cost of raw materials for production. Business owners need to monitor such events and develop subsequent plans to tackle them. Your ability to stay in business during any event that threatens your physical environment depends on how well you plan.

Environmental pollution includes air pollution, water pollution, soil pollution, etc. Air pollution is most peculiar to organizations that constantly emit pollutants, which are detrimental to human health and the planet in general. If your business poses a threat to the planet, then you should reevaluate your policies. You should also consider the potential health effects of a polluted environment on your employees, as poor air quality is a risk to employees' health, overall well-being, and ability to perform their duties judiciously.

Contaminated air can also affect your workers indoors as well as outdoors. So do not ignore indoor pollutants, as they can eventually lead to the loss of employees. And when this happens, you will be made to face the consequences of your action, which may lead to the collapse of your business. Make a conscious effort to guarantee the safety of your staff by ensuring they have quality air void of indoor toxins. No one wants to work for a business that cares less about the health of its workers.

A threat to your business is a threat to the economy and vice versa. This clearly explains the collective impact of employee health. Poor air quality can also affect the reach and growth of your business. Regions with above-average levels of air pollution are often seen as undesirable cities to live or work in. So, the chances of you attracting skilled employees and direct consumers are relatively low. Even with enough serenity within the company to retain, train and promote current employees, business growth could still be hindered.

A survey conducted by Bain and Company, and the American Chamber of Commerce in China, disclosed that 52% of American-owned businesses operating in China experienced difficulty in gaining senior-skill-level employees. And one of the biggest contributors to this shortage was the level of air pollution in the area.[42]

The negative impact of air pollution on business performance seems overwhelming. But an increase in public awareness can guarantee improved performance beyond the current state of things. You should invest in the working conditions of your staff, uphold good company morals, create growth opportunities, and improve your company's overall environmental position. Public awareness will also help you boost your company's image and credibility.

Note that modern technological advancements allow companies, individuals, and the government to detect the effect of pollution on health and the economy. And sooner than later, this detection will enable the tracing of these effects back to the source, revealing companies that are actively constituting havoc to the environment. You do not want your business or organization to be found guilty.

Natural resources

Availability of natural resources is an important environmental factor as most businesses have natural resources as their major raw material. Little or no natural resources can hinder the production and productivity of a company. While seeking to grow your business, identify places that have your required raw materials for production.

It is important to note that sometimes, your consumers' location may differ from where your raw materials are located. So, you need to strike a balance—devise plans on how you can reach your raw materials and still be accessible to your direct consumers. These plans may or may not be cost-effective. But the value of your business will determine how much you are willing to spend to get desired results.

For example, if your target audience is in Nigeria and raw materials required for production are in South Africa, you could seek for partnership with companies that supply those necessary materials. You can also find other ways to produce these raw materials for continued production.

Pandemics

Even before the outbreak of the coronavirus pandemic, the World Economic Forum has constantly warned about the adverse effects of pandemics on businesses through its publication, *Outbreak Readiness and Business Impact*.[43] It was like a premonition, a prophecy, which came to pass in 2020 with the Covid-19 pandemic which affected both the local and global economy. The pandemic also resulted in high mortality and caused many businesses to shut down. Many organizations that lacked a social media presence struggled to keep in touch with their customers. Others that could not integrate the internet into their business recorded poor sales.

From the Covid-19 outbreak, we could see that pandemics do not only affect health, but threaten the economies of nations, disrupt business operations, and limit day-to-day activities. Therefore, the world is adjusting one step at a time. Businesses are attaining sustainable models and diversifying their public approach. You should do it too. You should equip yourself by building a strong virtual connection with your employees. Ensure that they uphold basic work-from-home ethics when necessary, procure substantial health insurance for all, and organize virtual classes to equip them for the virtual era. Your workforce could also be made of remote and physical workers, especially if your business is not limited to a physical location.

You should also invest in digital marketing, social media marketing, and other remote methods to help you sustain the relationship with your customers. To be on the safer side, build your business framework to be formidable so it can outlive anything worse than the Covid-19 pandemic. In other words, endeavor to set long-term business goals.

Recycling

Recycling is one of the major environmental factors that supports a greener business environment. How does your business account for waste disposal? How often do you recycle waste materials? Instead of littering the environment with waste materials such as paper, glass, and plastic, do you recycle them for further production? Recycling waste materials provides alternatives to preserve virgin resources and keep the environment safe. It also saves you the stress and cost of purchasing raw materials.

Although there has been a positive trend towards recycling waste materials, many businesses still dump wastes in landfills. This affects consumers and workers and increases the cost of cleaning the environment in which the business operates. To create a balance, you should consider producing less waste, recycle them, and use them for further productions.

The attack is as important as the drawing board. It is like a footballer putting all he has practiced working in a real game. Never leave any stone unturned. Get the right knowledge. Forecast. Attack. Win.

Pledge to Action

I affirm that:

I am not afraid to attack.

I will launch every plan I have drafted on the drawing board.

I will leave no stone unturned.

I will use every qualitative knowledge, quantitative knowledge, and knowledge of causal relationships to my benefit.

I will not be caught unawares by any external variables.

I cannot wait to win.

So, I will attack right away.

CHAPTER THREE

The Strategy

"Strategy is about setting yourself apart from the competition. It's not a matter of being better at what you do – it's a matter of being different at what you do." — Michael Porter

Your strategy as an entrepreneur does not begin when you get to the battlefield; it begins the moment you conceive your vision. Many entrepreneurs make a mistake when developing a strategy—they seek to be better than the competition. This is not wrong *per se*, but it is limiting. When you aim to be better, all you are trying to do is improve on an already existing idea. And there is a possibility that your own improvement can also be improved upon. So do not aim to be better; aim to be distinct. This should be your primary strategy. One company that aims for distinction, is Apple.

In an exposition on Apple's generic and intensive growth strategies, Pauline Meyer noted that the generic strategy of the company is broad differentiation. It is a strategy that focuses on key features that distinguish the company and its IT products from competitors. Some of these key features include elegant design and user-friendliness of products, combined with high-end branding.[1]

Apple's sense of innovation and distinction made them the big leaders they are today in the smartphone market. When other phone companies like Blackberry were only focused on improving the software of their products, Apple became the first company to produce all-screen phones that were devoid of physical keyboards. Today we can hardly recall what a phone with a physical keyboard looks like.

Elon Musk didn't aim to be better by improving on gasoline cars; he strove for distinction. And that birthed Tesla cars. Tesla vehicles revolutionized the world of electric cars. Before their advent, electric vehicles had no market appeal. They were unsatisfactory, ugly, heavy, and took a long time to charge. But Tesla came with "the design of a sports car, the safety of a Toyota, and could charge in minutes rather than the hours it took earlier EVs to get juiced up."[2] For Musk, he didn't just create cars, he created "laptops on wheels."[3]

It is not enough to distinguish yourself from the crowd, you have to also maintain this distinction. Being different can come with its own challenges. For instance, your product may not be mainstream as you would like. But you need not worry as long as you know you are offering value no one else offers. iPhones are not as mainstream as Android devices. Apple controls just about 13 percent of the smartphone market globally[4], yet the company rakes in billions of dollars yearly. *Statista* reported that in the fourth quarter of 2020, the company generated $26.44 billion in revenue from the sale of iPhones.[5] Apple's strategy and company culture tells us that all we need is to provide top value to the world, and we would attract the right kind of customers who appreciate this value and are ready to pay for it.

When it comes to strategy, there are five key points you and your team need to know in order to sustain your victory. These key points, as outlined by Vu, are:

1. **Know when to and when not to fight.** As an entrepreneur, there would be times you would feel like going with the buzz in the industry. It may seem as though the competition is getting ahead. But do not panic. Do not rush in making decisions. Study the market and choose your battles wisely. If you panic, you may likely fall into the trap of doing what others are doing, and when this happens, you lose your uniqueness. You become just like every other business.

Before iPhones hit the market, Blackberry dominated. But Apple didn't just jump into creating a product to rival Blackberry. Blackberry stayed in the global market for over ten years and gained so much popularity. Now, the question is: Where was iPhone all the while? I want to think that Steve Jobs and the rest of the Apple team were busy observing and studying the market within that period. They probably investigated Blackberry's flaws by asking its users what they would want in a phone. They thought about the best innovation that would outpace and outclass Blackberry and other phones. Apple spent over ten years allowing Blackberry to rule the market. The company never launched an attack for over ten years. They chose when to fight, to attack. And when they did, it was a flawless victory abetted by Blackberry's lackadaisical approach towards innovation.

2. **Know how to use more troops.** As your vision and company expand, you would need more hands in your team. Never be afraid to try new hands (but that will be after you have taught them the company's vision, values, and culture.) Also, using more troops doesn't only mean utilizing human resources, it also means using new technologies. In this technological age, always try to be among the first to adopt new technology in your business or industry. Think outside the box. In fact, think as if there's no box . Study emerging technologies such as artificial intelligence, 5G, Internet of Things, serverless computing, biometrics, augmented reality/virtual reality, blockchain, robotics, natural language processing, and quantum computing to see how they could be relevant in your business. Be a pioneer. Let technology be part of your troops.

3. **Have the same goal and spirit in all ranks.** Once your team is in line with your vision, they would maintain the company's goal and spirit. I would want to believe that no team member from Apple felt like jumping ship when Blackberry was ruling the smartphone market. I would want to believe that every member of the Apple team knew that their goal was to be different, thus they weren't moved by their competitor's success. They knew that the success of their competitor didn't mean they were failing. I would want to believe that the goal and spirit of Steve Jobs were inherent in the team. They understood seasons and utilized every season to their advantage.

Many company owners are anxious about handing over because they know that some team members have ideologies and goals different from what the company was built on. But this should not be the case. When building a business, think perpetuity. Let your business outlive you. It is over nine years that Steve Jobs passed on, yet Apple has remained strong. The world has never had the cause to say that Jobs' death affected the company's performance. Some CEOs even cede control to another person while alive. Such CEOs understand that this new head of the company would maintain the goal and spirit they had set and built.

4. **A prepared army will always achieve victory over an unprepared army.** Be the prepared one. Be the one whose company positions itself to take advantage of trends and seasons. Be the one whose company aligns itself with emerging technologies. While your competitors are relaxed, prepare yourself. Watch. Study. Plan. Strategize.

5. **A talented general who is not restrained by the king would be victorious in battle.** Never allow anyone to stifle your creativity. Now, this does not mean you wouldn't ask for counsel, however, be smart enough to know which counsel would stifle your creative process and which would prune you to produce better fruits. Just as you shouldn't be restrained, do not also restrain your team. Allow them the freedom of expression, albeit within the confines of the company's vision. Allow room for mistakes and be prepared to correct them as often as possible. You will harness the maximum potentials inherent in your team if you give them the freedom to express themselves. No one wants to be caged, not even animals. This is why the moment they see an opening, they escape from their cages. We were not built to be caged—freedom of expression births groundbreaking ideas.

You can have all the human, financial, and material resources, but without a strategy—the right strategy—your vision would not go far. The best way to build the perfect strategy is by studying three things: (1) yourself and your company, (2) the market, and (3) your competitors. Little wonder, Sun Vu made the profound statement: "If we know the enemy and know ourselves, then we will not be endangered in a hundred battle engagements. If we know ourselves but not the enemy then for every victory gained, we will also suffer a defeat. If we know neither the enemy nor ourselves, then we will never win."

Pledge to Action

I affirm that:

I am not afraid of launching out because I have the right strategy for winning.

I will not just be the best at what I do; I will be different. I will be distinct.

I am innovative.

I know when to fight.

I choose my battles carefully.

I am prepared to use more troops—humans and machines.

I have the capacity to attract the best team.

A team that understands the goal and spirit of the company.

A team that can sustain this goal and spirit, and even transfer it to others.

I have a prepared team, a prepared army—an army marching to victory.

I am talented.

I am a wise general, a smart entrepreneur.

I have the right strategy.

CHAPTER FOUR

The Mystery

"The mysterious is always attractive. People will always follow a vail."
— Bede Jarrett

B y being different, you weaken your competition subtly. You make them struggle to keep up. This was Sun Vu's military disposition. He got victory by making the opposition miserable. He wrote, "We will entrench because we know we are in a position where victory is uncertain; and we attack because we have more than enough resources to win." With such a strategy, it would be difficult for the enemy to predict their moves. And nothing frustrates the soul like uncertainty.

Be a mystery, an enigma. Let your competition be unable to predict your next move. *Entrench* and *observe*. As you do this, always be prepared for victory. Vu put it this way: "The victory of great fighters is not famed for wisdom, nor is it known for bravery. Being prepared for every winning situation is what guarantees a certain victory." Vu went further to list four things a general must do in the place of preparation for victory to be guaranteed. They are range, measure, calculate and weigh.

- **Range.** Here, the general determines the terrain of both sides. As an entrepreneur, this means determining not just your terrain but that of your competitors. From the types of terrain we looked at in chapter one, you'd face stiff competition in the forest and most likely in the canyon. There is little or no competition in the desert, for no one wants to be in the desert. So observe your competition and know what they are doing to navigate the terrain. If it is in the forest, determine if they are among the tall trees or the short shrubs. If it is in the canyon, are they in the gorge, or are they atop the hill? Determine their range—and determine yours too.

- **Measurement.** After determining the range, the general measures both sides to determine how much resources to use. For instance, if you are in the forest and your competition is a tall tree, while you are a short shrub, then you would need more financial and human resources to elevate yourself and make yourself visible. You would need to be innovative, and resources are needed for innovation.

- **Calculation.** Sun Vu stated that the general has to calculate the number of troops on both sides. As an entrepreneur, do not only calculate the number of troops, also determine the quality of troops. Many entrepreneurs are moved by numbers. They see a company with many staff and they automatically feel afraid, yet those staff may be a bunch of figureheads.

I once observed two community pharmacies in my locality. One had just half the number of staff the other pharmacy had, yet their revenue was high. They restocked their shelves almost every week. The other with many staff barely had patients coming in. They had frequent stockouts. I would pass by the pharmacy and see boredom etched on the faces of the staff.

So it is not all about having a large number of people in your team. Employ people according to what you need in your company per time. Have efficiency and effectiveness in mind when creating a team. It may sound harsh, but if there is one thing the Covid-19 pandemic taught companies around the world is that they've been recruiting more hands than they need. For companies to lay off staff in their numbers showed that the pandemic was a drastic event that revealed where many companies were getting it wrong. Suddenly, these companies realized they could do away with some staff to cut costs. Could it be that if these companies had initially employed their staff based on need and efficiency, there would not have been the need to make employees redundant? Amazon never laid off any staff during the pandemic. As a matter of fact, they went on a hiring spree—employing 36,400 people as at the end of June 2020.[1] In 2020 alone, the company created 400,000 jobs, pushing its total number of employees worldwide to 1 million.[2] In your calculation, place quality over quantity. It is better to have ten excellent hands than a hundred mediocre hands.

- **Weigh.** After determining your terrain, resources, and troops, the next step is to weigh your company's strategy, strengths, and weaknesses and those of the competition. Simply put, at the point of weighing is where you carry out and implement your SWOT analysis. What are your strengths? What are your weaknesses? What opportunities do you have? What threats do you face? This analysis gives you a clue about the status of the competition because your area of strength may be your competition's weakness, while your opportunities may likely be their threats.

What will put you ahead of your competition is to be a mystery. Make people wonder how you do it. Always be prepared. Always be a step ahead. Determine the range of your terrain. Measure your resources. Calculate and evaluate the number and quality of the troops. Weigh your strengths, weaknesses, opportunities, and threats and use them effectively.

Pledge to Action

I affirm that:

I will be an enigma in my industry.

I will always dare to be different.

I will be a step ahead at all times.

I understand that my baby steps are valid.

I know that my steps will give me wings to fly.

I will study the range of my terrain and measure my resources.

I will determine the number and quality of my troops at all times.

I will weigh my strengths and weaknesses and opportunities and threats.

I am ready to employ my observations to get victory.

I know I will win.

Because I am a mystery.

CHAPTER FIVE

The Winning Team

"None of us is as smart as all of us." — Ken Blanchard

"If everyone is moving forward together, then success takes care of itself."
— Henry Ford

Throughout this book, I have emphasized the importance of building the right team. The statements of Ken Blanchard and Henry Ford highlights the fact that there is a limit to one's success if the *right* team is not behind a vision. The striking quality about teamwork is that its effectiveness is seen no matter where it is employed—whether for a good or negative cause. For instance, Unit 731 was a group of 3,000 researchers in the Imperial Japanese Army who carried out deadly experiments in northeast China between 1937 and 1945. Led by Lieutenant-General Ishii Shiro, the team vivisected prisoners without anesthesia; injected diseases such as syphilis, anthrax, and gonorrhea into subjects; raped female subjects to carry out tests on their fetuses; used prisoners as targets for grenades; burned people alive; and dropped plague-carrying fleas in Chinese villages to study how fast the disease spread. 3,000 to 250,000 people died in a single camp as a result of these experiments.[1] Such horrendous crime carried out by 3,000 persons could only have been possible through teamwork. If there was division in the camp, then maybe some team members would have attempted (and probably succeeded) in saving a large number of the human lab rats. Maybe some team members would have revealed this to relevant authorities so that appropriate action could be taken. But teamwork never let any of these happen. In one accord, 3,000 persons committed crimes against humanity and were never punished for it.[2] That shows us how powerful teamwork is.

Sun Vu classified an army into two types: the direct army and the indirect army. The direct army is what we have talked about so far in this book—human resources. But the effort of the direct army can be greatly amplified by the indirect army. Sun Vu advised generals to take advantage of natural elements like heaven and earth, rivers and oceans in a battle. Natural elements are the indirect army. And according to Vu, it is important to use them for two reasons: (1) "In combat, direct attack on the enemy is very obvious; but what brings about victory is the indirect attack on the side." (2) "A general who understands the use of indirect army has an infinite source of tactics [resources] like heaven and earth, like rivers and oceans, which will never run out."

So, what is the indirect army of the entrepreneur?

The entrepreneur's indirect army is classed into two groups: technology/innovation and climate.

Technology/innovation as an indirect army

Your competition would definitely know your direct army, but it would take a great deal of effort to discover your indirect army. Humans are tangible, social beings. They interact, and through their interactions, your competition would know they are part of your team. But when it comes to technology or innovation, especially software, there is a lesser tendency for your competition to know the technology you employ if you do not make it known. This is where trade secrets come in. Even if they get to know the technology behind your products, they would have to circumvent patent laws to replicate it. Technology/innovation has kept companies like Google, KFC, Coca-Cola, and New York Times ahead of their peers.

Google's search algorithm has been a top secret all these years. The algorithm is ever-evolving, but Google only reveals some of its changes.[3] This has kept the company ahead of other search engines like Bing and Yandex. According to Chuck Price, because of the algorithm, Google has transcended being just another search engine. It has become ubiquitous, a transitive verb, and a dominant online advertising platform that has amassed 87 percent of the global market share.[4]

Kentucky Fried Chicken (KFC) has a secret ingredient that was only known to Colonel Sanders. But before his death, he wrote down the recipe. The original handwritten copy is tucked away in a safe in Kentucky, and only a few employees—who are bound by a confidentiality agreement—know the recipe.[5]

Similarly, Coca-Cola has a secret ingredient. This confidential information is so important to the soda brand that it branded the ingredient a trade secret instead of patenting it since getting a patent would mean disclosing the ingredient.[6]

Trade secrets aren't only peculiar to consumables and information technology, it also applies to areas like books. The New York Times, which has the most influential book list, has not divulged its definition of what makes a book a bestseller. A book that has sold fewer copies can make its list, while a book that has sold more wouldn't make the list. The newspaper, which has won 130 Pulitzer prizes, has refused to share this secret because it fears that publishers would use the information to manipulate sales data to their advantage.[7]

These companies prove the importance of using technology/trade secrets as an army. These four companies listed above are the best in their respective industries because they've learned to use indirect armies their competitors can never know about. They go to prove Sun Vu's words: *In combat, direct attack on the enemy is very obvious; but what brings about victory is the indirect attack on the side.* Everyone knows Colonel Sanders was the brain behind KFC. KFC's competitors know that even though he is long gone, he is still putting them on their toes. That is the definition of direct attack. It is obvious and can be easily defended. Let's imagine that he never disclosed the secret ingredient before his death, KFC would have lost its place in the market. But a trade secret, an indirect attack, keeps putting KFC above the competition all these years.

Your competition understands the importance of your indirect army and wants to do everything they can to know about it. Thus, you have to protect your indirect army at all costs. This is why you shouldn't neglect your direct army. Your direct army can make your indirect army obvious to your competition. This almost happened to Co-ca-Cola. In 2006, a Coca-Cola employee alongside two accomplices stole the company's secret formula and tried to sell it to its biggest competitor, Pepsi. Being a reputable brand, the rival company alerted Coca-Cola's officials, and the culprits were arrested.[8]

So, I say again: think outside the box. Think up a technology that would distinguish you. This technology or innovation could either be applied to your input or process. It is difficult to employ trade secrets at the output level because at that level, the product or service is ready for distribution to the user. KFC's innovation is at the input—the blending of ingredients. Same as Coca-Cola, New York Times and Google have their innovation at their process—the method of selecting a best-seller, the method of optimizing search results.

Climate as an indirect army

In military warfare, Sun Vu recommended that an army use the elements of nature to their advantage. While you may not use the natural elements to your favor in business, you can use the sociopolitical or economic climate.

- **The sociopolitical climate.** Be smart and sensitive enough to use social issues to your advantage. Discourses on social issues like racism, feminism, domestic violence, and sexuality have gained so much momentum in recent times than before. A smart company would position itself around these issues to market itself. This is a strategy that *must* be applied subtly—because it would come across as insensitive to capitalize on such sensitive issues for the sole purpose of making financial gains. People are smart enough to know when a company is taking advantage of a situation for the sake of making a profit. Once people feel this way about your business, this strategy would backfire. So, show *genuine* concern towards these issues. True, boosting your exposure and profit should be part of your objective, but they should be secondary. Observe the issues that align with your company values and culture, and then offer value to society.

Paul A. Argenti in an article for Harvard Business Review[9], outlined three questions that a company must ask before lending its voice to a social issue.

> » *Does the issue align with your company's strategy?*

Argenti backs up what I said earlier. Your strategy is part of your mission and vision, thus the issue should align with what you already believe in and do.

> » *Can you meaningfully influence the issue?*

According to Argenti, you need to have the expertise and resources to make a difference; you need to be ready to put your money where your mouth is. Your inability to do this would make your efforts to be seen "as hypocritical or as 'woke-washing.'"

> » *Will your constituenci*es agree with speaking out?

You should ensure that your *key* constituencies are on your side, else you risk losing future businesses. In a case where your constituencies disagree, you must discuss and carefully analyze their relative importance to your company.

To provide a framework to guide a company's response to these questions, Argenti gave an instance using Starbucks. In 2018, a Philadelphia store manager of the company called the police after two Black men who were denied access to the bathroom refused to leave the store, which resulted in their arrest. After protests and online outrage, Starbucks apologized, issued a new bathroom policy, and shut down 8,000 stores for an afternoon of anti-bias training. According to Argenti, Starbucks' response checked yes for all three questions.

One, the issue aligned with Starbucks' strategy. In its mission, the company describes itself as "a third-place environment, where everyone is welcome, and we can gather, as a community, to share great coffee and deepen human connection." Hence, all customers must feel comfortable irrespective of race. Two, the company had the capacity to influence the issue. The anti-bias training, which instructed 175,000 baristas, was a medium to influence and ensure that people of color are treated well in the retail stores. Also, by shutting down 8,000 stores for the training, the coffee company demonstrated its commitment to the issue. Three, Starbucks's key constituencies—customers and community members—were outraged by the incident and supported Starbucks's response.[10]

The primary objective of Starbucks was to solve the issue of racial discrimination in its retail stores. However, it suffices to say that their response would appeal to people of color, and through that, they would gain more patronage. Solving a sensitive issue with such an approach would distinguish them from their competitors, especially if their competitors have never shown concern for any social issue.

- **The economic climate.** An entrepreneur can use a harsh economic climate to their advantage. It is logical for business people to protect their money in times of economic adversity, but is that always the smart decision? A harsh economic climate can be an indirect army for a company's growth and success. A perfect example of this was the coronavirus pandemic. In the cryptocurrency industry, some people speculated that the peak of the pandemic was a wrong time to invest in the digital asset, Bitcoin. Many people sold off their Bitcoin, crashing Bitcoin's price from about $10,312 in mid-February to $4,970 in mid-March.[11] But when people were selling off, smart investors were buying massively—using the rough economic weather to their advantage. And by December 2020, the same Bitcoin that people lost trust in rose to more than $23,000 (and is still rising as at the time of writing this). Those who sold regretted their actions, those who bought celebrated big wins. That is the benefit of using the economic climate as an indirect army.

When using an indirect army, be subtle. Use what I call "The Unpredictable Maneuver." I will elaborate on this strategy in chapter 7.

Let the competition be chaotic when you are calm, disorderly when you are organized, and weak when you are strong. Vu stated that "order or disorder is a product of the level of organization. Cowardice or courage is a product of position. Strength or weakness is a product of formation." Your company will be orderly if your organizational level is excellent, courageous if you position yourself to take advantage of economic adversity, and strong if you form a tenacious army. A tenacious direct army will readily spot and employ an indirect army even without you urging them to. This is why you need to select smart, talented hands as members of your team. In Vu's words, choose talented subordinates that can create an advantage position.

Pledge to Action

I affirm that:

I have the right team.

I have a direct and indirect army that will always put my business ahead of the competition.

I will take advantage of technological advancements.

I am smart enough to have innovations that will put me miles ahead of the competition.

I am smart enough to take advantage of the sociopolitical climate and add value to society and my company.

I will not be anxious about harsh economic climates.

I understand that there are opportunities in every bad situation.

And I am prepared to seize these opportunities.

I will build the right team.

I will have the winning team.

CHAPTER SIX

The Early Bird

"Always attack. Even in defense, attack. The attacking arm possesses the initiative and thus commands the action. To attack makes men brave; to defend makes them timorous." — Steven Pressfield

"Strike while the iron is hot" is an old saying, but the value of its message has never been lost. When it comes to establishing a business, you have no time to waste. Once the business idea comes to you, start immediately (after you have drafted your plan). As an entrepreneur, nothing is more rewarding than starting early in your chosen niche. Sun Vu wrote: "As a general principle, the troops that arrive first at the location of the battle and wait for the enemy will have initiative and will be at ease. The troops that arrive later to the battle position will be passive and exhausted."

The world does not wait for anybody, and unless you are a psychic, you cannot tell for sure what the economic or sociopolitical climate will be in the future and how it can impact your business. I have come up with four important reasons that should motivate you to strike while the iron is hot.

Reasons why you need to launch your business idea immediately

Market saturation

As I stated in the first chapter of this book, human minds are soils and one idea can be deposited into different minds simultaneously. The more you delay launching your business, the more populated and saturated the market becomes, and the less market share you'll get. People who arrive early in an industry have the advantage of grabbing a sizable chunk of the market before the industry becomes saturated. Let's say you had an idea to launch a social media app in 2008, but you deferred this idea till 2020. Do you think you would be able to compete favorably in a market with social media heavy-weights like Facebook, Twitter, Instagram, WhatsApp, LinkedIn, YouTube, Pinterest, Reddit, TikTok, and a host of others? For you to compete favorably, you must bring something different to the table, just like TikTok did.

TikTok was launched in 2016—twelve years and ten years after Facebook and Twitter, respectively—yet it got a sizable portion of the social media industry because of what it offered users. TikTok did not just offer its users a chance to create videos (YouTube had already given the world that); it gave them more. About TikTok and its unique selling point, Gary Vaynerchuk wrote: "TikTok provides a framework that makes it easier for people to create—especially if they don't know what else to do. TikTok is making it easier for them to become content creators. It 1) allows them to create content that they would not otherwise be able to make as easily on their own, and 2) gives them a framework they can play or create within. For example, the TikTok app gives people tools like filters, control over video speed, access to professional audio and more. Even if you're not the best lip-syncer, you can still create something fun on TikTok with a music background."[1]

So unless you can offer users what they have not been offered before, you may not do well if you delay launching your business. Bringing something new to the industry is an idea, and mind you, you are not the only one with that idea. Extant and prospective companies may have the same idea. Just like you are studying and researching the current needs of the market, other companies are also doing the same. They are seeing what you are seeing, hearing what you are hearing. This is why you do not need to delay. You do not have the monopoly of an idea.

Evolution of trends

Chapter one took us through the different types of trends a business can align itself with. But it is important to reiterate that no trend lasts forever. Even a disruptive trend evolves. This gives you, the entrepreneur, another reason why you need to launch your business early.

Sometimes, if not most, business ideas come to us from what we perceive in our physical, social, economic, or political environment. And our perception is a product of the *current* happenings or trends in any of these environments. Thus, a business idea may only fit into a particular trend. Once that trend is gone, the idea may lose relevance if it does not evolve. We will see how a business idea can lose relevance later in this chapter.

Studying the terrain and launching more attacks

By coming into an industry early, you have the opportunity of studying the terrain before it gets crowded and make plans towards scaling your business. It is more difficult to spot opportunities in a crowded place. There is a whole lot of noise to distract you. In a less crowded marketplace, you'd be able to spot gaps that need filling. Conversely, foresight and creativity would not be paramount objectives if you are coming into an already crowded space—a space where your competition had already filled the gaps you had intended to fill. Thus, your main concern would be how to get a portion of the market share—the crumbs from the table.

Same seed, diverse soils

I have mentioned this earlier. You do not have an exclusive right to an idea unless you implement it. As long as an idea is still cooling off in your mind, expect to see it being brought to life by another who is readier and more willing than you are. An idea is not yours for keeps. Inspiration can be deposited in *any fertile* mind. So, when you receive an idea, always bear in mind that at least a hundred people have received the same idea.

Despite these important reasons for starting a business early, many business ideas have failed to blossom because the owners of these ideas were not willing to take action. And two factors cause this unwillingness: fear and doubt.

- **Fear.** We have heard countless times that fear means false evidence appearing real. After drafting out a plan, some prospective entrepreneurs would become scared of their vision. They become scared of the market or industry, of existing competition, of the perception of others. They feel that the vision is too big for them to achieve or that the idea is laughable. Then they grow cold feet and remain in their comfort zones.

Fear has not only killed prospective businesses, it has also killed existing businesses. Fear has crept into the mind of business owners because of setbacks they faced in the past. I once had a story of a man who invested about 10,000 dollars in bitcoin. Then bitcoin dropped so much in value, which made the man lose his investment. Since then, he has never dared to invest in cryptocurrency even though the industry's resilience has been proven over time.

For you to have a setback as an entrepreneur, it only means one thing: you're making progress. And that is why a challenge is trying to draw you back. Challenges, as we all know, are a part of life. But after you've been drawn back, do not forget that you were on a journey, on a mission to offer value to the world.

Fear raises a false alarm—it tells you that things would always go wrong. But the truth is if you can overcome your fear and forge ahead, you would discover that what you feared did not even exist. So always be courageous so that you would not miss out on the rewards of your vision.

- **Doubt.** For other entrepreneurs, they do not suffer from fear but doubt. They doubt the potentials in their vision. They doubt their ability to bring the vision to life. They doubt their encouragers and believe the lies of their naysayers. Most times, people fall into the trap of doubt when they focus only on the big picture.

I know that many motivational speakers keep admonishing people to look at the big picture. It is good advice. But there is a clause they usually leave out. Before you can get the picture, you have to fit smaller pictures together. The big picture can be overwhelming. Looking at the big picture alone would make you doubt your capacity to achieve it. However, simplifying your vision into smaller goals and objectives would inject you with renewed zeal. Seeing yourself achieving these smaller goals would build up your confidence that you can achieve the big one.

Do not wait till everything is perfect before you launch your idea. Sun Vu pointed out that "if we wait to gather forces with adequate equipment before attempting to take advantage, we risk coming too late." However, we must also strike a balance. Do not, in a bid to arrive early, ignore adequate preparation. Ensure you have the needed resources to start with; resources that would satisfy your client even as a beginner; resources you can scale later on. If this is not done and you hurry to abandon the needed resources because you want to take advantage, you risk losing the abandoned resources.

Arrive early with just the right amount of everything you need. Do not delay yourself because you are waiting for more. Heed the words of James Clear, who rightly remarked: "Rome wasn't built in a day, but they were laying bricks every hour. You don't have to do it all today. Just lay a brick. That's how you build an empire."

The entrepreneur must eschew fear and doubt—they are two principal factors that delay success. Sun Vu stated that delay in combat would make the weapons rust and the soldiers lose their morale. This also applies to the entrepreneur, but unfortunately, many entrepreneurs do not consider the impact of delay on their business.

Do not let your weapons rust

Weapons signify ideas. Every idea has a timeline. And when you delay in implementing an idea, it "rusts." Rusting can happen in two ways: (1) The idea loses relevance. (2) Another person gets and implements the idea.

How can an idea lose relevance?

The earth is in constant motion, and as it rotates, developments happen. Every new development in the world requires innovation. And every innovation starts with an idea. When innovation is not birthed at the right time, a new development comes into play and phases out the old one alongside the innovation it would have thrived on.

Let's take, for example, the days of the Walkman. The Walkman was a portable media player manufactured in the late 70s by Sony. Music lovers could easily slot in an audio cassette into the device and listen to songs as they walked through the streets. Now imagine this: If Sony had delayed in manufacturing the product and decided to defer it by three to four decades, do you think they would have had a market for the product in this era of Apple Music, Audiomack, and Airpods? Definitely not. The idea of a Walkman has become an obsolete and rusty one. During the heydays of the Walkman (1979 – 2010), Sony sold over 400 million units of Walkman portable players for about $150 per unit.[2] Now, if we ignore inflation and other market forces, it means that within 30 years, the company made over $60 billion. Sony would have lost this revenue if they had delayed their idea. Also, if they had delayed their innovation, there is the possibility of another company producing the same device. This is the second way a weapon can get rusty.

Life abhors vacuum. Many things in life are not indispensable or irreplaceable. It is in the nature of life to always balance itself. Ideas are like seeds, and the human mind is a soil. So, nature does not just deposit a seed—an idea—in the mind of one person alone. It disperses the seed so that if a particular soil delays the seed's sprouting, there would be two or three other soil types that would favor the seed's growth. The story of Blackberry comes to mind.

Alexandra Appolonia, in an article for *Business Insider*, noted that at one time, Blackberry had 50 percent of the smartphone market in the US, and 20 percent globally.[3] But the company met its death because it was slow to change, while another company, Apple, was receptive to change. Blackberry held on to its old designs of QWERTY keyboards, while Apple launched iPhones without keyboards. By the time they wanted to get onboard the innovation, it was already too late.[4] Controlling a major share of the smartphone market should have made Blackberry flexible and receptive to ideas, but this wasn't so. The ideas that were meant to thrive on the soil of the then king of smartphones, thrived better on iPhones. Other phone companies now aspired to produce iPhone-esque phones, while Blackberry faded into history.

I wonder what went through the minds of Blackberry's staff as they watched the company's steady decline. It is possible that some of the staff would have suggested that the company go with the trend, but their suggestions were discarded. Many staff would have lost their zeal as they watched the company's steady descent into irrelevance.

Do not let your soldiers lose morale

You cannot run your company on your energy and drive alone; you need the fire of and in your team. This is why you should never let them lose zeal. Keep them motivated at all times. And one of the most veritable ways to do this is by executing ideas as soon as they are birthed. Everyone wants to be part of a success story. By executing your ideas and winning through them, you give your team a sense of fulfillment. You allow them to explore their creativity, and the results of their creativity would make them hunger for more wins. They would want to replicate their success over and over again.

If you keep deferring the execution of your ideas, soon your team would lose faith in you. Fear, doubt, and laziness are perceptible. Your staff can tell if you are afraid, doubtful, or just lazy. Once they notice any of these, they would stick with you just for their remunerations, not because they are motivated to work.

A demotivated team is a weakness and a threat to a company. Like Sun Vu said, if the enemy discovers this weakness, then an attack would be inevitable. It is easy for a rival company to poach a demotivated staff. And such staff wouldn't mind revealing the business secrets to their new company. This is one method through which an unexecuted idea is transferred to the next soil.

In a LinkedIn article, Victoria Ahl shared four stories of how different companies cleverly poached talent from rival companies. Two out of these four stories stand out for me. First is the story of MediConnect Global. The company bought an old truck and turned it into a mobile hiring center. They would park at the competitor's parking lot and hand out flyers to people walking by during lunchtime. The strategy worked. What was striking for me was what the CEO, Amy Rees Anderson, said when she recounted the experience to *Forbes*. She said that the ploy ended up being incredibly successful for her company. It engaged current employees, endeared them to the business, and *increased their sense of company pride*."[5] When a worker seeks company pride in another company, it means that that worker is no longer happy in their current company. Such a worker wants a fresh challenge and new wins, which the current company no longer offers because of reasons like failing to execute ideas.

A similar event occurred between Snapchat and Uber. A few years ago, Uber employees at their San Francisco office noticed a geo-specific Snapchat filter. The filter had the question, "This place is driving you mad?" and also had images of wayward taxis crowding the bottom of the screen, alongside a link to Snapchat's career page.[6] If an Uber staff clicked the link, it meant one thing: the company, Uber, was actually driving the staff mad.

Keeping your team motivated is very important. You should understand that you've got a bundle of talents working with you. Rival companies know that your success is tied greatly to your staff, so they desire what you have got. If they perceive a whiff of demotivation, they will do anything to keep the bundle of talents to themselves.

When you allow your team to be poached by the competition, the competition has used one of Sun Vu's many tactics on you. Vu stated that because of the cost of war, a wise general should forage and feed his troops with the enemy's food supplies. He wrote that "eating one "bushel" of enemy's food will save us the rigor of bringing along twenty." This is the mindset of your competition. It would save them both time and financial resources to poach talent from your company than carrying out a recruitment process to find that talent. Don't allow yourself to be played. Don't allow another company to strengthen itself with your human resources. So, motivate your team *always*.

A good way to keep your team motivated is by reiterating Sun Vu's words to them: "Anger must be the impetus to destroy the enemy and reward must be the stimulus to defeat the enemy." What is the enemy? Lack, financial stress, poverty. You should not be the only one motivated by the desire for financial freedom. This desire should be in every member of your team. They should understand that the company's success puts them a step ahead in their journey to financial liberation.

Let them be driven by the anger and frustration that comes with lack, with having a need and lacking the capacity to meet it. Let this anger drive them to provide value to their community and the world at large. Know this: There is wealth in this world, but it can only be accessed by those who offer value. It is an exchange system: give value, receive wealth.

While motivated by this anger, they should also balance and consolidate their passion with the knowledge of the reward they would receive at the end. Apart from the financial reward, let them think of the sense of fulfillment that comes with the knowledge that they were part of a creative process that offered immense value to the world.

You worked hard to get your team to believe in your vision, so do all it takes to sustain the fire. If you do not, you may lose them, and when you do, you may never get them to believe (in) you again. You don't want this happening.

Pledge to Action

I affirm that:

I am not just a talker but a doer.

I am not just a dreamer but an achiever.

I understand that nature hates vacuum, so I wouldn't willingly allow my ideas to be taken because I refused to act.

I do away with fear.

I do away with doubt.

I am a brave.

I have faith in my vision.

My vision is powerful and I cannot wait to show it to the world.

My team would not lose motivation because of me.

They will be ever-motivated and focused because they look up to me.

I spot ideas and act on them quickly.

I am the early bird.

CHAPTER SEVEN

The Unpredictable Maneuver

"Others follow patterns; we alone are unpredictable."

— Mignon McLaughlin

Do not let your competition know that you are not in line with their thoughts. Leaning on the ideas of Sun Vu, this is what I term "The Unpredictable Maneuver." Vu stated that maneuvering is the most difficult task in warfare. According to him, it involves turning a curved situation into a straight one and disadvantages into advantages. And you have to do this without the enemy being aware. You have to be subtle. Unpredictable.

When there is chaos, act as if you are also affected by the chaos. This is what Sun Vu meant when he wrote: "In the chaotic situation of the battle, our army may seem to be in chaos, but in reality, we cannot be chaotic. In a chaotic and tangled situation, the distribution of our troops may seem disorderly, but in reality, it is invisible. In this way, chaos clearly masks for real organization, cowardice masks for courage, weak force masks for strong force."

There are some points you need to take note of when employing unpredictable maneuvering. These points as outlined by Sun Vu include:

- **Victory belongs to the person who masters the combination of curvature and straightness.** Understand that in business, the path will not always be straight. Curves and bumps are bound to exist. Navigating these curves should not translate into a loss and a depressing moment for you. Learn to use these curves to your advantage. Let them be tools for your victory.

- **In battle, human voices are not strong enough to be heard, which is why we use gongs and trumpets. Our vision is not accurate enough, which is why we use banners and flags**. It is the same in business; you cannot attract attention to yourself through your voice alone. This is why you need effective marketing skills to amplify your voice. However, in this case of unpredictable maneuvering, you have to go beyond conventional marketing. In times of chaos, you have to get your customers to be your gongs and trumpets. And you would need to do this subtly. We can cite an example with the coronavirus pandemic. It was a moment of chaos. Everybody was physically and psychologically drained by fear. It was not the best of moments for companies to advertise their businesses, especially using the virus as a tool to promote their products. A bar in New Zealand came under fire for doing this. Their ad showed an image of two men in boiler suits and gas masks, each holding a bottle of Corona beer. The image had the caption: "CATCH SOME CORONA AT HOUSE THIS SUMMER."[1] It was a tacky promotion. Unfortunately, the bar did not see anything wrong with the ad.[2] It was a wordplay intended for humor, but it came at the wrong time. As at the time the promotion was released, over 360 people had died of the virus in Asia, and there were nearly 18,000 cases globally.[3] It was not a time for jokes. If the bar wanted to stay ahead of their competitors in a moment of chaos, I think they failed at it. It was a poor attempt at unpredictable maneuvering.

However, there were companies that employed unpredictable maneuvering effectively. For example, Coursera offered free courses to universities worldwide during the pandemic,[4] LinkedIn opened up 16 of its learning courses for free,[5] Dolce & Gabbana partnered with the Humanitas University to fund a coronavirus research project, and Giorgio Armani donated $1.43 million to four hospitals in Rome and Milan, as well as to the Civil Protection Agency.[6] The actions of these companies were unpredictable maneuvering at its best. They used empathy as their gongs and trumpets to amplify their voices, and charity as their flags and banners to demonstrate their vision and values[7]. These actions would leave an indelible mark on their beneficiaries, and these beneficiaries would love to be associated with these brands even beyond Covid-19.

- **Snatch away the morale of the enemy.** Always make the competition doubt their capacity. And the only way to do this is by getting the people on your side. While the competition is giving people what they want, give the people what they *need*. Once you give people what they need, you get them on your side and take away the enemy's morale. This was the case between Apple and Blackberry. Blackberry was busy riding on the wings of its elite status coupled with its popularity and multimillion-dollar deals and failed to innovate. Then Apple came with its keyboard-less iPhones, which were updated every year. Other smartphones copied iPhone's model, and Blackberry couldn't just keep up. Their morale was deflated—completely flattened.

Sun Vu pointed out that, "When an army first arrives at the scene, their morale is sharp and strong, after a while it becomes languid and lazy, and finally wants to return home." A similar scenario occurs in business. For some businesses, their morale tapers. They get comfortable with their current status and their current market share. They slack on their company culture; they stop aiming to become better. This was Blackberry's undoing, and iPhone capitalized on the opportunity to take over the smartphone market. Sun Vu advised the general to fight when the enemy's morale is low. While this may be a good strategy for warfare, it may not be completely healthy in business. Remember, we have emphasized so much on timing. Start early. Don't wait for the enemy's morale to get low before you strike. (What if the morale doesn't get low?) Take away the morale by intimidating the competition with your innovation.

- **Do not approach to fight with the enemy troops on a high hill.** Know your level. Fight at your level. Before competing against another company in your industry, make sure you are on the same level with them in finance, quality of human resources, and/or innovative ideas. You cannot be a newbie in an industry and decide to compete with industry giants. You can only aspire to be a giant, then become a giant, before competing with giants. In the world of smartphones, some names first come to mind before others. Apple and Samsung. Then others. These two companies are miles ahead of others in terms of market share, company valuation, quality of human resources, and innovation. Other phone companies like Huawei, Ericsson, and Nokia mainly compete among themselves.

As an entrepreneur, know your league. Knowing your league doesn't mean you wouldn't aspire to play in a bigger league. All I am saying is that you should not burn resources competing against companies that have the resources more than you. Bigger companies have the resources and know-how to create a lot of touchpoints. Say you are a new telephone company how would you compete with Apple's over twenty touchpoints—including their packaging, a clean website, store locations, personal set-up, software development kits, questionnaires on satisfaction, and number of employees?[8] It would be practically impossible to beat that at your level.

- **Do not press too hard with a desperate troop.** Never be the desperate company. The market is wide enough for everybody. All you need is patience. Desperation would lead you to make mistakes that may soil your company's reputation. Jeff Wiener shared a story of how a company, desperate to beat his company, resorted to copying everything Jeff's company did. The company copied their blogposts and primary web pages (including the typos). The only thing they changed was the company name. They even left the name of Jeff's company in their meta description and meta keywords.[9] That is how desperate they were.

Desperation will only hurt you *if you allow it to consume you*. I put that caveat because desperation helped a company like Nike. In an act of desperation to gain a competitive edge over Reebok, Nike signed Michael Jordan[10]—a deal that revolutionized the company. In 2019, the company made $3.14 billion from the Nike Air Jordan brand.[11] If you want to be desperate, then make healthy decisions.

Don't be reckless. Don't take unnecessary risks. Don't overwork your team just because you want them to meet up. You will only dampen their morale if you do that. Do not be the desperate one. Let the competition be the desperate company, then use their desperation to your advantage. Quoting Lior Arussy, Vivian Giang wrote in her *Forbes* article: "People do a lot of stupid things when they're desperate and if you can understand their level of confidence, you can exploit their weaknesses."[12] Vivian also advised that entrepreneurs should figure out what makes the competition desperate and become exceptional at what the competition lacks. "For example, if they are lacking in customer service, deliver an authentic and personalized experience to your own customers. If you're a smaller company, send your customers birthday cards and personalized letters," she wrote.[13]

A successful entrepreneur is one that is flexible and able to turn challenges into bright prospects. The competition will always be eager to know what's up his sleeves. That is the entrepreneur you should become. When the market or other uncontrollable factors take everyone by surprise, catch your breath and think out how to maneuver the challenge. Let your maneuver be smooth and subtle.

Pledge to Action

I affirm that:

I see opportunities and take advantage of them.

I will use challenges as raw materials for my success.

I am a master of curves and straights.

Therefore, I will not be caught unawares.

With my innovation, I will take away the morale of the enemy.

I am calm.

I am collected.

I am not desperate.

I know desperation would lead to mistakes.

And I don't need to make any mistakes while I engage the unpredictable maneuver.

CHAPTER EIGHT

The Contingencies

"One thing that makes it possible to be an optimist is if you have a contingency plan for when all hell breaks loose." — Randy Pausch

You may get everything right in your business—from planning to building your team to outpacing your competition—yet things would still go wrong. And it may likely be no fault of yours or your team. As humans, the only element of time we have full control of is the present. We can only predict the future; we cannot control it.

As a smart entrepreneur, it is important you prepare yourself for these contingencies. Do not be caught off-guard. Understand that these unforeseen events are bound to happen. This means that you should make provisions for them in your plan. Always ask yourself: What if this happens, what will I do? This does not mean you are a pessimist. On the contrary, it makes you a realist. You understand that it is in the nature of life to throw surprises at us once in a while.

Your ability to navigate unexpected challenges lies in your preparedness. Build your capacity. Have a high adversity quotient (I will discuss this later in this chapter).

Sun Vu advised the general to be prepared for changes that may happen on the battlefield. He didn't just inform the general of the likely events that may occur, he also taught the general what to do. And his lessons can also apply to you as an entrepreneur.

The Five Contingency Lessons from Sun Vu

Lesson 1: *If the terrain is not favorable, the force must not be stationed.*

One of the fundamental problems of the average human is the resistance to change. The average human would not want to take no for answer even when a yes may be detrimental. This should not be your story as an entrepreneur. As you draft out your plans on the drawing board, bear in mind that the real-life conditions for the business may not be favorable for you. Be open-minded enough to understand and *accept* this.

"If the *terrain* is not favorable, do not station your force." Terrain in this context is different from the types of terrain we saw in chapter one. The terrain in this context is *the* integral factor of the business. That factor is *you*.

You are the terrain. And yes, you can be unfavorable to your business. This may brew confusion in your mind, but hang in there. I know I have told you that you are the main repository of your vision. However, you should understand that things may be wrong with you. You may be toxic to your own vision. Don't forget you are a soil too, just like every other human being. And not all soils support every seed.

The good thing about starting a business is that it reveals qualities about you that you never knew existed. It takes you through a growth process. So you may have drafted your plans and when it is time to take action you discover certain traits about yourself that may be detrimental to your vision. Once this happens, do not station your force. Do not start the business.

What traits would you discover?

You may harbor a *lot* of traits that can be the little foxes that destroy the vine. In fact, Daphne Blake lists up to 100 of these traits. But according to Blake, these 100 traits can be grouped into eight major traits.[1] For each trait, I have listed certain questions you should use to assess if you possess any of the traits.

- *You are not cut out for entrepreneurship*

  » Am I motivated by money?
  » Am I motivated by fame?
  » Am I starting the business to escape from something?
  » Do I avoid difficult conversations?
  » Have I burnt all my bridges?
  » Am I confident and disciplined?
  » Do I know my strengths and weaknesses?
  » Do I have a vision for the future?
  » Can I accept and handle the possibility of failure?
  » Am I passionate about this business?

- *You are not in the right place in your life*

  » Am I caring for young children or aging relatives?
  » Do I have weak support systems?
  » Do I have other engagements (e.g., schoolwork) that I need to commit to?
  » Do I have physical or mental health challenges that would affect my work?
  » Will my business affect my emotional/romantic relationship?
  » Can I give up sleep to get the work done?
  » Do I have a free time in my schedule?
  » Do I have the opportunity to travel?
  » Do I have good outlets for stress?
  » Am I willing to give up my hobbies?

- *You have a personality problem*

  » Do I want or love routine?
  » Do I hate networking and motivating others?
  » Do I always want to be in control?
  » Do I lack focus and organization?
  » Am I obsessed with perfection and hate being wrong?

» Am I creative?

» Can I handle failure?

» Am I given to learning?

» Can I self-evaluate?

» Can I complete projects?

- *Your finances are not in order*

  » Do I have a low credit score?

  » Am I in debt?

  » Do I have huge financial obligations?

  » Do I need a steady salary to survive?

  » Am I totally dependent on bank loans to start my business?

  » Do I have a budget?

  » Do I have other funding plans aside from venture capital or angel investors?

  » Do I understand that crowdfunding may not be successful?

  » Do I have an insurance plan?

  » Do I have a backup plan?

- *You have a faulty business idea*

  » Am I in love with my idea that I cannot let it go even when it is not feasible?

  » Am I scared to tell others my idea because they will reveal its weaknesses?

  » Am I starting this business because a friend or relative is into it?

  » Is my idea devoid of innovation?

  » Do I lack the resources to bring my vision to life?

  » Do I understand how my idea can be profitable?

  » Do I have a compelling business proposition?

  » Have I done a pre-launch market testing to ascertain the demand for my offering?

  » Can I withstand the competition in the market?

  » Do I understand the market or industry I am getting into?

- *You don't know what you are doing*

  » Do I hate customer service?

  » Do I hate data and analyzing them?

  » Will I be uncomfortable firing underperforming staff?

  » Do I have a problem scaling a business?

  » Do I have a wrong definition of success?

  » Do I understand how entrepreneurship works?

  » Do I know how to delegate duties?

  » Do I know how to recruit staff and set KPIs?

  » Do I understand cash flow?

  » Do I know how to value and price my products?

Assessment Guide 1: *For you to be an entrepreneur, your answers to the first 5 questions should be negative, while the remaining 5 should be positive. If your score is less than 60%, then you are not cut out for entrepreneurship.*

- *You don't know how to sell*

  » Do I know how to attract customers?

  » Do I understand the difference between features and benefits?

  » Can I give a compelling value proposition?

  » Do I listen to my customers?

  » Can I sell my vision to mentors, investors, and stakeholders?

  » Can I get a partner or co-founder on board?

  » Can I motivate my team?

- *You can't handle risk*

  » Can I handle uncertainty and surprises?

  » Do I know how to manage and minimize risks?

  » Do I have mentors?

  » Do I have a plan for handling lawsuits and negative press?

Assessment Guide 2: For you to be an entrepreneur, your answers to all the questions above should be positive. If your score is less than 60%, then you are not cut out for entrepreneurship.

Provide honest answers to these questions. And once you see that you do not have what it takes to be an entrepreneur, once you see the terrain is not favorable, do not deploy forces. Retreat. Get things right. Then try again.

Lesson 2: *Do not linger on a barren land.*

Sayings like "Never give up" and "Winners don't quit. Quitters don't win" have made many remain in businesses that are not profitable. Your decision to leave an unprofitable business is *solely* at your discretion. I say this because there are popular businesses that are not making profit yet are still in business. Examples include Snap Inc., Uber, Lyft, Airbnb, Dropbox, Soundcloud, YouTube, and others.[2]

The question that may be going through your mind is this: *If these companies aren't profitable and are still in business, why should I close shop?* Know this: These companies are still in business because they make revenue and are also backed by investors. They are global brands. They add value to their customers. The only issue is that the business doesn't give them any profit to enjoy. Now, we cannot term these brands barren. They witness *consistent* growth.

- Does your business experience consistent growth?
- Are you making enough sales to cover the operations of the company?
- Is the business sustaining itself without your personal funds?
- Are you still physically and mentally fit in spite of the demands of the business?
- Are your key employees still with you?
- Are customers (still) impressed with your product?

Your honest answers to these questions will tell you if you are wasting time on a barren land or not. If you gave a negative answer to more than 60% of these questions, then you are lingering on a barren land. Move.

Lesson 3: *If besieged, you have to think straight.*

One of the questions asked in Lesson 1 was: "Do I have physical or mental health challenges that would affect my work?" This question is vital because you need to be physically and mentally alert in times of unexpected drastic events. A wrong decision made in a moment of panic can ruin your entire business. Events like lawsuits, natural disasters, and fire outbreaks can be a heavy blow to your belly. They can make you lose air . You see everything you've worked for (almost) destroyed in a wink.

These moments are tough. Sometimes these moments would determine the life or death of your business. Sun Vu advised that in moments of life and death, you have to take risks. But be careful not to make any hasty decisions—take calculated risks.

You have to maintain composure and grit for yourself, your team, and your customers. In his article for *Life Hack*, Tanvir Zafar noted that to defy existential crises as an entrepreneur, you have to understand your purpose for being in business in the first place. It is this understanding, this conviction in your identity, that will help you withstand challenges.[3] Zafar echoed the words of Christian T. Russell, the president of Dangerous Tactics: "You have to know your purpose for running your company in the first place! Why does your business exist? Who do you serve? What do they need most from you, right now? 99% of business owners do not take the time for this introspection."[4]

Be part of the 1% of business owners that have time for this introspection. Your challenge shouldn't be the end of your business.

Lesson 4: *There are roads you should not cross.*

There are different routes to a destination, but depending on your position, you must not go through every route. In good times, in times where your mind is not muddled by unexpected events, it is easy to know and choose the routes to follow. However, when you become anxious due to events that take you by surprise, you may take the wrong routes.

There are two roads you should not take in times of anxiety and uncertainty. They are: The Road of Impatience and The Road of Non-delegation. These two roads may seem appealing, but they may be detrimental to your business.

The Road of Impatience. When unexpected events happen, we want to get out of them as soon as possible. And we may want to take the quick route, even when it is not the right route. This is why you need to have a high adversity quotient. Adversity quotient measures your ability to withstand challenges without breaking. Impatience or haste is the extra force that pushes you to your breaking point. But if you can withstand just a little more, you will get the logical and perfect solution to the challenge. No matter what happens, follow through the process. You will see the light at the end.

The Road of Non-delegation. In times of adversity, we lose trust in people, in our team. We feel that it's because we didn't do something right that's why things went wrong. So, in seeking a solution to the challenge, we would want to handle everything ourselves because we don't want things to go wrong again. This may seem understandable, but it is unhealthy. During the times of challenges, that is when you need to do two important things: *seek help* and *release control*. It is a time you need all the help you can get. It is a time you need to consider other perspectives. It is a time to delegate tasks. Surround yourself with think-tanks, mentors, and trusted employees who are committed to ensuring that things become normal again.

Lesson 5: *We sometimes do not fight the enemy*

This may seem like a contradiction, but it is ideal. The enemy here is your competition. And there are times when you don't fight the enemy. There are times you need to collaborate with the enemy, because the enemy may have what you need. Perrie Kapernaros noted that competitive collaboration is a "healthy and viable" road to take in your business.[5] This corroborates what I stated earlier about an entrepreneur not taking the road to non-delegation. You cannot do it all alone. And sometimes, your best allies would be your competition. We see, or we've seen excellent competitive collaboration in Microsoft and Intel, Pfizer and Merck, Vimeo and YouTube[6], even Samsung and Apple (Samsung supplies screens to Apple).[7]

Before you fight the enemy, think of collaboration—because, according to Kapernaros, it can help you increase profits, improve brand awareness, and attract your target market.

These are the likely unexpected events you may encounter in the battlefield of business. Asides these five events, there are also five mistakes or drawbacks you must avoid. When you handle unexpected events well enough and go ahead to avoid these mistakes, you set yourself on a path to become a successful, well-rounded entrepreneur.

The Five Dangerous Drawbacks

"Recklessness, greed, anger, self-conceit, a men pleaser. These five are common mistakes and catastrophes to the successful conduct of the war."
- Sun Vu

Throughout this book, I have given you strategies for success in business. The strategies are not foolproof. Did I shock you with that statement? Of course, they are not foolproof because of one factor: you. You are human—an emotional being. And your emotions can interfere with these strategies and mar them. A human being has a total of 27 emotions.[8] Therefore, it is impossible to apply these strategies without interference from your emotions. For example, in chapter six, I highlighted how *fear*, a human emotion, can limit you from launching your business on time. Apart from fear, Sun Vu listed five dangerous emotions or traits that can drastically affect your business. But before we look at these emotions or traits, we will look at an overview of emotions—what they are and how they differ from feelings.

What are emotions?

Simply put, emotions are involuntary responses to external or internal stimuli. Our body processes sensory information—sight, smell, sound, taste, and touch—received from our external environment. For instance, if you are walking on a lonely path and you see a lion, you will feel afraid. You would tremble, your heart would beat faster, you would have a dry mouth, you would be mentally and physically alert to take flight. All these are your body's way of processing the information it received from your sense of sight. This means that emotions are physically expressed.

Not only does the body use emotions to process information from our external environment, it also uses them to process information received from our internal environment; our mind. Our mind, which is the seat of our memory and thoughts, can trigger an emotion. For example, if you lost a loved one, you would feel sad whenever you remember that person even a long time after their demise. That is the body using an emotion—sadness—to process internal information, a memory. Remember, emotions are involuntary; we have no control over them. No one chooses to be afraid when they sight a lion. No one chooses to be sad when they remember a dead loved one. These emotions overwhelm the human body because they are a product of physiological processes, we have no control over. And this is where emotions differ from feelings.

Many often confuse emotions with feelings (and vice versa), but they are different, even though they are related. So, what are feelings?

Feelings are our reactions after we have processed and understood emotions. They are simply the feedback we give after an emotion. While emotions are physically expressed, feelings are mentally expressed. They counterbalance the physical responses we express as a result of our emotions. For instance, if you see a lion on a lonely street, you can choose not to *feel* threatened (although it would take a lot of courage to do that). Unlike the emotion, fear, which you could not control, you can control what you feel. Instead of feeling threatened, you can make the conscious effort of feeling calm. The same thing applies when you feel sad because you remembered a loved one. Instead of sadness, you can choose to feel happy, holding on to the belief that they are in a better place.

Emotions and feelings are often seen as the same because there is a quick switch from emotions to feelings. The line dividing the two is too thin that it is imperceptible. We often don't know when we have transited into feeling from emotions.

We have to understand the workings of emotions and feelings because the inability to neutralize a negative or inappropriate emotion with the right feeling may cost us a whole lot. Now, let us see the five emotions/traits/actions that can be catastrophic to your business.

Recklessness

"Reckless disregard for death will actually lead to death." - Sun Vu

Entrepreneurship is all about risks. This risk stems from the inability to accurately know what the future holds. We go into entrepreneurship with a blend of predictions, history, and hope. The market dynamics are not subject to our dictates, thus we position ourselves according to the market dynamics, hoping that our position will favor us. If we can accurately know the future, then it would be easy for us to know what or what not to do. It is this uncertainty that makes business risky.

Now, some people have interpreted risk as recklessness. You'd hear them say things like, "Life is all about risk." This is true. But it is quite different for business. Business is not all about risk, but *calculated* risk. Just like Sun Vu said, if you interpret risk as recklessness, and have total disregard for the life of your business, then your business would definitely meet its end.

There are countless books and articles that tell motivating stories of people and/or businesses that took risks and succeeded. But there are hardly any stories of those who took risks and failed. These businesses went into oblivion and are not remembered because they mistook recklessness for risk.

The reason why people become reckless is that they cannot control an important emotion: excitement. The general who is reckless with his attack may be excited about his troops' strength or number, his weapons, his strategy, or the enemy's supposed weaknesses. The reckless businessman is excited about the prospect of huge profits to be made, his team's strength, financial acumen, or the competition's supposed weaknesses. This excitement strips off his thought process. He doesn't analyze the market. All he thinks about is taking action. Such a businessman is headed for doom. He would plow his resources into the venture, only for him to hit a brick wall. This is why you should avoid being reckless at all costs. Now, the question is, how do you do this? How do you know you are moving towards recklessness instead of (calculated) risk? To answer this question, I would borrow the ideas of Gwen Moran, a Business and Finance writer and author.

In an article for *Entrepreneur*, Moran outlined four traits for entrepreneurs—risk-takers—to watch out for. For me, these traits are signals that would alert you when you are crossing the thin line between risk and recklessness.

- **Sensation-seeking.** Some people become reckless because they love the adrenaline rush that accompanies recklessness. They are entrepreneurial daredevils. Moran stated that people who naturally crave sensation and seek out risky adventures like skydiving might transfer this trait into their business. They want to thrive where the atmosphere is chaotic or where they are engaged in high-stakes decision making.[9] If you are such a person, it is expedient you dampen this excitement and think things through before acting. Move beyond emotions and transcend into feelings. Although you are excited and pumped-up, choose to feel calm. Choose to be calculating. Choose to be analytical.

- **Unconcerned about consequences.** People who are unconcerned about consequences are the people to whom Sun Vu directed the saying, "Reckless disregard for death will actually lead to death." These businesspeople simply do not care about the outcome of their actions. And I wonder why this is so. If you wouldn't be bothered about the longevity of your business, why start up the business in the first place? Some erroneously define this unconcern as bravery. Being cautious is not cowardice. It only means you value your business and resources that you wouldn't want to jeopardize them. When you notice that you are unbothered about the outcomes of your risks, then you should know you are approaching recklessness. However, in the words of Moran, "That's not to say you should be paralyzed by fear, but you should understand what could happen if the outcome of your action or decision is not as you'd hoped and have an idea of what you'll do in that situation."[10]

- **Impulsiveness.** When you are about to take a risk, ask yourself: Did I think this through, or am I just being impulsive? You can get an answer to this question by analyzing past decisions you have taken. Is there a pattern? Do you fail to carry out adequate research each time you're to make a decision? Do you regret your actions later? These questions are necessary because, just as Moran noted, "People who have issues with willpower and who tend to make decisions quickly without doing the necessary research or investigation are typically more prone to making reckless decisions than those who are more disciplined."[11] Quoting Steven Mundahl, co-author of *The Alchemy of Authentic Leadership*, she added that such people are "the type of people who will follow a plan for a while, but then will throw it all away with a decision that looks good at the time instead of keeping the big picture in mind."[12] This tells you that a moment of impulsiveness can ruin everything you did at the drawing board.

- **Denial.** This is another trait to watch out for. Many reckless people fail to accept the reality of life. Sometimes, a reckless person knows they are reckless, but they keep believing a lie because of the anticipated reward. In Moran's words, "They prefer not to face the reality of their choices. Instead, they ignore fallout or make excuses for why a particular decision didn't work out. They also make light of the potential for failure or choose to disregard it entirely. People who have trouble facing a situation's facts are more likely to make decisions that are not grounded in the best interest of the company."[13]

These signals do not only prevent you from being reckless, they also help you ask the necessary questions for taking calculated risks. Questions like:

- Why do I want to do this?
- Is this actually good for my business, or am I just looking for a thrill?
- What are the possible outcomes of this decision?
- Is this venture sustainable?
- Does this venture have a solid roadmap?
- Am I unbothered about the consequences of my actions?
- Do I feel that this venture is foolproof and I do not need to think about it?
- Am I facing reality or shielding myself from it?
- Am I only motivated by prospective gains?
- Do I love my vision so much as not to jeopardize it?

Greed

"A greedy general will be captured." - Sun Vu

Greed is just as drastic as recklessness. In fact, greed is one of the causes of recklessness. Don't be a businessman that doesn't know when to stop. There is a difference between aspiring for more and being greedy. When you aspire for more, it means that you want to scale your business without losing sight of your vision and core values. It means that you want to grow based on what your business needs, not what you want. On the other hand, when you are greedy, you have the *excessive* desire to want more—even more than what your business needs.

Often, greed is a product of impatience. In a bid to rise quickly, some entrepreneurs seek and inject so much funds into their business and in the end, suffocate it. You may be wondering how this is possible. I hear you ask: "Thẩm, I thought funding is what every business needs to thrive?" That's true. But there is also the popular saying that too much of anything is bad. Anastasia Belyh explained three ways in which too much funding can be detrimental to a business.

First, too much funding, especially as a startup, will raise your company's valuation so high. While this may seem like a good thing, "gathering high valuations initially can lead to expectations that may be out of the reach of a company that has only just begun operations. Companies that are new market entrants might not have the market knowledge to achieve targets that come coupled with high value funding,"[14] Belyh wrote.

Second, driven by the desire to inject funds into your business, you may likely not be selective about the type of investors you want in your business. This would result in you having numerous investors, which would, in turn, affect your business. Belyh rightly pointed out that many investors are difficult to manage, thus it is better to have a few investors who understand your business than to have many whose ideologies do not align with yours. Belyh cited an example: "Let's say a small business has sixty investors (a large number for a small business) this means that when making decisions, the business proprietor will need to take into account sixty opinions and sixty expectations."[15]

Third, apart from having too many investors, having low-quality investors could also be detrimental to your business. Don't be so funds-driven that you do not care about the type of person(s) investing in your business. When all you are concerned about is who has the money, you would not care if they understand your company's mission, vision, unique selling proposition, and core values. For this reason, Belyh advised that your number of investors should be small and well informed because it cuts back the time it takes to explain menial things to the investors. She further added that: "When you are scanning and filtering investors for quality, choose those who have had experience investing in your respective industry. They can provide helpful information and explain some of the workings of the industry to new industry entrants."[16]

Grow your business based on what it needs and not based on your greed. Sun Vu said that the greedy general gets captured. When you are greedy, you become ensnared by the poverty you were trying to escape from. And Kayla Matthews noted that this could happen in 10 ways. I have highlighted 8 out of these 10 ways, which I consider too important to ignore.[17]

1. **You look for ways to make money, and not to improve.** This means that you sacrifice quality on the altar of an excessive desire for wealth. You forgo excellent customer experience. You are only concerned about cutting costs and gaining more wealth.

2. **You make bad personnel decisions.** You may overlook the flaws of your team members as long as they are making you money. Matthews stated that an employer might ignore sexual harassment perpetrated by one of his managers because that manager is his top salesman.

3. **You don't spend money making your employees happy.** If you are a greedy entrepreneur, not only would you be unconcerned about your customers, you would also be unconcerned about your employees. A business that cares less about its employees is a dead business already. In Matthews' words: "Happy employees make for good businesses, because they are the bridge between you and your customers. When employees are unhappy, they

won't do their best for you, and that can actually lead to a decline in sales."

4. **You forego vacations to work.** In a bid to make more money, you are likely to burn yourself out. You would only be concerned with work, work, work. You might even make your teamwork without vacation—an action that can leave harmful consequences on your team. Greed would tell you the lie that you don't have the luxury of taking a break. It would tell you that while you're resting, your competitors are moving miles ahead of you. But as I said, these are all lies. You would need to take a break. If you do not take a break, then you'd break down. And that would likely end your business.

5. **You take on more clients than you can effectively manage.** You want all the money to yourself. So, you keep taking orders even when you know that you are choked already. This will result in you delivering a shabby service, burning yourself out, and ultimately denting your business's image. Matthews put it better when she wrote: "If you stretch your staff too thin with your workload, [your] clients will not be happy with your work. Worse yet, word may leak out to other potential clients that you're not meeting deadlines or producing good work."

6. **You squander your clients' trust.** As a follow up to the previous point, when you keep delivering a shabby job or fail to meet up with clients' expectations, you'd lose their trust. Trust is a pillar that upholds your business, and once this pillar is gone, your business begins to collapse gradually. On the issue of trust, Matthews wrote: "When it becomes clear that you only care about making money, you risk losing even the most loyal clients. They want someone working for them who sees them as more than just a dollar sign."

7. **You alienate your employees.** A greedy employer would overwork his team, get them to make money for him, and then give them a remuneration not commensurate with their effort. This can deflate the morale of your team. And when this happens, they wouldn't mind selling you out to your competition.

8. **You're not mentoring anyone.** Many do not know this, but mentorship is vital for a business. Beyond money, mentorship helps you expand the value you add to the world. Your mentees become outgrowths of you. Steve Jobs mentored Mark Zuckerberg. Warren Buffett mentored Bill Gates. Christian Dior mentored Yves Saint-Laurent.[18] As a successful mentor, you would look at what your mentees have built and feel a sense of fulfillment that money cannot buy. However, greed has the power of denying you this. According to Matthews, many entrepreneurs nurse the thought that there is no monetary reward for mentoring, so they shove it aside. But for Matthews, it is a foolish thought "because great mentors produce great workers who can carry on your business for years to come — and ultimately make you more money to boot."

Avoid greed. Be patient. Build gradually. Feed your business with only what it needs. And you'll definitely win. You'll see.

Anger

"The angry general is easily provoked into taking superficial action." - Sun Vu

As an entrepreneur, it is almost impossible not to get angry at certain situations or people. Remember, anger is an emotion, and we cannot control emotions. Why would you get angry as an entrepreneur? The answer is simple: things will not always go your way. They wouldn't always go as you planned them. I stated earlier that entrepreneurship is all about history, prediction, hope, and patience. There are times when your predictions wouldn't be correct. It is normal to get angry and frustrated in those times, but you have to choose how to respond to the anger.

As an entrepreneur, there are five elements that you are likely to get angry at. They are life, your market/industry, your employees/team, your competition, and yourself.

- **Life**. It is often said that life doesn't give you what you deserve, but what you demand. But the process of demanding often takes a long time. The process of making a demand on life is quite frustrating and exhausting. You begin to wish that life was a bit lenient. You wonder why things are not going as planned when you have done everything right on the drawing board. You have gotten sufficient capital. You have gotten the right team. You are innovative; you are confident in the quality of your product. Yet, for no fault of yours, things are just not working out. It is in times like this you feel like punching the wall or throwing a flower vase.

- **Your market/industry.** Sometimes, life may not be the culprit. The industry you find yourself in has a way of playing games with your mind, and this can get you angry. Entrepreneurs in the financial niche experience this a lot. One day the market is bullish, the next day it is so bearish that their portfolio is greatly affected. They would then sell off their assets to cut their losses, and immediately they do, the market becomes bullish. This is just an example with financial markets like the stock and cryptocurrency industry. Every industry has its peculiarities that can leave entrepreneurs angry.

- **Your employees/team.** Human beings are difficult to control. Your team comprises different individuals with different backgrounds, ideologies, experiences, skills, goals, and so on. It is a huge task to streamline these diversities in one direction. In your quest to do this, a member(s) of your team would still want to deviate from the cause. This can be upsetting.

- **Your competition.** Your competition is always out to get on your nerves. Everything they do is a subtle message informing you that you are in a war with them. An instance that readily comes to mind is the Coca-Cola vs. Pepsi Cola war, in which the two companies always take a jibe at each other with their ads. For example, there is this Pepsi commercial where a little boy buys two cans of Coke, only to step on them for height to reach for the button to get a can of Pepsi. In another ad, a Coke truck driver tastes Pepsi for the first time and refuses to share the drink with anyone else. These are just a few examples where the Cola Wars have gotten messy. Coca-Cola is not exonerated; they have thrown their fair share of blows, though mostly as a response to Pepsi's commercial. The bottom line is this: Your competition can get you angry through different forms. They would try to elicit a negative response from you. Do not give in to their antics.

- **Yourself.** There are times when you'd get angry at yourself. You'd get angry at the mistakes you made. You'd get angry at failing at a venture. You'd get angry for missing a business opportunity. You'd get angry for employing the wrong hand. You'd get angry for purchasing the wrong equipment. You'd get angry for not starting early. Sometimes, your anger would morph into sadness. At other times, frustration. And at other times, recklessness because you are trying to meet up with what you think you've lost.

No matter the reason for your anger, never let the anger control you. Remember, *the angry general* (read: entrepreneur) *would be provoked into taking superficial action*. Superficial action here means an action or decision without depth, without a solid foundation. An action that is bound to crumble and probably take the business down with it. So, choose to respond to the anger positively. Use anger as a raw material to build a solid business. Neil Patel, a former contributor for Forbes, outlines different ways to use anger as a raw material to build a solid business.[19] I will use Patel's ideas as solutions to handle the five areas of your life and business that can get you angry.

What do you do when you are angry at life?

Neil suggested that you should **be more perseverant**. These were his words: "I know I've felt deflated and defeated on more than a few occasions because things simply weren't going my way. However, I've found that anger is perhaps the best emotion for pumping me back up and giving it another go." This means that you should channel your anger into demanding what you want from life. Get angry with the state of things and determine to change them. Let anger be your spur to have a better life, a better business.

What do you do when you are angry at your market/industry?

Still persevere. Remember that the market moves in trends and cycles. What goes up would surely come down. The market is a sinuous wave of highs and lows. In your anger, persevere, be patient. You will surely win.

In addition to being more perseverant, use your anger to **eliminate fear**. You get angry at the market because you fear you are going to lose your investment. It is a chain: fear births anger, anger births desperation, and desperation births carelessness. Neil stated that anger helps slash through his anxieties. It helps him take action instead of focusing on the hypotheticals. According to him, it is scientifically proven. Citing *Psychology Today*, he wrote, Anger causes levels of the stress hormone cortisol to drop, suggesting that anger helps people calm down and get ready to address a problem -- not run from it.

What do you when you are angry at your employees/team?

Your anger can be effective in two ways. First, use it to **improve communication** with the team. Sometimes, we need anger to express how we truly feel about a bad situation. Some people get angry yet find it difficult to express themselves because they do not want to hurt the offender. But this shouldn't be so. Neil pointed out that letting the anger come through would help you communicate how you are feeling. He added that "Getting a little pissed now and then allows you to cut through the BS and tell it like it really is."

Also, your anger can **aid in negotiation**. Remember, we are talking about your employees *or team*. Members of your team include your investors, partners, and other people or organizations tied to your business one way or another. So if you, according to Neil, find yourself "getting the short end of the stick, getting a little pissed is sometimes all you need to put your foot down and negotiate like a boss. This ensures that you're nobody's doormat and gives you the courage to do whatever it takes to get your needs met."

What do you do when you are angry at your competition?

The answer is simple: When they go low, go high. Be the one to get them angry by not responding the way they want you to. **Show your humanness** in all its entirety. Being angry is a part of being human, but after getting angry, be the bigger person. Do not try to pull the competition down even though they are trying to play a dirty game. The world is watching, and the customers know who is offering real value. Don't allow the competition to get you into taking superficial decisions that would only hurt you and your business in the end.

What do you do when you are angry at yourself?

This is where the bulk of the work lies. Everything about your business may not continue and end with you, but it will definitely start with you. And the beginning of a venture is important for its sustainability and success. There are five things you can do when you are angry with yourself.

First, you can **achieve hyper-focus**. At that point of anger, kill the emotion and birth the feeling. Anger comes with muddled thoughts. That is one of the physiological responses it produces. But you can counter this with your feelings. Choose calmness. Neil wrote that when he's angry, he becomes obsessed with the source of his irritation. But he overcomes this and all the obsession melts away. He becomes "like a horse with blinders dead set on accomplishing whatever goal is at hand." Use your anger to gain clarity of purpose, to be more focused on your goals.

Second, use your anger to **boost your confidence**. Recall that fear births anger. Just like anger can be used to conquer fear, it can also be used simultaneously to boost confidence. Quoting Evans and Foster, Neil wrote: "Get mad and the automatic rush of adrenaline heightens your senses and reduces your inhibitions."

After this, you can now **ignite your passion**. Fear can take away your zeal towards your goal, and one veritable way of getting your passion is through anger. Use your anger to (re)ignite your passion. Neil pointed out that "it's hard to only be lukewarm about something when you're in a fit of rage," but using anger intelligently helps you approach a task or a goal with zest and zeal, which would ultimately lead to great results. It also gives you the assurance that you can take on any challenge and leads you to the fourth thing to do: **take action**.

Let your anger be your spur. This time let your anger not make you punch the wall or throw away a flower vase. Take bold steps towards getting what you want for yourself and your business. On taking action, Neil had this to say of himself: "For me personally, a little bit of good anger makes me feel like I'm ready to take on the world. If I was only half-invested in a project beforehand, getting angry can be the catalyst for me actually getting it done."

Then, after all these, let your anger **provide self-insight**. Neil said he uses anger as a means of personal reflection to shine a light on his imperfections, and it has helped him grow and progress. Like Neil, use anger to analyze your situation. Understand why you got angry in the first place. What went wrong? Was the fault from you? How can you make things better? How do you ensure that there is not a repeat of whatever went wrong? Anger is a good motivation for going back to the drawing board.

Self-conceit

"Self-conceited generals are easy to shame." – Sun Vu

Sun Vu's quote above summarizes the danger of self-conceit. Undue arrogance does not pay. In this era, many confuse self-conceit with self-confidence. They are not the same. Self-conceit is simply arrogance. Merriam-Webster Dictionary defines it as an *"exaggerated* opinion of one's own qualities or abilities."[20] Same dictionary defines self-confidence as "confidence in oneself and in one's powers and abilities."[21] And the word "confidence" means "a feeling or consciousness of one's powers or of reliance on one's circumstances."[22] Notice that these words have similar meanings, but what separates self-conceit from self-confidence is the operative word, "exaggerated."

It is good to be confident of your abilities and qualities. This is why we have egos—to give us the sense of worth we deserve. But when this confidence becomes exaggerated, then we are crossing a very dangerous line. Do not overestimate your worth to the point of dampening the worth of another. There is a difference between saying, "We are the best online school in Europe," and "We are the best online school in Europe, unlike ABC school and XYZ academy, which do not have the capacity we have." The former is you having an opinion about your ability and quality (confidence), while the latter exaggerates that ability and quality by pulling down the ability and quality of others (self-conceit).

Sun Vu rightly pointed out that the arrogant or self-conceited general (or, in this case, entrepreneur) is easy to shame. This was the case of one of the favorite examples in this book—Blackberry. *The*

Economic Times stated one of the reasons for Blackberry's fall was "institutional arrogance."[23] Institutional arrogance is "offensive and incorrect certainty of correctness by an entity or person with artificial power within a narrow space of influence."[24] Mike Lazaridis and Jim Balsillie, The CEOs of RIM, makers of Blackberry, felt that Apple and Google's innovation couldn't bring down Blackberry. "Balsillie and Lazaridis believed it was far too soon to seriously entertain the idea of putting a computer on a phone, and Apple and Google were able to outmaneuver them through simple technological superiority."[25] Simply put: Apple and Google easily shamed Blackberry.

People pleasing

"General who loves the people easily gets troubled." - Sun Vu

Know this: You cannot please everyone, no matter how hard you try. This is one of the major reasons many have failed in business. Some entrepreneurs want to be tagged, "The (wo)man of the people," so they go out of their way trying to please everyone—from investors to employees to clients. What hurts about being a people pleaser is that most times, the people you are trying to please do not really care about you or your business. They just want you as a medium to meet their desires. And once that is granted, they move on.

Being a people pleaser is never rewarding. Like Sun Vu pointed out, it only leaves you troubled. You end up giving up what is best for your business because you are considering what is good for everyone. Your product or service cannot satisfy everyone. This is why you have competition. Healthy competition is good for the market or industry because, one way or another, each company is meeting the specific needs of the clients in the market. You have your target market; those who love and value your product. Those are the people you should be concerned about.

Also, when you are out to please people all the time, you end up burning yourself out. Your mind becomes a rowdy marketplace filled with thoughts of how to satisfy everyone's needs at the same time. This would tell on your mental and physical health. And the truth is: you cannot keep up with this behavior. Therefore, the best thing to do is to stop it completely. Investors, employees, and clients will have more regard for you when they know that you are kind yet firm, empathetic yet uncompromising, especially when it comes to your business. Being a smart species, humans can perceive when you are always out to please them, and since they love the attention, they will milk the opportunity and take you for granted.

So, don't get yourself into trouble. Do not sacrifice your personal values or that of your company on the altar of wanting to be the good (wo)man to and for everyone. You cannot do that. No one can.

Act right in times of uncertainty and also avoid the five drawbacks at all costs. These drawbacks are dangerous because they deal directly with you. It is easier to rectify drawbacks that stem from other factors like your staff, investors, or competitors, but one drawback from you could destroy everything you've built in a flash. You are the foundation of the vision. You have to protect yourself. Your business, and everything attached to it, needs you to function optimally.

Pledge to Action

I affirm that:

I will make room for contingencies.

I understand that they are part of life.

I understand that I am a terrain, so I avow to be a favorable one so that I can station my forces.

I will not linger on a barren land.

I will think straight at all times.

I will not cross the roads of impatience and non-delegation.

My competitors can sometimes be my collaborators and partners.

I am prepared to work with them if it is necessary.

I will not be reckless with myself or my company.

I let go of greed.

I let go of anger.

I will not puncture the ego of others to inflate mine.

I am confident in my abilities.

I am committed to treating my employees and customers with respect.

I will not be a people-pleaser.

I understand my worth.

I will not make mistakes at times of uncertainty and despair.

I know how to handle contingencies.

CHAPTER NINE

The Resilience

"Resilience is accepting your new reality, even if it's less good than the one you had before. You can fight it, you can do nothing but scream about what you've lost, or you can accept that and try to put together something that's good." — Elizabeth Edwards

Entrepreneurs are the lifeblood of commerce and the cutthroat world of business. The business realm is fiercely competitive all over the world. Therefore, business owners should arm themselves with everything that brings about positive business ideals. One of such ideals is resilience.

Markets are bound to experience downturns. Think of the Asia financial crash of 1997. The dotcom bubble of 2000. The economic meltdown of 2008. And the Covid-19 crash of 2020. Businesses that will win in the long run are those that are resilient enough to withstand harsh market conditions. As an entrepreneur, you should learn to come up with decisive actions that would boost business resilience.

Business resilience is the positive ability of a company to adapt to the consequences of catastrophe. It is like the adversity quotient for businesses. Other factors embedded in business resilience include crisis management, business continuity, risk assessments and management, and the ability of an organization to adapt, thrive, and survive in a new environment.

Resilience strategies are crucial to businesses because unless they are in place, most businesses would not be able to thrive or recover from unexpected changes or disruptions in the market. Business survival and ultimate business success are tied to business resilience. According to Eleanor Murray, a senior fellow in management practices at the University of Oxford Saïd Business School, the creation of resilience is an iterative learning process.[1] It is continuous. It is a trait that should be consciously and continuously developed.

This means rather than trying to bounce back to where the business was, you cultivate new ways to take it forward. For instance, according to Murray, businesses learn from previous disruptions and incorporate the learning process into their businesses as they move forward.[2] Most business schools focus on the financial growth of a business, which isn't particularly surprising, considering that financial performance, is perhaps the most famous metric used to gauge business success. The repercussion, however, is that most entrepreneurs do not prepare adequate resilient strategies for the future.

To spearhead a thriving and flourishing business in times of uncertainty is one of the most daunting tasks entrepreneurs face. Our world today is highly dynamic and unpredictable. Business systems are constantly being stretched to breaking point. This is why it is necessary to create new fundamental approaches and models for businesses. And these approaches must incorporate interdependence, systems thinking, and new perspectives.

Resilience must analyze risks that are not easily seen or prepared for, and it must consider the changes in the immediate environment of the business, and how they can be used as an advantage for the business. It requires new levels to critical thinking, and the ability to conduct proper analysis beneath the surface of things.

The *Harvard Business Review* outlined six principles by which businesses can develop resilience.

One: The business must learn the art of adaptation. Adapting means learning to survive in spite of circumstances. It requires some level of diversity, and it can be attained through natural or planned experimentation. Adaptive processes and structures are established so that businesses can learn how to be flexible and diversify.

Two: The business should have diverse ways of responding to new disruptions or stress levels in the business environment. The advantage of this is that all systems that propel the business do not fail or collapse. Diversity also involves hiring different people from different backgrounds who have distinctive skills and cognitive abilities. It creates new ways of thinking and new methods of doing things.

Three: Redundancy is yet another resilient structure. It is a sort of protection against uncertainty. It is created by duplicating elements (for example, having many factories that produce the same product) or by having different elements (both human and non-human resources) working towards the same goal.

Four: A modular system allows certain aspects of the business to fail without the whole system falling and collapsing. If the business can be divided into smaller parts, then it is more understandable and can be recalibrated during a time of crisis.

Five: Prudence is another resilience strategy. It operates on the principle of caution and creates scenarios of possible situations that have incredible consequences on the fate of a business. Contingency plans, working out scenarios, monitoring signals early, and constant analysis of the business systems are ways to institute prudence in business resilience goals.

Six: The business must align its goals and activities with broader systems. Business corporations are positioned within several elements—from supply chains to business ecosystems, economies, etc. Therefore to develop resilience, businesses need to have clearly defined purposes for contributing effectively to society. When a business venture is a friend to society, it is unlikely that it will have any disruptions, and even if it does, it can easily be propelled back to the top. For instance, Google, Apple, Amazon, Tesla and Netflix are businesses that are positively interwoven into society.

Another key way of building business resilience is to intermix the business portfolio. It also involves taking risks that are educated and calculated. It involves the ability to spot opportunities from afar. Having a diverse portfolio helps a business from falling in times of adversity. Also, collaboration and cooperation are veritable ways by which business resilience can increase. Through collective resilience, businesses can have shared assets that provide insurance through investments. They can also access new capabilities, new skills, and professionalism. Powerful alliances have always proven to be prime assets in the long run, for ages. Remember competitive collaboration.

But before resilience can be built into a business, one important factor must come into play first—and this, your resilience.

The Role of Leadership in Resilience

A business can only be resilient if you are resilient. You are the powerhouse of the business both in good and bad times. To maintain business resilience in times of adversity, you need to learn how to act, adapt, and anticipate.

You need to be at the top of your game. You need to be informed about everything that can affect your business. This is where qualitative knowledge, quantitative knowledge, and knowledge of causal relationships come into play. You need to ask key questions like: How can we tackle upcoming challenges? What strategies are in place for the survival of the business? How can we turn a challenge into an advantage? These questions need to be critically analyzed if you are to make informed decisions.

You must learn how to think quickly on your feet and act with decisive action if you want to adapt fast to new business climates. New strategies would have to emerge in all spheres—from branding to employee performance to team building.

It is also your responsibility to diversify business networks and create opportunities for other capabilities and skills to thrive. The world has transcended into the era of digital communication, so people with the right skills in that field should be brought on board to work if your business still slacks in that area.

Business resilience can be developed from three key areas. I have termed these areas the pillars of resilience. They are Vision, Productivity, and Assets and Liabilities.

The Pillars of Resilience

1. **Vision:** The number one pillar of business resilience is Vision. Everything else written above would be highly impossible if they aren't envisioned in the first place. The resilience of your vision

translates into the resilience of your business so as you develop your vision, you must ensure that such vision is strong enough to withstand forthcoming challenges. Ask yourself these questions:

» Am I tenacious?

» Does my vision align with my tenacity?

» Can my vision thrive in every environment?

» What are my ambitions? Are they well laid out?

» Is there a consistent drive to accomplish them?

2. **Productivity:** A resilient leader will build a resilient team, and together they will build a resilient business. You need to review employee productivity and teamwork from time to time.

» Do the employees share the same goals and vision?

» How much fire and dedication do they have towards the growth of the business?

» Are they ready to work tirelessly and relentlessly to build business resilience in uncertainty?

3. **Assets and Liabilities:** The ability to have invaluable assets that can see a business through thick and thin is perhaps the most intricate part of business intelligence.

» How diversified is the business?

» What kind of assets or network does it have as a sustainable strategy?

The survival of a business depends solely on how much work has been put into making it resilient over time. The only way your business can flourish and blossom is when you think about it in a futuristic sense.

Pledge to Action

I affirm that:

I am a resilient entrepreneur.

I will build my business to be resilient.

My business will withstand every storm that comes in the market.

I am strong.

My team is tenacious.

We are productive.

Together, we will build a resilient company.

CHAPTER TEN

Using Spies

"You can only get ahead of your competition when you know things they don't know and do things they don't do." — Tham Trong Ma

Spies are important in battle. They offer intelligence to the general. They inform the general about the enemy's plans, weapons, strategies, strengths, weaknesses—everything. Spies are valuable to the general but detrimental to the enemy.

In business, it is necessary you use spies. There are information or perspectives you cannot access unless you have certain people around you who offer this information. Your goal is to win as an entrepreneur, and you need all the information you can get to stay ahead in the game.

Now, spying in business is not new. In fact, it goes by different names—"corporate espionage," "industrial espionage," "economic espionage," or "corporate spying." The activities under corporate espionage or spying include trespassing a competitor's property, accessing files without a competitor's permission, posing as a competitor's employee in order to learn confidential information like trade secrets, hacking a competitor's computers, wiretapping a competitor, or instigating a malware attack on a competitor's website.[1]

These are all criminal activities backed by desperation and malicious intent. I would *never* recommend that. However, Josh Fruhlinger noted that there is form of corporate spying that is not illegal (at least according to the companies that practice it). This form of spying is called "competitive intelligence." It involves gathering and analyzing information that is mostly public but that has the capacity to affect competitor's fortunes such as mergers, acquisitions, new government regulations, and so on. For instance, a company may research an executive in a rival company to try to understand the executive's motivations and behavior, and use this information to predict the next action of the company.[2] This may sound simple, harmless, and legal, but I would not recommend it either for a reason: you may not know when you cross the divide between legal and illegal.

So the question is: If I don't recommend corporate spying because it is illegal, and I also do not recommend competitive intelligence because it may become illegal, what then do I recommend?

I have developed a concept of spying on your competitors without actually spying on them. My method will allow you to get information about a rival company without even getting to know their trade secrets or any confidential information. If used effectively, my method will also give you access to information your competitor *may* not know about. This method is nothing elaborate. It is a simple means of obtaining intelligence you may even have thought about. I have termed it "The Strategy of Indirect Spying."

Before I go into this method, I need to state a fundamental point: Legal or true spying or espionage should only try to gain information about the products in the market or the market itself. Once spying or espionage crosses the line of obtaining confidential information about the competition, then it becomes a problem.

The Strategy of Indirect Spying shows you two ways you can obtain information about the products in the market or the market itself. The information gotten through this strategy can put you miles ahead of the competition.

The first method is to *become a customer*. Get into the market and blend in like a customer. You can do this or members of your team could do it for you. Interact with other customers and middlemen in the market. By doing this, you would get undiluted information about the strengths and weaknesses of not just the competition's product, but your product as well.

Before a customer commends or lays a complaint to a company, that customer has most likely aired their opinion to more than two end users. The customer may not register their commendation or complaint exhaustively when they reach out to customer care due to the formal atmosphere around such conversations. Customers or end users bare their heart in the marketplace—among other end users.

So, get into the marketplace. Be active on social media. Listen to what is said about your product or your industry. Engage social listening: monitor social media channels for mentions of your brand, competitors, products, and so on.[3] Tony Tran noted that social listening differs from social monitoring. In social monitoring, you track metrics like brand mentions, relevant hashtags, competitor mentions, and industry trends. Social listening is much deeper—you track the mood or sentiment behind these metrics.[4] And it is this information that can distinguish you from your competitors. This is why Warren Buffet got the name the Oracle of Omaha. He didn't just use numbers to predict price movements of stock, he understood the emotions, sentiments, and psychology of the market.

With social listening, you can get information about your competitor without using corporate espionage or competitive intelligence. Tony Tran wrote: "Social listening is more than understanding what people say about you. You also want to know what they say about your competitors. This gives you important insights into where you fit in the marketplace. You will also learn what your competitors are up to in real-time. Are they launching new products? Developing new marketing campaigns? Taking a beating in the press? Social listening allows you to find out about these new opportunities and threats as they happen, so you can plan and respond accordingly."[5]

So why go through the negative route when there is a positive one? This means that the Road of Corporate Espionage is another route you shouldn't follow, especially in moments of crisis when you may be forced to take *desperate* actions.

While you are in the market as a customer and engaging in social listening, you can proceed with the second method of the strategy of indirect spying.

Be part of a premium community. Not every information about your industry or market is available on social media or on Google. You have to be part of a *premium* and *exclusive* community to gain access to such information. This is a lesson you can pick from investors or traders in financial markets like the stock market, cryptocurrency market, etc. Advanced investors or traders often belong to communities where they get information about a company or the industry before such information is made public. This is why they buy assets at low prices and sell at high prices when the information has hit the market and driven up the asset's value. This is why they also sell out assets early when they get news of a possible market crash.

As an entrepreneur, you cannot underestimate the importance of belonging to a premium and exclusive community if you want to be on top of the food chain.

You can only get ahead of your competition when you know things they don't know and do things they don't do. A veritable way to do this is by spying—a different kind of spying.

Pledge to Action

I affirm that:

I want to win at all times.

But I wouldn't take any illegal route to win.

I will win by hard work.

I will win by getting access to the right information.

I will win by empathy, by understanding the customer needs.

I will win by joining the right community.

I will win by using the right spies.

CONCLUSION

E ntrepreneurship is a fierce battleground. The battle never stops. You would always be in a constant battle with yourself—trying to be better than who you were yesterday. You would be in a constant battle with your team—trying to get them to align with the vision. You would be in a constant battle with your competition—trying to outpace them.

Warfare is never easy. But some armies and generals have a record of never losing a battle. Sun Vu was one of them. And I have replicated his strategies for you to use in your business. I believe the ideas in this book are all you need to be on a constant victory march as an entrepreneur.

Because you have read this book, I know you are not afraid of entrepreneurship's many battles. I know you have the assurance that you are on a pathway to victory. Bask in this assurance always. I hope to see you at the top soon.

INSIDE THE WAR ROOM

25 Winning Strategies for Politics

INTRODUCTION

Apart from being renowned philosophers and political strategists, Niccolò Machiavelli, Sun Tzu, and Miyamoto Musashi had one thing in common - they understood the idea of winning and doing so by any means necessary.

These three men in the prime of their lives wrote three books, each that have become the pinnacle for military strategy from old to present. However, one could not be more wrong to assume that the books' strategies are only limited for use during wartimes because they were written for warring medieval laws.

Life is a battlefield, and each day brings a new opponent for you to challenge. If you live on a battlefield, then each obstacle thrown at you becomes an enemy that you need to overcome. To overcome your enemy, you would need a warring strategy to ensure you win at all costs. Essentially, if you can break down the strategies written in each book, you can pick out enough points to create an effective winning strategy for life.

However, because we have a culture that expects us to treat everyone fairly, be democratic in our approach towards issues, cooperate with other people, and, importantly, fit into a standard, our approach towards fighting these wars may be somewhat limited. The few people who step out of the fold to do what they find necessary always pay a heavy price for it. For example, Machiavelli to date still has a reputation of being a devious, cunning, dishonest, deceitful, and unscrupulous person because of some of the strategies he advised in his book.

It was so bad that an adjective was created solely to describe the kind of person he was. However, he was a preacher of "the end justifies the means" in his book. In a way, if people around the world find something that resonates with them inside his books and use them to their advantage in real-life scenarios, maybe he is not so far from the truth.

Sometime within the 5th century, in what was known in China as the Age of Warring States, Sun Tzu rose to fame and power as the general of an army that won many wars using interesting methods. He then wrote *The Law of War* to hand down the wisdom and knowledge he had gained from his many battles. The strategies shared in the book have been employed in many famous battles and shaped events of history. Along the same vein, Miyamoto Musashi wrote *The Five Spheres* as a five-part letter to his students and followers to teach them summaries of his strategies for winning sword fights.

On the surface, these books look like a "how-to" material on martial arts and armed militia, but they are so much more than that. The essence of these books, which are still studied by millions of people worldwide, is to provide tips on how to have a competitive advantage in life. Beneath the surface, these books are a practical tool for enhancing competitive success.

The values of cooperation, harmony, and unity at the forefront of this positive culture we imbibe are instilled in us in both overt and subtle ways. You read about them in books that are supposed to teach you how to get ahead in life, see them play out in the political correctness that has saturated any public space - both physical and virtual, as well as in the somber exterior that people present to the public.

However, there is one thing that these books or the culture do not prepare you for - the ruthlessness of the ongoing war in the real world. The same can be said about politics. Before Machiavelli, politics was strictly governed by ethics, at least if not in practice but in theory. There was a clear distinction between tactics employed by the military and those employed by politicians - one had leeway for ruthlessness, and the other didn't.

In fact, tracing the history of this ancient history back to Aristotle, politics was grouped as a subset of ethics. Ethics was defined as the moral principles that govern a person's conduct or behavior. Politics was defined as the moral principles that people in organized communities or social groups hold.

Machiavelli was one of the first people to divest politics from the shackles of ethics with his book *The Prince,* which has then gone on to redefine what the word means. What stands out the most from Machiavelli's treatise to rulers is how looking at the world from a de-moralized view opens up a different perspective for actions. You will also pick up this same from reading Sun Tzu's *The Law of War* and Miyamoto Musashi's *The Five Spheres* (although the last two were more military strategies than political).

This brings me back to the purpose of this book. This war that we have to fight in life exists on many fronts. The world has become even more ruthless and cutthroat, even in business, arts, and politics. The most obvious detractors we have to challenge are our rivals that stand in opposition. We challenge opponents that will not hesitate to do anything if it means getting an edge over you every day.

Even more troubling and perplexing than the battles we have to fight with your rivals are those you will have to fight with the people who appear to be in your corner. Those that will outwardly play at things that are in your best interests, those who are very charming, agreeable, and friendly on the outside, but behind the scenes are plotting against you and sabotaging your efforts to serve their own self-interests and agendas.

These are harder to spot than your outright enemies and the most capable of creating destruction. They play subtle mind games of passive aggression. They use every secret weapon within their arsenal to weaken you from within, including guilt-tripping, manipulation, and offering help that never comes. On the surface, it looks like you have found your community to support your dreams but just below it, is every person for themselves - each tearing at the other to be the one to enjoy the results of it all.

While our culture will have us pretend or deny this reality by promoting a calmer picture of gentility, it would be foolish of you to make the same mistake. Human beings are base creatures governed by their self-interests. Any play at being a community will only last as long as that self-interest isn't threatened. So, you see, we cannot afford to live up to the ideals of selflessness, fairness, cooperation, and peace that society would have us.

If you do not look out for your self-interest first, someone else will find the opportunity you are missing and use it against you. It is either you strike first or be struck, eat or be eaten. Gone are the days of turning the other cheek in the hopes that your neighbor will extend you some goodwill not to repeat the same offense. If you turn your other cheek to someone who slaps you, rest assured that they will do it again.

What we need is not the seduction of peace, selflessness, and cooperation that human beings will never attain. That is just idealistic nonsense that gets nothing done. However, the blatant, if somewhat painful, realism and unrestrained truth that these men preached about in their books because they offer practical insight, knowledge, and strategies for dealing with the daily conflict and battles we have to fight.

Strategy is a way of life. It is the art of acting the right way even while under pressure to combat the most difficult situations. It involves developing ideas and thoughts that can modify already existing principles to fit life's ever-changing situations and apply that knowledge to real-life scenarios.

When handled properly, one can even say that conflict is a great tool for solving problems and reconciling differences. As the case may be, the amount of success or failure that you have in your pursuits can be linked to how well you handle the inevitable conflicts that you will face. As expected, our culture only prepares us to be reactive towards conflict and not proactive. When faced with situations we cannot handle, we lash out in emotion or try to avoid them. In the long run, all of these solutions are counterproductive because you cannot control the outcome of events, and often, they end up making things worse.

Strategy is about controlled planning. You already have an idea of what your end goal is. All that is left are the strategic steps that will bring you to that desired end. Strategic warriors are proactive, not reactive. They plan ahead towards their end goals, determine what fights are worth fighting and which are inevitable, and more importantly, know how to control and master their emotions so that it doesn't get in the way of their goals.

If they have to fight for their goals or defend themselves from threats, they do so indirectly and with subtle moves that make their machinations hard to trace. That way, they maintain the peaceful exterior that society, and politics at large, seems to love.

The idea of controlled fighting in political settings comes from organized warfare, such as those described in *The Five Spheres* and *The Law of War*, where the art of strategy was created and refined. Before then, war was a brutal, senseless machine for violence with no strategic ending. Humans formed clans and tribes that fought both with each other and within themselves in a brutal, ritualistic kind of violence for individuals to assert their dominance or heroism. However, as these clans and tribes began to evolve and grow more into cities and states, it became clearer that war came at a great expense. They could no longer afford to fight blindly as it led to self-destruction, exhaustion, and loss - even for the winner. The need for controlled and rational wars arose, and human beings have adapted to creating strategic moves that will have the least cost.

To that effect, I have compiled 25 strategies that everyone interested in politics should have in their arsenal - all taken from the strategies these three authors listed in their above-named books. Please note that the idea behind this book is not to teach or educate you on how to outsmart your opponents but to share the strategies that these men have already created.

Also, the knowledge shared in this book is not about getting anything you want forcefully or defending yourself against perceived threats. Rather it is knowledge about how to be more strategic and rational in your political moves when it comes to handling conflicts, managing people, dealing with opposition, and using your natural impulses to your favor instead of repressing them.

Suppose there is an ideal image you need to create for yourself. In that case, it should be one that shows you as a strategic warrior that manages difficult people and situations very deftly and intelligently, rather than an impulsive person that just reaches for the things they want without planning for the possible repercussions.

PART ONE
Offensive Strategy

Chapter One

Planning To Do Battle

"War tactics should follow the principle of deception." - Sun Tzu.

The most important aspect of any battle you will have to fight in war is creating a plan. Without a proper plan, all your aspirations could unravel in the blink of an eye. You can only go so far by being good or being capable. If you lack a proper plan of action to win or bring the results that you desire, you may end up losing out to someone less capable but with an airtight plan.

The same thing is applicable in politics. Each election, we hear complaints and arguments about seemingly capable people losing out to their less desirable counterparts because they didn't prepare properly for the race. It is easy to lose sight of what's important, and that is where a concrete plan comes into place - to act as a guide to bring you back on track when you begin to lose focus.

The key to staying one step ahead of the game is adequate preparation and proactiveness. Before you can test whether or not you can put out fires, you have to first make sure that you are fireproof. Proper planning will also make sure that you are not wasting your time on things that won't yield or contribute to the results you desire.

One has to be careful with how they invest their time, or you will find yourself spread too thin to focus on the important things. According to Sun Tzu, a winning army first ensures victorious planning before engaging in battle, while a defeated army is one that fights first before victory is sure.

A strategic plan brings razor-sharp focus and clarity, which ensures that its execution is effective and efficient. With a strategic plan, everyone knows what the end goal is, what roles they play, the outcome of their different roles, and what to fall back on when they experience difficulty. That way, resources, times, and actions do not go to waste.

That is what Sun Tzu means by saying that a winning team first creates a winning plan to assure their victory before taking the first step, while a losing team will first venture head-first into an enterprise before scrambling to create a plan to match whatever situation they find. Obviously, you can already tell who is more prepared to win between the two. If all your resources, energy, time, and allies are not channeled in the same direction, you end up going in circles, chasing after your own tails, and frustrating everyone in the process.

"In the aspiration of victory, there are five important key elements to observe:

1. Know when to fight and when not if it's going to lead to victory or not.
2. Know how to use more troops.
3. Having the same goal and spirit in all ranks will lead to victory.
4. A prepared army will always achieve victory over an unprepared enemy.
5. A talented general who is not restrained by the king will be victorious in battle."

- Sun Tzu.

To rewrite this in terms of politics, what Sun Tzu was saying in essence was:

1. Choose your battles well. Know when to fight and when to cut your loss and regroup. If you are setting goals for your political career, they must be realistic and attainable. There is no point in reaching for something that you know that you cannot achieve. Instead, focus your attention on goals that are attainable and assure you of victory.

2. Know when to bring in more people to your team. You have limitations and blind spots that other people can cover. Learn how to delegate responsibilities to people who are well-suited or have expertise in them.

3. Clearly communicate your goals and objectives to everyone on your team so that you are all on the same page. Also, develop a system to better coordinate all internal activities. A united team with the same goals and mindset is already assured of success.

4. Preparation will always put you one step ahead of all your opponents and the game of politics. When you have made provision for all the steps you plan to take and created alternatives for when those don't work out, you can easily adjust to situations without losing momentum.

5. Micro-management can upset the balance of things. Once you have gathered experts on your team, give them free rein to do the job assigned to them without micromanaging every step.

Before you fight, you must first know your strength so you can properly compare yourself and your team to your opponent's. That way, you can easily determine if it is worth fighting before you begin. These five points will help to understand where your strengths and weaknesses lie so you can plan properly towards your strategy.

"War has five determinants that we must plan. We must understand their correlations. One is righteousness. Two is the atmosphere. Three is the terrain. Four is the general. Five is martial law." - Sun Tzu.

Righteousness, in this case, is the cause that you are fighting for as a politician. It is the mandate that the people can get behind and give all support. Righteousness is the unifying factor that makes people rally behind you to be the one to represent them.

The atmosphere is the season and time. If you wanted to be literal, it could mean just that - the four seasons (whether hot or cold), time (whether night or day). But if you wanted it to be more of a metaphor, it could mean the situation of things on the ground. What is the general temperament that the people have? Are they happy or sad? Do they think it is time or change? How do they feel towards you? Warm and affectionate, cold and scornful, lukewarm and indifferent?

Like the atmosphere, if you wanted to be literal about the meaning of the terrain, it could be the topography of the area—high or low ground, smooth or rough roads, near or far distance. However, metaphorically, it could signify your path towards your goals. What are your chances of winning? Do you have a smooth way towards it, or are there many bumps that you would have to maneuver? How far would you have to go to reach your goals? Do you have a high ground to stand on, or are you the underdog?

The general, in this case, is yourself. A great leader is one that leads by example and inspires others with their actions. Can people count on you? Does your leadership inspire people to throw their lot in with you? Do you exude confidence in your dreams? Are you strategic, focused, strict, courageous, and, importantly, kind?

Finally, martial law signifies the pooling and organization of your resources, including mental and physical manpower, funding and finances, weapons, and tools, as these will be your weapons. Basically, martial law is putting together and managing everything you would need to ensure your victory.

Anyone serious about politics must know all five points listed above and how to interpret them. If you know, then you will win, but if you do not consider them, then you are on the path to failure.

To that effect, Sun Tzu says that you must compare the following situations based on the definitions above to determine which team would lose and which will win, and in turn, determine if it is still worth fighting.

1. Who has the more righteous cause?
2. Who is the most skilled or talented general?
3. Who stands to benefit more from the current atmosphere and terrain?
4. Who follows martial law?
5. Who has the most sophisticated weapons in their arsenal?

6. Who meets their team more frequently to improve on their game plan?

7. Who has the fairest methods for reward and punishment to ensure the cooperation and loyalty of their team?

The answers to these questions will tell you who is more prepared to fail or win. When using the answers to these questions to plan for advantage, you must also take advantage of solutions that are beyond the expected line of action. The best-laid plans have been improved on to reflect and grasp the situation of things firmly but flexibly.

Sun Tzu insists that your tactics should always be unexpected to leave your opponents unprepared to counter. If you have the power to challenge them, pretend to be weak, so they become arrogant and careless. If you want to hit them very close to where it would hurt, misdirect them by acting like your target is far away from what they think is important. If you want to get close to them, then act like you are retreating, and they will lower their guard, leaving themselves wide open for your attacks. When they are disorganized, find a weak spot and attack. If your opponent is guarded on all ends, then be prepared for them. If they are strong enough to go head-to-head against you, evade them. If they are temperamental, harass them until they lose their temper and make mistakes due to their hotheadedness. If their camp is united, divide and conquer. If they are at rest and enjoying peace, cause unrest and unsettle them. Attack when they are not prepared and appear where they least expect it.

Let surprise and deception be the key to unraveling your opponent. They must never be able to predict your next move, or they will be prepared to counteract. Be like the magician that uses sleight of hand to misdirect his audience - while their eyes are distracted following the fake trail you give them, let your actions wreak damage in their camp.

These are the basic strategies towards creating a plan that assures you victory over your opponent. Before you make any move, you must first create a concrete plan that assures you of complete victory. A sketchy plan will at best bring the occasional battle win, but in the big picture of the entire war, such a plan is bound to fail. Your degree of preparedness based on the analysis above will make it easy to determine if you will win or lose once you make your move.

Winning Without Fighting

"The ultimate achievement is subduing the enemy without fighting."-
Sun Tzu.

According to Chapter 3 of The Law of War, Sun Tzu found it prudent that the ultimate achievement of war was to subdue your enemy without fighting. In Sun Tzu's time, cities grew and became wealthy not from engaging in commerce but from warfare and statecraft. Soldiers waged wars and went on campaigns to capture other cities and take their loot. Political and military alliances were created and discarded as the need arose. Warfare and diplomacy were the crutches by which most cities stood on, and they deployed either to vie for more territory, wealth, and growth.

However, if there is one thing that we have learned from the history of the wars ever fought, warfare brings not only more wealth and loot but also waste and burdens. For instance, the two world wars had a devastating effect on countries all over the world, with millions of avoidable deaths and aftereffects that left much of Europe and Asia devastated. Even the apparent winners of these wars were not left unscathed, as many were left poorer and weaker than when the fighting first started. We can still see this play out in many of the other wars that have been fought since then and even before then.

War is an expensive business. It comes at a very high cost of lives, psychological and social well-being, businesses, economies, and cities. Sun Tzu believed that when it came to taking on an opponent, winning without damaging them is better than ruining it because the ultimate goal of war is not to win every battle fought without considering the casualties.

When planning an offensive attack against your opponent, Sun Tzu advises thirteen things.

1. *In military maneuvering, the supreme art of war is to keep our nation intact as a superior policy; taking over an undamaged enemy nation is more appropriate than breaking it. Keeping our army whole is the best policy. Capturing all the enemy troops is better than killing them …*

Surely, it is better to win over a group of people united to your cause than one divided between you and your opponent. There is nothing profitable about winning over your opponent and having to deal with people that are hostile or frown against the actions used. This is why whatever methods you must apply in beating your opponent, ensure that you will still have the support of the people at the end.

2. *By applying this principle, we can understand that winning a hundred times in a hundred battles is not the ultimate achievement. The ultimate achievement is subduing the enemy without fighting."*

It is exhausting to constantly fight with your opponent, especially if you are fighting to win. Aside from ensuring that everyone in your camp is working towards a unified mission, you have to look out for your opponent's camp to counter every move they make. It is an exhausting, time-draining, and energy-consuming process that could demoralize your camp and affect your long-term goal. However, everyone enjoys it when you use methods that break down your opponent's resistance without unnecessary scheming and battles.

3. *Therefore, the highest form of war is having a broader strategy than the enemy, followed by breaking allies of the enemy, then defeating the enemy in battle. The lowest is to besiege the enemy's city.*

Even more important than fighting your opponent at every turn is creating a broad strategy that thwarts their plans. The next best course of action is to divide and conquer by breaking down the allies and camp of your opponent. Then you can match them head-on on the battlefield and be assured of winning. However, the worst strategy to follow is attacking your opponent in their stronghold as this is their home advantage, and any mistake from your end could spell doom for your plans.

4. *Siege wars should only be waged if unavoidable. Siege time is very expensive. It takes up to three months to craft and prepare weapons to attack city walls. It takes another three months to build the mounds of construction around the enemy walls.*

You should only attack your opponent where they have the home advantage if it is unavoidable. Attacking your opponent from a well-defended front will take too much time and resources before you begin to see results. At that point, while distracted with trying to break down their defenses, you leave yourself and your team exposed to their counterattacks.

5. *If the general is impatient, he will launch his men to the assault like swarming ants around the citadel so that our troops could lose one-third of the casualties while the town still remains untaken. These are the dangerous effects of a siege.*

Control your emotions. In politics, every rash decision that has altered the course of history has been the result of one uncontrollable emotion or the other. Anger, impatience, irritation, lust, greed, frustration - all of these are dangerous emotions to be the basis of your actions because they cloud your judgment. Remember that a strategic warrior is proactive, not reactive. Acting based on your emotions is many things but proactive. Rash decisions will make you lose every advantage that you have already gained.

6. *Therefore, a skillful leader does not need to use the battlefield to subdue the enemy. He captures the enemy's city without having to attack.*

As said before, a skillful leader knows how to strategize to win the war without having to fight. A great leader out-strategizes, out-plans, out-classes, and out-maneuvers the opponent, such that when they see that they are out-matched, they are forced to concede defeat without fighting or suffer a humiliating defeat.

7. *He destroys enemy countries without putting his troops at great risk. All is to preserve the force by making use of strategy. Therefore, there is*

no wear and tear, and still, there is a great benefit. This is the strategy of offensive art.

As said before, strategy is the key to winning without having to fight. Constant battles reduce the resources available to you and, as a result, reduces the number of wars you can wage on your opponents. If you, however, use very few resources when engaging your opponents by avoiding a fight, your team can defeat every opponent and the obstacles they throw at them with very little additional cost.

8. *When deploying the army and we discover that our soldiers are ten times larger than the enemy, then we encircle them. But if we are five times larger, we attack straight up. We divide our troops if we are twice as large.*

Keeping along with the theme of winning without having to fight, once you notice that you have outplayed, out-manned, and out-matched your opponent, force them to concede defeat and end the war. However, if you have a strong team but there are still a few loose ends to tie, go on the offensive before your opponent gets the opportunity to regroup. If you know you have enough resources, split them so that you can attack from multiple points at the same time.

9. *However, if the forces are equal, we make plans to defeat the enemy forces. In situations where the enemy soldiers are more than us, the best thing to do is to avoid direct attacks. If the enemy is too crowded, we retreat completely. So a small army should persevere rather than be defeated.*

However, if you and your opponent are equally matched, you can fight until the best-prepared team wins. If your team is outnumbered or out-resourced, then you must avoid direct attacks from the opponent. However, if you are completely out-matched, cut your losses and restrategize. The underdog should live to fight another day with a better plan than to display bravado and be completely destroyed and broken.

Chapter Three

Employing Subterfuge

"For what allows a leader and a general to attack decisively and successfully, where ordinary people fail, is foreknowledge." - Sun Tzu.

When challenging a formidable opponent, the surest way to ensure a decisive victory is foreknowledge. Throughout the course of history, wars have been won based on vital information that spies collected from the opponents. Political espionage began to gain popularity and spread during the middle ages.

Genghis Khan lived and breathed the teachings of Sun Tzu in the *Law of War*. He and his generals preserved the teachings in the book by practicing and improving on all the strategies Sun Tzu describes, reshaping the history of Asia and Europe in the process.

Genghis Khan was able to rule his Mongol Empire alongside Subutai, his primary military strategist, by employing subterfuge, including spying and scouting in advance for any signs of invasion from his enemies. Before the Mongol invasion of Europe in the 13th century, Subutai spent a decade sending out scouts and spies to gather as much information as they could from the continent.

The spies were well trained to observe details about the enemy that could be important in conquering them including their military strengths and their defenses. They switched between three to five horses to cover large distances and maintain speed, ensuring that intelligence got back to their base faster than the enemy could account for or imagine.

Then, Khan and Subutai could make their assessments based on the information gathered. They made maps of the Roman roads, established trade routes, and made educated guesses on the ability of each city to withstand attack and resist capture. When they had gathered enough data to create a strategy, they attacked.

1. *Foreknowledge allows you to forecast the likely behavior of your opponents. It shows you their weaknesses, their strengths, and their plans so that you can create yours to counter them. At the center of all strategic decisions is intelligence. Cold, hard information beats guesswork when creating plans.*

Concerning using spies to gather intelligence, Sun Tzu had the following to say:

2. *Foreknowledge cannot be found by consulting with the divine being or by comparing similar situations. Nor could it be found by measuring the movements of heaven and earth.*

If we are factual, there is no divine being that will confer foreknowledge about your opponents to you, and you cannot make accurate strategies using conjectures and deductions alone. When making war strategies, you cannot rely on gut feeling alone. Lives are on the line and too precious to stake on a risky gamble.

In the middle of the American Revolution in 1776 at the Battle of Trenton, George Washington led his men in a surprise attack against a group of German mercenaries fighting for the British. After the battle ended and they rounded up the survivors and dead, they found an unopened letter written by a loyalist to warn of the coming attack in the pocket of the mercenary commander.

Here you can see the importance of foreknowledge play out. Had that letter been read, the mercenaries would have prepared a counterattack or avoided the attack rather than rushing in head first to their defeat. Making decisions based on wrong information or no information at all can have damning consequences.

Foreknowledge can only be obtained from people who have accurate knowledge of the enemy's situation. In this respect, there are five types of spies that we can use: local spy, internal spy, counterspy, suicide spy, and reported spy. If we use all five types, no one can understand our scheme. It is a type of sacred organization and the greatest treasure of a wise ruler.

In every political camp, there are different levels of people that have access to different classes of information. One level of information may not make any difference, but when you combine information from all the levels, it is enough to create a vivid picture for your strategy.

Recruit local spies from your opponent's locality and allow them to feed you information about your opponent's popularity among the people and the public actions they make. These are the easiest spies to make, especially if they already have an ax to grind with your opponent.

Cozy up to higher members of your opponent's political team and make them your internal spies to feed you vital insider information. You can convince them to spy for you with financial reward or fan the flames of malcontent they already have against your opponent.

One other thing you have to account for is that your opponents will have their spies in your camp just as you have yours in theirs. You can misdirect them by using their spies against them. Fish out the spies and use them as counterspies. However, be careful of using these double agents as they cannot be fully trusted and will double-cross you as soon as the need arises.

Another form of spying is using suicide spies, aptly named because they are dispensable. You deliberately feed them false information about your team to give your opponent. It involves openly doing certain things for the purpose of deception and allowing the spies to report what they have seen to your opponent.

Reported spies are the ones who focus on bringing enemy information to us. They may go deep undercover in the enemy camp and gather all the information you may find to bring down your opponent. For example, in 1976, the FBI planted Agent Joe Piston as a spy with the alias Donnie Brasco to infiltrate the mafia and acquire information that they would never have had access to. What was intended to be a 6-month operation extended into several years, and

Joe was able to gather enough evidence to put away over 100 mafia members.

If you play your cards right, using espionage could be an effective way to soundly beat your opponent and ensure complete victory.

3. *So in the whole army, no one is closer to us than spies. No one is more rewarded than spying. No secret is more closely protected than the spy network. Spies must be used wisely and treated with kindness and virtue. We must use the utmost subtlety to ensure accurate reporting from spies. Subtlety is the key.*

Your spy network is a great resource for you and should be your well-guarded secret so as not to compromise them. When handling your spies, treat them with kindness and benevolence but be straightforward and do not accept anything less than what you deem proper from them. Remember that spies can bring down your camp with as much ease as they would your enemy. The same virtues that make them a perfect asset for your plans will make them the perfect weapons against your plans.

Apply utmost ingenuity and due diligence when sifting through the intelligence gathered by spies to ensure they don't pass on weak, incomplete, or false information. Verify information to ensure you have accurate information and that your spies are not working against you.

4. *Whether we want to destroy an army, attack a city, or assassinate someone, the first important thing is to determine the name of the commander-in-chief, trusted people, assistants, gatekeepers, and his bodyguards. We have to order the spy to find out this information.*

During the American Civil War, Elizabeth van Lew acted as a spy for the Union army. She freed all her slaves and used them to build a network of spies and informants behind the confederate lines. Nobody would have suspected such a seemingly unimportant woman of running a superior spy ring. The intelligence she gathered for the Union army was so good that General Ulysses S. Grant later attributed it to be a major reason they won the war.

On a political mission, do not overlook anyone - even the seemingly unimportant people - because they could have a role to play to the end of your mission. As a matter of fact, you stand a lot of intelligence to gain from people who are not seen or heard but hear much. These people can be convinced to help, or perhaps, not interfere in the way things play out. However, be careful with your dealings with them as they may also see or hear something from your camp that they will report elsewhere.

5. *When we discover the spy of the enemy who is watching us, we bribe them, take care of them wholeheartedly and release them freely. That way, we can use them as counterspies. Through these spies, we can recruit local spies and internal spies. Through them, our suicide spies will provide false reports to the enemy. And also, through them, our reported spies will be able to act as needed.*

If you have the good fortune of catching one of your enemy's spies, don't yet destroy them but look for a way to convert them to your side and make them counterspies. Intelligence gathered by counterspies can be instrumental toward creating a well-oiled spy machine. Through them, you know what people to use as internal and local spies, can pass false reports from your suicide spies, and collect information from your reported spies.

Chapter Four

Employing the Spirit of the Void

"Through emptiness, people naturally enter the right path."
- Miyamoto Musashi.

Avoid is a place of emptiness - a barren wasteland where nothing exists - and as such, scares most people. People like to deal with predictable situations. They want to know and be able to calculate the risks and rewards of a venture, so they can effectively plan. Going into a void is like losing your eyesight as you run into a tunnel or cave. You cannot see your front to advance or behind you to retreat, entirely at the mercy of whatever is at the other end. Most people would find that intolerable.

However, according to Sun Tzu, that is a very good strategy for offensive attacks in war - lure your enemy into a void, so they cannot see where your attacks will come from. He says:

Therefore, for those who are good at fighting, the enemy will not know where to defend. Those who are good at defending, the enemy won't know where to fight. Delicate instead! So subtle we can make ourselves invisible. Secret instead! So secretive that we can move without making a sound. That's why we keep the fate of the enemy in our palm. We attack, but the enemy cannot stop because we fight without people. We retreat, and the enemy can't follow because we escape quickly.

The spirit of the void allows you to be secretive and subtle with your attacks while your opponents are scrambling to figure out what is going on and how to protect themselves. They cannot attack because they don't have a target, and retreating is out of the question because you are there, in the shadows, poking at all their weak sides. Their inability to attack, defend or retreat will do one of two things - tire them out or cause them to make a huge error they have no hope of recovering from.

When talking about how the warrior could employ the way of emptiness to their advantage, Miyamoto Musashi gave the following tips:

1. *The fifth is the Emptiness scroll. In this scroll, I talk about emptiness — that with no beginning or end, that with no depths or shallows, nothingness. This means that once you understand the principles of the Way, you'd have to let go of them.*

The emptiness scroll was the last of the five scrolls. Before then, he had talked about using all the four elements like the way of the warrior to your favor - earth, water, fire, and wind. So it seemed counterproductive to make the last scroll a void that asked you to forget everything you had learned. But the first four scrolls gave the warrior almost rigid predictability that could be countered by any other opponent, especially one versed in the same skills as you.

2. *As a warrior, you'd become free and gain extraordinary strength. You'd understand the right rhythm for any moment and spontaneously attack and hit your opponent. This is the Way of Emptiness. Through emptiness, people naturally enter the right path.*

One of the reasons why he advised warriors to embrace the spirit of the void was so they could have an extraordinary advantage over their opponents. The void makes you flexible and free to attack and win your opponent without fear of retaliation.

In the 19th century, the business world was rocked by a mini-war between Jay Gould and Cornelius Vanderbilt called the Erie war. However, these business moguls were unmatched at the business war front because Jay Gould employed elusive means to goad the highly temperamental Cornelius into making several bad decisions after the other.

He created disorder in the markets that he could exploit to push out his competitor for the control of Erie Railway Company which managed the Erie Railroad. He would push his connections in the New York State legislature to create laws that would negatively affect Cornelius' businesses. According to American historian Gustavus Myers, members of the legislature would take money from both parties - one to support a bill and the other to oppose it. Jay Gould personally showed up at Albany with $500,000 that was rapidly shared among the members. On one occasion, an investigating committee disclosed that one senator accepted $75,000 from Cornelius and $100,000 from Jay Gould to vote towards a bill. He kept both sums and voted in favor of Jay Gould.

He would also plant anonymous articles in the paper that would smear Cornelius, but instead of looking away, his hot-headed opponent would take the bait and reply. In the process, he would give the article more publicity with his name attached to it, and Jay Gould's name would be free from all controversies. He kept Cornelius distracted like this with so many petty wars as a smokescreen so he wouldn't see what he was actually doing.

In 1866, Cornelius decided to buy a major part of Erie railroad stock. However, one of his board members, Daniel Drew, conspired with Jay Gould and James Fisk to sell spurious Erie railroad stock, thereby watering down the stock and reducing its value. In the end, Cornelius Vanderbilt lost over 7 million dollars to the scheme. After Jay Gould returned a large portion of the money to him under threat of litigation, Cornelius had to pass off the ownership of the stocks back to the trio that tried to swindle him. In the end, Gould won.

The strategy behind employing the spirit of the void is psychological. Once you know what exists, it helps you to infer what doesn't. The trick is to take away that knowledge of what exists, so your opponents are completely clueless about what doesn't. Once you have upset their strategic bearings, they become easy pickings for you and your team.

3. *In the world, if you see things the wrong way, you cannot understand things like "emptiness." We don't see it physically, but it is there in existence.*

As you work to understand your opponent, you must deny them the same advantage by making yourself as difficult to read and formless as you can. Since they will only be able to make conjectures and educated guesses, they will be easy to deceive. Be unpredictable. Throw them crumbs that lead nowhere, and they will not be able to defend themselves from you or counterattack.

PART TWO
Defensive Strategy

Chapter Five

Build a Formidable Presence

"Anyone who fortifies his town well, and manages other concerns as outlined before, will never be attacked without caution. Humans are always averse to obviously difficult circumstances, and it will be seen as not easy to attack one who governs a town that is well fortified and a people that don't hate him." - Niccolò Machiavelli.

One of the best ways to defend yourself against an opponent is not to have them attacking you in the first place. Human beings would rather avoid difficult situations, so when sizing up their opponents and they find you powerful, they will think twice before making the first move. On the other hand, if they think you are weak, it gives them extra boldness to attack. Play on their natural inclination towards fear and anxiety to prevent them from testing you.

According to Machiavelli, here are some of the tricks involved in building a formidable presence, it deters enemies from attacking you first.

1. *German cities are completely free; they own very little of the surrounding countryside and only obey the king's orders when it suits them. They are not afraid of this or any possible power around them because they are fortified in such a way that everyone thinks that taking it by the direct attack would be tedious and difficult.*

The trick is to build a presence so formidable that your enemies will think twice before going against you. Create a reputation that gives you more power than you really have; let your opponents think that crossing you would be a suicidal effort. However, cement this reputa-

THE GAME CHANGERS SERIES

tion and make it more credible with a series of random ruthless acts. Make it random so that your opponent cannot peg the exact action that could set you off. That uncertainty works better as a subtle threat than any overt threat you could make. Unless your opponent is completely crazy or an absolute risk taker, they wouldn't want to start something when they are unsure of how you will react.

2. *This is because they have strong fortifications, with sufficient artillery and enough supplies in public warehouses to eat, drink, and fight for a year. In addition to this, in order to keep the people alive without wasting money, they always create jobs for the community with city-building works, and from this, the people are well-fed and supported. They value military training, and more than that, they enact many laws to support it.*

There are many people like that in life that will be stronger, richer, more resourceful, and more ruthless than anything you manage to build. Some of these people will be not only crafty but also unscrupulous, and any engagement with them will leave you on the losing end. There are like sharks circling around a prey - any sign of weakness or faltering is a signal to attack. The only way to deter them is by making yourself an unpalatable prey. You do this by creating a formidable reputation for yourself as someone who can go head-to-head with sharks and not lose.

One of the keys to creating a formidable presence is by giving the illusion of being well-prepared with enough resources at your disposal to independently counter any attack launched against you.

In 1474, King Louis XI, to the surprise of his courtiers in attendance, launched into an irate tirade against Galeazzo Maria Sforza, the Duke of Milan. Part of the surprise was because the king was usually unflappable, cool, and calculative, so his impassioned speech was out of character. Although the Duke's father was a friend, he claimed not to trust the son, accused the Duke of plotting against France to break the treaty between both countries, and threatened to. To the horror of everyone present, right in the middle of the speech, the Milanese ambassador to France, Cristoforo da Bollate, walked out. The king seemed to have forgotten about his presence at court.

His bold and irrational proclamation could create a diplomatic mess for France to clean up, so he invited the ambassador to his private rooms. While in the middle of a seemingly harmless discussion, the king began to feel out Bollate to find out what he had heard, and he confessed to having heard the whole speech and tried to convince the king that the Duke of Milan would never do any of the things he suspected him of. The king, in turn, told him that he had valid reasons to feel that way and would appreciate it if none of his words got back to Sforza. To make Bollate forget the whole experience, they tried to butter him up with the best accommodations and experience that France had to offer.

Of course, this was a ruse as the king had deliberately set out to give the Duke a subtle warning. He knew that Bollate would not hesitate to report everything he had said word-for-word, and he needed someone to pass on his threats without taking away from its severity.

You see, if the king had challenged Sforza directly, he would have fervently denied all allegations, and he wouldn't have been able to do anything about it. The same thing would have happened if he had taken a diplomatic approach with Bollate - they would have made the king and his wild suspicions appear crazy. So he had to warn the duke of what would happen if he continued down that path. It worked because the fear kept the duke in line for the next few years and made him the most pleasant ally to France.

From this story, we can pick out several things that the King did that were in line with building fortifications, as Machiavelli suggested.

1. Become unpredictable: The king was known to be cool and collected, which meant that his reactions were predictable. As a cool, collected person, it was expected that he would take the direct approach to make inquiries about the Duke's action, and they could have effectively managed him. However, his irrational outburst made Ludovico pause to consider if he knew the king at all.

2. Capitalize on people's natural instinct to avoid trouble: King Louis chose to send a message that made Ludovico think, rather than an overt one, this way, he could draw his own conclu-

sions. Fear that comes from an open threat is not as powerful as the one that comes from talking yourself into it from a subtle one. When you coax your opponents into thinking they have unlocked a more sinister version of yourself, their imagination runs wild with it, especially if you don't give them hard, cold information to work with.

3. Turn the threat around: Sforza threatened to sabotage Milan's treaty with France, and King Louis retaliated by threatening to hurt him with something he valued. This move brought a new side to the king, and with a hint of ruthlessness that showed that Louis was not afraid of the Duke, he backed off.

The purpose of building a formidable presence is to prevent your opponent from attacking you. However, be careful with how you use this strategy, so you don't rile up the wrong person. This should only be used as an act of defense, not offense, and only when absolutely necessary. Constantly passing on threats may either throw down a challenge or make enemies out of the people you have pushed to the limit, which will undo everything you have worked hard for.

Chapter Six

Choose Your Battles Well

"To understand the situation, it is necessary to grasp and understand the conditions of the terrain and the condition of the enemy."
- Miyamoto Musashi.

You cannot always rush in headlong into every battle your opponent calls. It is exhausting to the mind and body of the people who have to fight, not to mention draining the resources that could be better spent somewhere else. There is a limit to how much you can handle at the same time. There are only so far your skills, connections, and available resources will take you. Part of being a skilled strategist is recognizing where your limitations lie and where the strength of your opponent is.

You can always expect that it will end badly for anyone who overestimates their limits or underestimates the strength of their opponent. It is dangerous to allow some attractive promise of a prized conquest to trick you into overextending your limits, or it will leave you exhausted, vulnerable, and weak. Political war is expensive - even the victor incurs some hidden expenses. You lose time, energy, resources, political goodwill and instead gain an embittered enemy who will probably seek retribution.

Miyamoto understood that there would be times when you will have to navigate through tight spaces, and he had this to say about planning your journey:

1. *Through the course of one's life, there are many cases where you'd have to "cross the ford." When you are about to journey at sea, you need to*

know the location of the places you want to go, understand the capac-
ity of a boat, and consider the weather carefully.

Before you engage in any battle, you must first weigh the costs in-volved. Choose your battles carefully. Sometimes, it is prudent to wait or attack using more subtle means than a head-on attack. If you feel that you have too much to lose by going head-to-head with your opponent, abandon that line of action and look for one with more bearable consequences. If you cannot completely avoid the battle, ensure you fight on your own terms and not on your opponent's. That way, you can afford to choose methods that will cost you less.

Your strategies, in this case, should be the ones that stretch your opponent to their limits while affording you the flexibility to use your strengths. Make the cost of battle high for them and cheap for yourself, explore their weaknesses, and poke holes at them. With this method, you can outlast anyone no matter how formidable they appear.

2. *To understand the situation, it is necessary to grasp and understand the conditions of the terrain and the condition of the enemy. Under-stand if the conditions are floating or sinking, shallow or deep, strong or weak. By continuously practicing with the "measuring cord," the situation can be assessed on the spot. See and act at the right moment, and you would win, whether at the front or at the rear. This needs to be deeply considered.*

In 1558, when Queen Elizabeth I ascended the throne of England, she inherited a country that had been ravished. She set about cre-ating a peaceful country and rebuilding the economy as she under-stood that England could not hope to compete against the other world powers like France and Spain at that point - not at war and certainly not by financial powers.

However, Philip II, the King of Spain, had other plans. He wanted to restore England to a Catholic country and fought against the Protestant rebels, determined to crush them. His short-term goal was to have Elizabeth assassinated and get her catholic half-sister, Mary Queen of Scots, to the throne, and if that failed, he planned to amass enough armies to invade England. Either way, war was loom-ing on the horizon, and England was not ready.

Queen Elizabeth's advisors suggested sending an army to help the rebels push back at the Spanish, which would cause Philip to divert his attention and resources there and distract him from England. While Elizabeth agreed to send small troops to assist the rebels, she didn't agree to anything else. If she was going to fight Philip, she wanted to do it on her own terms and after weakening her opponent.

So she chose her battles well, defying her advisors and choosing to maintain peace with Spain by any means necessary. This move bought her enough time to gather resources to begin the creation of the British Navy. While maintaining the outward appearance of peace between the two nations, Elizabeth was secretly plotting to destroy Spain by exploiting their weakness - their finances.

She had studied the situation, understood the strengths and limits of her opponent, weighed the cost of doing battle, and chose a method that would bring the least consequences to her while dealing her opponent with the greatest damage possible.

3. *You should think of your body as the opponent. Whether you are dealing with someone who has retreated into a protected place, or a very large opponent, or someone who is well versed in strategy, you should think about the weakness in his mind. If you are not aware of the enemy's mind, you may mistake a weak person for a strong one, a person with no skills for one that is competent, and a small opponent for a dangerous one. The enemy may capitalize on this mistake. So become the opponent! You should analyze this carefully.*

One of the biggest contributors to Spain's wealth and economy at that time was the profit they made from their empire in the Americas. However, because it was so far away from Spain, they depended heavily on shipping. Philip had a large fleet of ships which he maintained with heavy loans from Italian banks, using the gold he shipped from the Americas to build credit with them. It was a weak system of operation. If anything were to happen to those ships, the Spanish economy would be sunk, literally.

Elizabeth understood this and exploited it by unleashing one of her captains, Sir Francis Drake, to act as an independent pirate, robbing the Spanish of their precious gold. With every shipment Philip lost, the interest rate on loan skyrocketed until the Italian bankers were increasing the rates not because he lost his ships but because of the threat of Sir Francis. Philip was supposed to unleash his army against England in 1582, but because of his money issues had to delay, buying Elizabeth more time to wreak havoc in the process.

Rather than making adjustments to his army according to his financial limitations, Philip decided to borrow more money to pump into it. He had been enticed by the promise of his prized conquest of England and by his holy crusade. On the other hand, Elizabeth used the little resources she had to build an impressive spy network to spy on Philip's every move and report back to her. That way, she knew how large Philip's army was and when he planned to attack, so she wouldn't waste what resources would be better used somewhere else, maintaining an army that wasn't ready to fight.

When Philip launched his army, he sent 128 ships full of soldiers on the way to England with a planned detour to pick up some of the soldiers fighting rebels. Elizabeth, already warned of their plans, sent a small fleet to disturb the progress of the Spanish. First, they sunk the Spanish supply ships, then when they docked at Calais to pick up their remaining soldiers, the English set fire to dozens of Spanish ships. These losses destabilized and demoralized the Spanish soldiers that they called off the invasion. In a bid to avoid further attacks, the Spanish sailed north instead of south, planning to sail around Ireland and Scotland. The rough waters and weather dealt with what ships the English did not destroy in their attacks. By the time they got back to Spain, Philip had lost 44 ships, and the rest were not seaworthy either. He also lost two-thirds of his great army while England escaped with minimal damage.

Queen Elizabeth had successfully stretched King Philip to his limits while affording herself the flexibility to use her strengths. After weighing the cost of going head-to-head in battle with Philip, Elizabeth chose the path of least resistance - one that would bear little to no consequences to her and her country. In the end, the cost of fighting England became too high for Spain to bear, and Philip called off his crusade. That was how, even from a place of limitations, Queen Elizabeth I outlasted King Philip in battle.

Chapter Seven

Counterattack

"If you think there is going to be a deadlock, give up your intention immediately and use some other advantageous tactics to win."
|- Miyamoto Musashi.

The mistake that a lot of people make is thinking that there are only two positions to assume - attack and defense. A strategic warrior does not see battles in binaries, as there are many maneuvers that can be done in between that do not exactly classify as a complete attacking or defensive method. One of them is employing the method of a counterattack.

Whoever makes the first move and initiates an attack puts themself at great risk because you are showing your cards and telling your opponents what you planned. The way that battle progresses from there depends heavily on the way that your opponent decides to take your move and spin it. Rather than leaving yourself at the mercy of your opponent's strategy, why don't you become the player that has all the cards that could decide the game?

This strategy is particularly important when you and your opponent are almost equally matched or plan to use the same methods against each other. If you keep going at each other like that, the battle becomes unnecessarily drawn out because you are at a stalemate. To tip the odds in your favor and claim a resounding victory, Miyamoto Musashi suggests this:

1. *In large-scale strategy, if you sense a deadlock, that is, the spirit of "four hands," do not try to advance as that would make you lose many*

of your men. Quickly re-strategize and achieve victory using tactics that the enemy cannot think of. This is extremely important.

Allow your opponents to make the first move. Let them show you the cards they plan to play so that you have more flexibility to counterattack. Just like you would a high-stakes poker game, call their bluff and bait them into making a mistake that takes all the power from their attack. Dangle the smell of victory in their noses and allow their eagerness to strike while you seem weak to throw them off balance or break them down.

2. *Similarly, in hand-to-hand combat, if you think you will fall into a "four-hand" stalemate, change your approach immediately. It is important that you improve the way you assess your opponent's attitude. Use a completely different tactic to win. You must be able to judge this.*

Being enslaved to your emotions will cause even the most fool-proof strategies to fail, and that's because emotions push you to make rash decisions that may upset the outcome of your plans. You can use your opponent's emotions against them and force them to make rash decisions. Hold back and wait for the right moment to turn your weakness into your gain.

If your opponent is an aggressive, temperamental person, bait them to lose their temper and act in anger. If they are impatient, use their eagerness to weaken them. If they are greedy, allow their greed to cloud their judgment. If they are overconfident, let it be the foreboding of their downfall. The best way to do that is to study your opponent and learn their behaviors.

Miyamoto did not just teach. He walked and lived his teachings too. One of the reasons he won his duels was because he never backed down from a fight. Rather, he found ways to adapt his strategy for each opponent he faced. He depended on the element of surprise to launch a counterattack against his opponents and took them down when they were unguarded.

In the thick of the Napoleonic wars in 1805, Napoleon was in one of the biggest binds of his military career. Both the Austrians and Russians had joined forces against him. In the south, a faction of the Austrian army attacked the French occupying Northern Italy, and in the east, another Austrian troop attacked, with a sizable Russian Army coming to join them in the east. The plan was for the Russians and Austrians to merge in the east and head towards France. The Germans, seeing that Napoleon's forces were stretched thin, were also considering joining the alliance.

Napoleon found himself boxed in by the machinations of his enemies. Any move towards fighting on any of his sides posed great danger for him, his troops, and France at large. It seemed like the only possible way out was for him to retreat with his army. Even his generals advised him to go take that route.

Meanwhile, the Austrian and Russian leaders were thrilled that they had Napoleon just where they wanted him. The Austrian emperor offered him a ceasefire, but in reality, it was a ruse by the Austrians to buy time to completely surround the French army. Anyone in Napoleon's position would have quickly swooped in on that deal - anyone except Napoleon because he was a formidable opponent who knew how to take risks. So it came as a shock to the Austrian Emperor and Russian Czar when he accepted to listen to their terms.

At first, they were suspicious, but Napoleon began to make erratic battle decisions that made it look like he was confused and afraid. The Czar sent an emissary that reported Napoleon's apparent agitation and distraughtness. The young Czar, chomping at the bit to get his first victory against Napoleon, could not allow this golden opportunity to waste, so he launched an attack.

However, because his decision was spurred by impatience and heightened excitement, the Czar rushed his troops to attack the break-in Napoleon's line. This move left his own center exposed to attacks. By the time his general noticed this mistake, it was too late to turn back. The tables turned, and Napoleon became the aggressor. Some French troops had arrived for reinforcement, and they attacked the Russians.

The best position to disguise an offensive attack is using a defensive maneuver. As I said before, war tactics do not have to be an either/ or option. You do not always have to choose between an offensive or defensive strategy. In fact, you stand a risk of boxing yourself in using that method. Being offensive as a rule of thumb creates more enemies and increases the risks of making costly decisions, while being defensive corners you into a position your opponent can exploit. Either way, your actions, and responses are predictable - remember that Miyamoto won most of his duels by using the element of surprise.

When it looks like you have been cornered and there's no way out, do not accept defeat just yet. You can turn almost any situation around if you learn to act like Napoleon - play weak to trick your opponent into making rash decisions from overconfidence, then catch them off guard by launching an unexpected counterattack. This way, what appeared to be your weakness becomes your strength.

Another person who was famous for using this method of baiting and switching was President Franklin Roosevelt. He had a habit of retreating into himself and his opponents, thinking that it meant weakness, would go on a rampage trying to tarnish his name and attacking his methods. Each time, he would wait for them to exhaust all the negative things they had to say about him and would pick a strategic moment to use their words as ammo against them. It always worked.

On September 23, 1944, he made his famous Fala speech because his Republican opponent accused him of using the taxpayers' money to care for his Scottish Terrier, Fala. He said:

These Republican leaders have not been content with attacks on me, or my wife, or on my sons, that they now include my little dog, Fala. Unlike myself and my family, who don't resent these attacks, Fala does. Fala, being a Scottie, was furious to learn that the Republican fiction writers had concocted a story to say that I had left him behind on the Aleutian Islands and sent back a destroyer to find him at the expense of two, three, eight, or twenty million dollars to the taxpayers. He has not been the same dog since. While I am accustomed to hearing malicious untruths about myself, I think I have the right to resent and object to libelous statements about my dog.

The speech was well-received by the audience to the eternal embarrassment of the republicans because he used their words as a counterattack against them. He allowed them to make the first move, exposing their strategies and blindspots. He used their aggression and impatience against them by goading them to speak rashly. In the end, that speech became instrumental towards his win in the elections because it endeared him to many people.

Your retreat should be a means to an end and not an end itself - the former is a strategy towards winning while the latter is a surrender in acceptance of defeat. Retreat with the mindset that it is temporary, and you may have to turn and fight back.

Chapter Eight

Retreat To Advance

"When we get to dangerous grounds first, we will be able to occupy high, sunny places where it will be easy for us to observe and wait for the enemy. If the enemy goes there first, we should not fight, and we should retreat." - Sun Tzu.

Sometimes, you will find yourself in a tight spot that makes victory over your opponent unattainable. When you have weighed the pros and cons of forging ahead and taking some space to regroup and the latter looks like the better option, do not be ashamed to retreat. Sun Tzu goes on to say:

1. *Don't move unless you see a clear advantage. Do not use soldiers unless there is something to gain. Do not fight if we are not in danger. The king cannot mobilize the army because of personal anger. The general cannot engage in battle because of personal outrage. Only mobilize the army if it is beneficial for the country, otherwise do not move.*

Another reason why a retreat might be the best course of action for you to follow is that you sometimes lose perspective of the war while in the thick of battle. Miyamoto Musashi defined perception thus:

2. *There are two ways to see - perception and sight. Perception means concentrating strongly on the opponent's mind and terrain of the battle place. It also involves observing the situation of the battle and seeing how the advantage changes. That is the way to win.*

He goes on to say:

3. *In small and large-scale strategies, there is no reason to gaze at minute things. As I mentioned before, if you focus closely on specifics, you*

would forget the big things. You would lose your perspective, and victory would elude you.

You can get so sucked into the thrill of winning, the exchange of wit and parrying shots that you forget why you need to win or how you intend to win. Perception is very important in battle - once you lose sight of important things, you are well on your way to losing the battle already.

When you notice that you do not see things as clearly as you should, take a step back to regroup and detach yourself from influences that may be narrowing your sight.

Retreating in the face of impossibilities is not a sign of weakness but one of strength. We all love a good underdog story - the one who rose against all odds to gain complete victory over their opponents. However, out of the underdogs that made it, there are thousands more like them that failed before they got the chance to find their feet.

If your circumstance does not give you firm ground to plant your feet, do not risk everything you have on a gamble. There is a popular quote from Napoleon that goes:

4. *Strategy involves the use of both time and space. I am less concerned about the latter than the former. You can recover space but cannot recover lost time.*

Space in this sense is the battle area. The space where you battle should afford you an advantage over your opponent - you should be able to face them and attack with both long-range and short-range strikes. Time, on the other hand, is the window of opportunity you have to respond quickly and decisively to your opponent's attacks.

Revisiting Napoleon's quote, if you lose the space to battle an opponent because you cannot find any advantage in it for you, you can always find another space more suited for your needs for a rematch. However, if you miss the window of opportunity to respond swiftly to an attack or launch one, you may never get it back again.

Retreating affords you the luxury of sacrificing space for time. It does not mean you have completely given up, but if you choose not to fight, you are buying yourself time to find the perfect window of opportunity to act.

If your enemies mistake this for weakness, let them. If they advance, allow them and evade every attempt they make to draw you out. Remember, time is more valuable than space. Allow your perceived weakness to feed their arrogance or your perceived nonchalance to feed their aggression. Sooner, rather than later, they will make a mistake that will give you the perfect opening to act.

Time reveals all things and balances the scale, sometimes, without even any input from you. The summary of Murphy's law is that anything that can go wrong will go wrong. Buy yourself time until everything that can go wrong indeed goes wrong.

The Chinese have a concept called Wu Wei, which plays an important role in her statecraft and Taoism. Wu Wei simply means action through inaction. It describes knowing the reality of any situation, accepting it, and conserving your energy. In other words, it means taking control of your situation by not trying to control your situation.

When you try too hard to fight your circumstance, you could make things worse for yourself than it already is. Sometimes, the best course of action is to lay low and do nothing, and as Murphy's law states, anything that will happen will.

If your situation calls for you to retreat, but you fight against it by continuing to advance towards your opponent, you might think you are making progress, but the reality is that you are marching towards your doom.

When Frederick the Great ascended the throne in 1740, he could only be called the King *in* Prussia because his territories were scattered all over, and his kingdom was only a portion of Prussia. So he set about acquiring the rest of the kingdom so he could be called the King *of* Prussia.

However, there was one problem. Some of the territories he sought to reclaim were under the control of Habsburg, which was ruled by Maria Theresa of Austria. This led to several wars and hostilities between Prussia and Austria. After the first Silesian war, Frederick suspected that Maria Theresa would launch another attack to regain the city, so he formed an alliance with France and invaded Bohemia. At the same time, the Saxons joined Austria to push back at Frederick's army. However, his army claimed so many victories that Austria was forced to sign a treaty to hand over Silesia to Prussia and ensure peace.

Although the treaty was signed, Austria still remained in several wars until they signed another treaty in 1748. Less than a year after signing it, Maria Theresa was back to seeking an alliance with France and Russia to beat back Prussia. In 1756, in the bid to forestall England from financing a Russian army to Prussia's border, Frederick also gained an alliance with England.

So that when the Seven Years' War began between the British and the French in 1756, both Prussia and Austria had switched allies from the original ones they formed during their own wars. In the thick of war, Frederick found his army battling an alliance of enemies made up of Austrian, Russian, Swedish, Roman, and French troops, his only support being Great Britain and her allies, Brunswick, Hesse, and Hanover.

His situation became worse in 1761. After having gotten what they wanted from the Indian and American colonies, the British stopped their financial support for Prussia and left Frederick in quite a bind. Frederick, whose usual style of fighting was an aggressive, offensive attack, had to revert to defensive methods to protect himself. His new strategy involved maneuvers that would buy himself and his army enough time to slip through the net that his enemies had laid in wait for him. He did this dance of retreat for years, barely managing to avoid disaster and waiting for when he would have a window of opportunity to turn the tables around.

Fortunately for him, Murphy's Law happened, and the ruler of Russia, Czarina Elizabeth, died which led to the succession of her German nephew, Peter III. Peter was sympathetic to the Prussians and completely enamored of Frederick that he pulled Russia out from the war, returned the Prussian lands that Russia took, and offered his army to Prussia to fight against Austria.

This event became aptly known as the Second Miracle of the House of Brandenburg. Right at the point where he needed it, a window of opportunity landed on his laps that led to his success in the war. Had he rushed in headlong with fake bravado or completely surrendered, he would have lost more than he already had. Instead, he waited and didn't make his situation worse by fighting it.

By disengaging and retreating from your opponent, you do not run a loss in the long run. Instead, it buys you time to rethink your ideas, consider your circumstances, and shuffle things around. Time is your biggest ally - it settles things into place. When you sacrifice space for time, it buys you the power to act.

PART THREE

Solo Warfare

Chapter Nine

Gaining Power Through Merit or Fortune

"One does not need genius or good fortune to attain civil power, but rather fortunate intelligence." - Niccolò Machiavelli.

T here are two ways to gain power - you are either born into it, or you work into it. Like wealth, it is easier for people born into power to recreate it. They already have access to the right tools, know all the right people, and the right procedure to follow.

However, for the common person who was not born into power or was not raised in close proximity to it, it is an entirely different ball game. The journey from commoner to political elite is a long one with several challenges involved. Machiavelli, when describing the ways by which an ordinary person can rise to power and hold on to it, had the following to say.

1. *Now it is clear that for an ordinary person to rise to the position of a prince either by his ability or luck, one of these will help to mitigate difficulties to an extent. However, those who depend on luck the least will come out stronger.*

According to Machiavelli, there are two ways by which an ordinary citizen can gain political power - through their abilities or through luck. Either one of these things can help to ease your way as you do your socio-political climb.

However, of the two who depend on luck and abilities, the one who depends on the latter will always thrive over the other. The reason is easy enough to infer. Luck is beyond your control. You cannot influence or manipulate it to always be in your favor. Relying on luck alone is like building a sandcastle and hoping the weather remains kind enough to leave your structure standing.

2. *Territories that rise too quickly, like all things in nature that are born and grow rapidly, cannot lay the proper foundations and groundwork fixed in such a way that the first storm does not destroy them.*

There are many things that you can control to make your construction last longer, such as the kind of material you use and where you build it, but you cannot control the weather. If you choose not to lay the right foundations, follow due process, or use the right materials, one day the weather will turn against you, and all your hard work will be for nothing - blown away by the wind, never to be recovered.

When you depend on luck to build your political career, it is not a matter of *"if"* it will but *"when"* it will. If you are not prepared to flow along with the changing tides, you will be left behind with only the ruins of your career to keep you company.

3. *Those who become princes from commoners through good fortune have little difficulty rising to the top but find it hard to remain on the throne. They experience no hardships on the way up because they fly, but once they get to the top, they have many. Such goes for people who acquire a state by buying it or by the favor of one who bestows it. The same thing also applies to rulers who, by the corruption of soldiers, came into power.*

When Machiavelli spoke of fortune, he meant luck, favor, goodwill, fate, chance, or opportunity. Fortune has so many advantages, especially for people starting out with no prior experience. It smoothes the way and makes the journey easier. You ride to the top faster without a hurdle in your way. However, one of the disadvantages is that it hardly prepares you for the real work you will face when you hit the top. That is why it is hard to find someone who got to the top solely by luck and maintained the position using that same means.

4. *Unless, as noted, those who suddenly become princes have great abilities that they know they have to be ready at once to hold on to what*

luck has given them. They must understand that they need to lay a solid foundation for their status, like others that had come before did.

An example of one who rose to power through fortune is Cesare Borgia, the illegitimate son of Pope Alexander XI. Cesare was originally groomed to have a career in the church. By the time he was 15, he already became the Bishop of Pamplona, and with his father's elevation to Pope, he became a cardinal at 18.

His older brother, Giovanni, was the one originally groomed for political office, but he died in 1497, leaving the family hopes of having a political position to Cesare. In 1498, Cesare resigned from his cardinalate to join the military, and that same day, the French King, Louis XII, made him the Duke of Valentinois. Thus began Cesare's political ambition.

He got his first position as goodwill from the King due to his father's machinations and alliance with France. Pope Alexander, seeing an opportunity to push Cesare to an even better political position by carving out a state for him in Northern Italy, propositioned the King for Romagna and was granted it. However, Alexander's bid to uplift his son had many challenges.

The only territories he could give his son were those owned by the church. If he did that, he knew he would be opposed by the Venetians and the Duke of Milan. Also, the only army that could have helped was controlled by people who would not want the church to acquire more power. He decided that the best course of action was to disrupt the state of things, and while the powers that ruled Italy were scrambling in confusion, he could take what he wanted for Cesare. So, he brought King Louis to Italy and caused a disruption. When the King invaded Italy in 1499, and Ludovico Sforza had been ousted as the Duke of Milan, Cesare accompanied him to Milan.

However, this was where things began to turn sour for Cesare. King Louis appointed him as the commander of the papal armies, which were made up of Italian mercenaries, 300 cavalries, and the 4,000 Swiss infantry he sent.

Cesare began to suspect that his troops were not loyal to him, and he couldn't do anything about it because they had the support of the King. He was also afraid that the Orsini mercenaries he used would betray him. He tried to acquire more territories, but the King stopped him from attacking Tuscany. At that point, he knew that he couldn't trust any of these people and decided to rely only on the goodwill and armed forces of other people for his plans.

Cesare brought in good policies that improved the lives of the people in the regions he ruled. Therefore, it was hard for his enemies to remove him from power, but it didn't stop them from plotting. Understanding how tenuous his situation was because everything he had, he could only keep on the goodwill of the Pope, Cesare decided to do four things before his father passed.

1. He had to kill all the families of all the lords he defeated so they would not come back to seek revenge or a claim to his territories.

2. He had to gain the loyalty of all the powers in Rome so that they would support him, not the new Pope when his father died.

3. He would gain the support of the College of Cardinals.

4. He would have gained so much power and stability that he could push back the first wave of attacks when his father eventually died.

He had already worked his way through the first three items on the list and was on the fourth one by trying to invade Tuscany when his father suddenly died. When Alexander died, Romagna was the only city held by Cesare that was settled. He only had a tentative hold on every other place.

The new Pope, Pope Pius III, supported Cesare, and for a while, it seemed like all was well. Unfortunately, after only twenty-six days in the papacy, he died. His successor, Pope Julius II, was an old enemy of Cesare's that tricked him into supporting his papal ambition by offering him money and continued papal backing for his ambitions. After Pope Julius won by unanimous decision, he promptly disregarded his promises. Upon realizing his mistake, Cesare tried to remove Julius from the papal seat, but he failed at every turn. Having lost the goodwill of the only thing keeping his ambition together, Cesare quickly hurtled towards destruction.

5. *As stated above, any prince that does not lay his foundation may be able to do so after with outstanding talent, but with so much trouble and danger to the building.*

Although Cesare gained power through fortune, he tried to change the foundation of his power to his abilities and, in the process, hurt a lot of people that became his enemies. During the conversion, his position was made extra dangerous as a result of this. But the final nail that sealed his coffin was that he ran out of good fortune and everything he built came tumbling.

When talking about men who came into power by their own merit and abilities, Machiavelli had this to say:

6. *When considering their actions and lives, we can see that they do not owe anything they achieved to luck beyond the opportunity that gave them the material to mold into any shape that best suits them. Without that opportunity, their abilities would have been wasted, and without those abilities, the opportunity would have been in vain.*

An example of an ordinary citizen that rose to power through his merit was President Andrew Jackson. Born to Irish immigrants, Andrew Jackson lived his early life in abject poverty and hardship. Different circumstances led to the death of every of his immediate family members until he was the only survivor. After a series of false starts, Andrew finally made headway with his life by becoming a wealthy Tennessee lawyer. In 1812, Andrew fought in the war between the United States and Britain. He earned national fame as a war hero through his leadership and conduct during the war. This reputation gave Andrew the opportunity to become one of the most influential political figures in American history, and he seized it.

In 1824, he contested against three other nominees for the presidency in one of the tightest presidential races in American history. All of these men were from different parts of America. However, of all of them, Andrew was the only non-elite - a simple worker from the other side of the tracks that worked his way up into affluence and influence. He won the majority of the popular votes, but since there was no majority winner in the Electoral College, the House of Representatives decided the winner of the election. One of the presidential hopefuls, John Quincy Adams used his political background to convince Clay into supporting his claim to the presidential title.

However, Andrew did not give up and contested in the next elections where he soundly defeated the incumbent, Adams, to become the seventh president of the United States. Andrew Jackson's merit as a military hero won him the presidency. His accomplishments during the war sparked pride in the voters who lovingly called him *Old Hickory and the Hero of New Orleans*. Apart from his achievements, he remained in the mind of the people as the leader who rose from nothing - an ordinary citizen.

7. *Those who, like these men, become princes from brave deeds acquire territories with difficulty, but they keep it with ease. The difficulties they face in acquiring it arises partly from the new rules and methods they are forced to enforce to establish their government and secure it. It is important to remember that there is nothing more difficult to solve and more dangerous than the adventure of creating a new regime. This is because the founder will meet enemies who have enjoyed many privileges under the old regime, and lukewarm supporters, in those who enjoy the new laws, will not actively protect the new collaborators.*

This fits Andrew's story to the last letter because, throughout his eight years in the office, he claimed to represent the interests of common white Americans, especially those from the South and West, over the country's powerful and wealthy elite. His proclamations did not endear him to the powers that were because they undermined all the privileges they were enjoying before he came into office. This later led him into a series of bitter political struggles to maintain his position.

Chapter Ten

Be Present

"As long as the prince resides there, it will be very difficult for others to take the throne." - Niccolò Machiavelli.

The biggest mistake you could make is by imagining that after winning over your opponent, the war ends. Politics is a continuous war with different battles fought every day. Before you gain office, your battle is with your opponent, but once you get the seat of power, your battle is against anything that will seek to take that power from you.

One of the hardest offices to take over is one that has different laws, agendas, customs, or languages from what you are used to. It can be hard to keep everyone together to ensure you all have a common goal. Machiavelli believes that the way to do this is to remain present.

1. *Managing acquired territories in countries with linguistic, custom, or legal differences is difficult and requires a bit of luck and a lot of effort. One way to work around this is if the prince decides to live in the territory to secure his position. While staying there, he can spot problems immediately and fix them. If he doesn't live in the territory, it might be easy to overlook problems until they become too severe to fix.*

As Machiavelli stated, being present in a new area you are governing allows your position to remain secure because you can easily spot problems before they escalate and take measures to curb them. It allows you the freedom to control, regulate, or repress whatever situations come up as you deem necessary.

Establishing your presence, especially as a politician that will have to deal with opposition from think tanks and political opponents or bureaucracy from committees and state departments will protect your administration from being tossed around by people, pushing different agendas or people with different goals and allegiances than your interests.

When you notice these situations do not align with your goals crop up, nip them in the bud to prevent them from blowing up all over your face. Your presence should not be irregular or off/on the thing. Be hands-on; let people feel your presence.

2. *Another benefit of having the prince reside in his acquired territory is that it prevents the officials from abusing his new subjects and the easy access keeps the people satisfied. The prince needs to give his subjects many reasons to love him while still maintaining their fear. Any foreign state that wants to attack this territory must also be very afraid. As long as the prince resides there, it will be very difficult for others to take the throne.*

Another reason why you should make your presence felt is to curb the excessive actions of your staff or cabinet against your constituents in your name. It will not end well for you if members of your team harass, mistreat, abuse, or hurt the people you are supposed to lead in your name. One of the ways that you can hold on to power is securing yourself in the mind of the people as having their best interests. As long as the people love you and as long as your presence serves them well, it will be hard for anyone else to try to take power from you.

However, it is understandable that with so many responsibilities, both national and international, you might not be physically present everywhere that you are needed. Since you cannot be in more than one place at the same time, being present in today's context would mean remaining informed on the daily progress of your political mandates and engaging your community. Every political leader has to be available when needed and be ready to show others how to follow. Failure to do this encourages behaviors that could spell doom for your political aspirations.

Some of the most promising politicians have had their careers affected because while playing the long game, they forgot to keep their eyes on the ball. It is easy to get carried away about the future. You have dreams to change the world, and you plan to begin with the office that you manage. However, your priority should be to effectively manage the present while making plans for the future. You shouldn't sacrifice the here and now for the future. If you don't manage your present well, none of those visions or dreams that you have of changing the world will ever see the light of day.

3. *Whoever causes others to become powerful is ruined because that power is due to either cleverness or force, both attributes that are not trusted by those who have been raised to positions of power.*

In Machiavelli's book, *The Prince,* King Louis XII made several mistakes that cost him Milan. One of those mistakes was not inhabiting the state after he had conquered it. When Louis XII made another grave mistake by bringing in a foreign power to rule Milan, instead of protecting his newly acquired state from the influence of foreign powers, many of her citizens were unhappy with him and allied themselves to the Pope. The hatred they felt towards their current ruler because they felt he didn't have their best interests at heart caused them to rally behind Pope Alexander VI.

Instead of securing his place, his absence allowed Pope Alexander VI to grow more powerful until King Louis XII became alienated from his subjects, and his power among them weakened, which made it easy for Pope Alexander to oust power from him. He did not live in Italy, so he could not quickly see these issues as they were starting until they became too severe for him to handle. In the end, he lost all his territories.

A modern-day example of a politician who allowed his absence to send his career and constituency to deterioration is Nigerian's president, Muhammadu Buhari. In May 2017, reports came in that he had left the country to the United Kingdom for unknown medical reasons and for 90 days, nobody in the country could say for sure where he was or what ailed him, nor could they ascertain when he would return or who was in charge of ruling the country. Before then, he had just returned to the country in March after nearly two months away in London.

His continued absence sparked outrage among members of the Nigerian community, both online and offline. Many Nigerians were worried about how effective the president was and who took critical time-sensitive decisions in his absence as the country was experiencing several economic uncertainty and difficulties caused by delays in making vital policy decisions.

As a result, the country split into two factions, with one group calling for the president to either return to his duty or resign and the other defending his right to seek medical care overseas if he so wished. People took it as far as storming the streets to demonstrate the president's absence. He eventually returned, but the damage had already been done. He had lost the trust and confidence of a large portion of his electorates.

Remaining present or letting your presence be felt is a great way to build confidence among the people you lead and to prevent confusion and division among them.

Gaining Cooperation: Is It Better To Be Feared or Loved?

"It is safer to choose being feared over being loved."
- Niccolò Machiavelli.

O ne thing about politics is that the people you lead play a role as important as yours as the leader. Without them, your position is practically useless. It is every politician's dream to have the support and cooperation of the people, whether they have the same ideologies or not. You can either win their cooperation through the love they have for you or force it through their fear of you.

On the topic of being loved or feared by the people you lead, Machiavelli gave some interesting points that should bear mentioning.

1. *Coming down to the other qualities mentioned above, I say that every prince should expect himself to be seen as benevolent and not ruthless. However, the prince must be careful not to allow his mindedness to be abused.*

Popularity is a major factor in the success of a politician or political party. Every politician wants to remain popular among the people. They want the people to see them as accessible, thoughtful, generous, considerate, caring, compassionate, and friendly. They want every news story to capture their more human side, to show them caring for people, helping their community, serving in happiness, and reaching out to local charities.

Public relation is very important, and that's what Machiavelli high-lighted in the quote, *"every prince should expect himself to be seen as benevolent and not ruthless."* The kind of reputation you have is very important. However, you have to be careful not to go overboard with it, or you will find that people will not hesitate to use your kindness against you.

2. *Is being loved better than being feared or feared better than being loved?" I will tell you immediately that a prince ought to strive for both, but because it is difficult to combine them both in one person if he had to choose one, it is safer to choose being feared over being loved.*

Machiavelli insists that concerning treating your constituents with kindness or cruelty, it is best for a politician to strive for the balance of both love and fear. However, it is almost impossible for humans to both fear and love the same person. If you had to choose between the two emotions, he believed that it was better for a politician to gain the fear of the people than their love, and we would get into his reasons for that in a moment.

Politicians always have to make the hard choices that their constit-uents would not want to make. It is part of the responsibilities of being a leader. Your policies cannot please everyone. So if you had to make the hard choice of choosing between sacrificing one for the greater good of the world or saving one person to the detriment of the world, you should understand which of these courses would bring less pain in the long run.

An example of this would be comparing the responses that Jacinda Ardern, the Prime Minister of New Zealand, and Jair Bolsonaro, the Brazilian President, had towards the COVID-19 pandemic. In the first half of 2020, when the disease was still under investigation, and not a lot of information was known about it, the WHO recom-mended lockdowns as part of the means to reduce the spread of the disease and buy more time until a cure could be found.

Understandably, this recommendation had a lot of pushback from people who were worried about the possible implications it will have on the economy, as most businesses would be affected by the ban, as well as its social and psychological impact. Some people felt that the risk of a few infections was not worth plundering the whole nation into compulsory isolation and others felt that if the result was fewer infections and deaths, lockdowns were worth exploring. While this argument was going on, valuable time was wasting, and world leaders needed to act fast to curtail the spread of the disease and reduce the alarming to the WHO recommendation was a hard decision to make, as either of the options would have angered some people. Some leaders, like Jacinda, were proactive in imposing the lockdown and banning flights into and out of the country. After sensitizing her people about it, she gained their cooperation and put the whole country on lockdown while working with scientists to create a more feasible solution. The result is that New Zealand has one of the lowest infection and death rates worldwide.

On the other hand, Jair Bolsonaro refused to place the country under lockdown because he didn't think the disease was deadly enough to place the country's economy in stagnation. The result is that Brazil has the second-highest infection and death rates in the world. The irony is that the economic suicide he was trying to avoid in the beginning still happened because the Brazillian economy shrunk by 5.8% in 2020, and World Bank predicts another recession for the country. At this point, even the people that supported him when he decided not to place the country on lockdown because of the negative economic implications would have changed their stance.

Two leaders in the same situation with two choices to be made, one chose to make the tough call that might cause temporary discomfort but less pain to the citizens in the long run while the other didn't, and the results were markedly different.

3. *The reason for this is that people are generally ungrateful, fickle, false, cowardly, and greedy. As long as you remain successful, they will remain with you, willingly offering their blood, properties, lives, and children when need is far away. However, as soon as the need arises, they will turn their backs against you.*

Human nature is fickle. They will accept anything as long as it serves their selfish purpose. Machiavelli warns that people who appear to support you because of the favor they stand to gain from you will not hesitate to turn against you if the tides turn against you and the favors they used to enjoy stop coming.

4. *Therefore, the prince, as long as he keeps his people united and loyal, should not be bothered about the reputation of cruelty. With only a few examples, the prince will show himself to be more benevolent than those who, through too much mercy, allow riots that lead to killing and looting to arise. Such incidents are capable of hurting a large population, while the executions that could have quelled them would only affect a few individuals.*

According to Machiavelli, as long as whatever policy you are about to put in place ensures that your people will be satisfied, happy, and at peace, you don't have to bother yourself with earning the reputation of cruelty. Most leaders would show too much compassion and consideration to the point that it will cripple whatever tough call they have to make. In the bid to not estrange or disappoint the people they lead, they end up worsening things by causing more problems, disorder, and turmoil.

Once they taste benevolence, people will always want more from their leaders, but since they hate discipline, only one taste of it will maintain peace and restore order. Machiavelli points out that although cruelty may be necessary, you shouldn't overdo it. Just use a few people as scapegoats for well-used discipline or cruelty, and the rest will fall in line to avoid being punished.

Just like love, it is quite easy to overuse cruelty, and that defeats the entire purpose. Choosing scapegoats to take the brunt of your cruelty rather than punishing the entire population is an economical and efficient way to get your message across.

People who choose to be overly compassionate in the bid to remain loved are often not strong and assertive. Once you walk down that path, it can be hard to turn back. Once you have earned yourself a reputation of being kind, it boxes you in, and more people will expect you to behave that way. The moment you don't, people will see you as being mean, indifferent, and even tyrannical.

However, when people have a reputation for being cruel to do something compassionate, no matter how little, people appreciate it more. It is better to have a bad reputation and do the occasional good thing than to have a good reputation and do something occasionally bad.

The former is seen as an improvement, while the latter is seen as a blemish.

Too much compassion can lead to overindulgence, while too much cruelty leads to hatred. It is best to use them both sparingly.

5. *Out of all princes, it is impossible for a newly crowned prince to avoid the reputation of cruelty. This is because new territories are full of dangers that need to be checked. Nonetheless, the prince must be slow to believe or act and should not show fear. He must act calmly with concern and empathy for his people, such that overconfidence does not cause him to be careless, and too much caution does not cause him to be suspicious and intolerable.*

Machiavelli adds that of everyone that will find it hard to avoid having a reputation of being cruel, a newly elected leader is top on the list. Usually, when people elect new leaders, they do so because they expect to see change. It is never easy to change things because, unlike what they will have you believe, people don't like change, and they will resist it. You will ruffle a few feathers in your line of work, especially newcomers that will have to fight hard to establish their position and reputation in their offices. Therefore, since you cannot avoid the reputation of being cruel, you might as well not bother trying.

However, Machiavelli did not promote unnecessary and extreme cruelty towards your people. In fact, he criticized leaders who were overly cruel and misused their power because it bothered on the line of mistreatment and abuse. As mentioned before, too much cruelty will not lead to obedience, cooperation, support, or loyalty - only hatred. If you are going to use cruelty, let it be justified, and the benefits have to be worth it.

6. *Any prince that completely believes their promises and neglects to place other precautions would be completely destroyed. This love is caused by the things they stand to gain and not by sincere or noble feelings. It may be earned but is often insecure and cannot be relied upon in times of need. People are less afraid to offend the one who is beloved than one who is feared. This love is held by a chain of obligation that, due to the fickle nature of man, would break at any opportunity for their advantage. The fear of severe punishment, on the other hand, never fails.*

Love is a powerful motivator, so is fear. While love creates a feeling of obligation or duty, fear instills obedience and discipline. The fear of punishment, imprisonment, social stigma, and retribution is what motivates people to obey laws. If people did not fear the consequences of flouting laws, people would act without discipline and control.

Every city and its inhabitants need a reasonable amount of fear for order to exist. Hoping that people will be well-behaved because they love you or because it is their civic duty is futile as none of these are firm enough to compel obedience.

7. *However, the prince should inspire fear in people in such a way that, even if he doesn't win affection, he cannot be hated.*

While there should be a price to pay for stepping out of line, it should be within reasonable limits. If you set them too high, it will encourage resistance, rebellion, and overt disobedience. If you set them too low, the price is not worth encouraging obedience and becomes useless. The price should be high enough to encourage obedience without crossing the line into abuse and mistreatment.

8. *His reign would endure without being hated, which will continue as long as he does not steal his subjects' properties or their women. When it becomes necessary to take someone's life, he must do it on proper justification and an obvious reason for it. Above all else, he must keep his hands off the possessions of others because, while people can quickly forget the death of their father, it is harder to forget losing possessions.*

Machiavelli listed some of the limits of cruelty; he said that in dishing out punishment, do not take your people's properties, jobs, offices, or honor for yourself. Don't attack their staff or their family members. It is understandable if you have to get your hands dirty while fulfilling your duties - that's what sets a leader apart. However, if you need to act, don't dally with it.

According to Machiavelli, people are more inclined to forget the death of a parent quicker than they would the loss of their properties. In modern times, we can call property reputation, honor, and any other thing people consider more valuable than family. If you tamper with any of these, the victim will never forget or forgive you, and these are the worst kind of enemies to have.

9. *Returning to the question of being feared or loved, I have come to a conclusion that, because people love according to their will and fear according to the will of the prince, a wise prince would do well to establish himself on that which is under his control and not in the control of others. However, as noted, he must endeavor not to attract hatred.*

Machiavelli concludes by saying that while people may admire or love good leaders, they obey and respect strong ones who make all the hard decisions. People will love you according to their discretion but will fear you according to your behavior. You have no control over other people's emotions, but you can definitely control your behavior. It is best for a politician to base his administration on things that are within his control.

Chapter Twelve

Making Promises: Is it Better To Be Generous or Miserly?

"Nothing disappears as quickly as generosity because even while you are exercising it, you are quickly losing your power to do so." - Niccolò Machiavelli.

I n line with the behaviors that a politician should be notorious for, there is a question of whether they should be generous or miserly. Should you donate to charity or not? Should you ask for credit or recognition when you do or not? Do you take the cameras along or leave them behind? Machiavelli answers these questions in his book.

1. *Of the two qualities above, being generous is better. However, generosity is done in such a way that brings you the reputation for it harms you. If a person is genuinely generous and is not known for it, such a person would not be able to avoid the criticism of being the opposite.*

He said that generosity was better than being miserly; however, being benevolent for the sake of it without it being known is a waste of money and does more harm than good to your political career. If you are a big anonymous donor and nobody gets wind of this generous streak, you will live your life with the reputation of being a miser when the reverse is the case.

If you must do a good deed, don't let it be anonymous, and there must be a purpose behind it. Be sure to get a photo op, at least, of your generosity. However, be careful with what methods you choose to show your benevolence.

Barack Obama is one of the most charismatic politicians in recent world history. Part of his charm was his generous streak. While he was the president of the United States, some of his most memorable generous acts to charity include the $50,000 donation he made to the charity organization CARE and his Nobel Prize, which provided ten different charities a total of $1.4 million to share.

Other charities that enjoyed Obama's generosity include the United Negro College Fund, the Appalachian Leadership and Education Foundation, the Hispanic Scholarship Fund, Africare, the American Indian College Fund, the Central Asian Institute, which promotes the education of girls in Afghanistan and Pakistan, and the Posse Foundation which helps non-traditional high schools get a college education.

If you look closely at all of these charities, they have a common theme - helping the disenfranchised communities in both the United States and the world at large. This theme served the purpose of further endearing him to all of these communities. It fulfilled three of the requirements that Machiavelli gave - let it have a purpose, let it be known, and be careful about choosing them.

2. *Therefore, anyone who wishes to maintain a reputation of generosity must be outlandish in his display of generosity. A prince who does this will use up his fortune on such acts and, in the end, would be compelled to unduly burden his people by taxing them and doing everything possible to make more money. This will soon make the people hate him, and when he becomes poor, he will be worthless to everyone.*

However, he pointed out that too much generosity will ruin you as human beings are insatiable and will always want more. You cannot meet all the needs that they will keep dropping at your feet. However, if you are the type that wants to maintain the reputation of being generous at all costs, you will have to give out more to maintain the degree of satisfaction that your good deeds used to bring.

The downside is that you will soon run out of personal and public funds living this way. To offset this decline, most politicians will tax the people harder to make more money to meet their needs. As with the previous chapter, people want to enjoy good things without having to pay for them. So you will discover soon that they will resent you for taking this route.

3. *It is either you are already a prince or on the way to becoming one. In the first instance, generosity is dangerous, while it is very necessary to be known as being generous in the second.*

During election campaigns, you can always expect politicians to give several promises to convince their electorates to vote for them. This is understandable because campaigns are a fight to earn a seat at the political table. Having a reputation for being generous is one way to get people interested in you. Politicians will make promises to cut taxes, build new facilities, provide better services, grant favors, etc.

4. *Also, if anyone should reply, "Many people have become princes and have done great things with the military and remained very generous," I would say, "Either the prince uses his own money or that of his subjects, or that of others."*

However, when they get into office, it becomes difficult for them to meet up with those promises, and that's because they quickly discover that while funds are finite, needs are not. Most politicians cannot afford to make good on the promises they make, especially if they also want to keep the promise of tax cuts, as the only available source of funds is your personal money or the taxes from your electorates.

5. *With his generosity having offended many but rewarding little, he will be affected by every trouble and run into risk at every sign of danger. Once he recognizes this and wanting to avoid this problem, he will be criticized for being miserly.*

When you run out of gifts or good deeds to give to the poor, they will turn against you. One, because you have outlasted your usefulness and have no worth to them anymore. Two, because your acts of benevolence will only benefit a few as they will, more often than not, target a small part of the community or special interest groups.

However, breaking the big promises you made, like increasing taxes to fund your little acts of benevolence, will offend many. People who don't benefit from them will be angry at you for using the taxpayers' money to fund things they consider frivolous. For example, if you build a new football pitch, the scientific society may see it as a waste of funds that could have gone into more research. If you construct a new park, the literary society may view it as an affront because they needed more libraries. If you repave a bad road, people on the surrounding streets may complain about not being considered. If you create a scholarship fund for marginalized demography, others may complain about being neglected.

You see, these are good deeds, but once you start doing them for one group of people, others will also expect you to do the same for their needs. But there's only so much money that can go into fulfilling all these needs. When you realize the hole you have dug for yourself and try to find safe footing by cutting expenses, people will call you miserly, and your hard-earned reputation ends up in shambles.

6. *If he is wise, then he should not be afraid of being labeled as miserly. With time, the prince will be appreciated more than if generous because it would become clear that the economy is in abundance, that he can defend himself from all attacks, and that he can carry out his projects without burdening his subjects. Therefore, it happens that the prince exercises generosity towards the many who are his subjects and miserliness to the few who he does not give.*

Machiavelli believes that a smart politician should not be bothered about making generous promises. If that earns you the reputation of being miserly, so be it. However, if you can manage to keep the economy stable enough for everyone to benefit from it, and you can carry out your projects without placing the burden on your electorate, people will come to appreciate you better in time. That's because a large majority of your community will enjoy the rewards, as against selected minorities.

In 1988, when George H.W. Bush made his presidential nomination acceptance speech at the Republican convention, he made a promise to his electorate:

I am the one who will not raise taxes. My opponent, on the other hand, claims that he will raise them as a third or last resort. However, when a politician talks like that, just know that is the only resort he will have.

My opponent will not rule out raising taxes, but I will. Even if Congress pushed me to raise taxes, I won't. When they insist, I will say to them, "Read my lips, no new taxes."

As Machiavelli predicted, when Bush became president, he found it hard to keep his promise. On June 26, 1990, he admitted that he would need to implement several measures to improve the stalled U.S. economy, including increasing tax revenues. The newspaper headlines went wild the next morning. One very interesting one from the New York Post said, "Read My Lips, I Lied!"

It was not Bush's fault that he had to raise taxes. He and his team had been working hard to cut down out-of-control spending to generate more revenue, but, in the end, the only thing he could do was to renege on his promise and raise taxes. He had failed to do the one thing he promised the people he would do, and it hurt his chances at his re-election bid in 1992 when both his primary opponent, Pat Buchanan, and his election opponent, Bill Clinton, repeatedly reminded voters of the promise he failed to keep.

George Bush was not the only United States President to make campaign promises during the heat of the moment that he failed to keep. Throughout American history, you will find those failed promises littered.

1. Woodrow Wilson, in 1916, ran for re-election using the slogan, "He kept us out of war." Barely 30 days into his new administration, he asked a joint session of Congress to declare war against Germany, using Germany's broken promise to halt unrestricted U-boat warfare and an attempt to talk Mexico into forming an alliance against the United States as his reason. Two days later, Congress granted his request.

2. Herbert Hoover in 1928 promised everyone prosperity, including "a chicken in every pot" and "a car in every backyard." Less than eight months in office, the stock market tanked and plunged the country into an economic recession called the Great Depression.

3. Franklin D. Roosevelt in 1932 criticized his opponent, Hoover, for his deficit spending and promised to put the nation back to work. While Roosevelt's New Deal policies did place the na-

tion back to work, it also increased the deficit spending more. In an unheard-of bid for a third term in 1940, he also promised the electorate, "Your boys are not going to be sent into any foreign wars." When Pearl Harbor was bombed in 1941, Roosevelt asked Congress to declare war on Japan, sending boys to fight another foreign war despite his promise.

4. Lyndon B. Johnson became president in 1963 after John F. Kennedy was assassinated. While running for re-election in 1964, he painted his opponent as a war hound and promised not to "send American boys 9 or 10 thousand miles away from home to do what the Asians should be asking their boys to do for them." He failed to keep his promise when he sent combat troops to Vietnam and caused the war to escalate with his interference. He was forced to pull out of the 1968 presidential race after public opinion turned against him.

5. Richard Nixon in 1968 promised to end the war and find a way to make "peace with honor" in Vietnam. His aides went as far as telling reporters that he had a secret plan to end the war. However, in his first six months in office, the United States combat casualties increased. He was not able to end the war, and it dragged on, even after Nixon was re-elected in 1972. The last American soldiers did not leave Vietnam until 1975 after Nixon left office.

6. During his campaign in 1976, Jimmy Carter promised to solve the energy crisis, deregulate the oil and gas industry, increase the gas tax, and even pursue alternative sources of energy by installing solar panels on the White House. However, once he got into office, he couldn't find anyone to support or sponsor any of his initiatives, and the energy crisis worsened under his administration.

7. In 1980, Ronald Reagan promised to pass a constitutional amendment that would allow voluntary prayer in public schools. Although he did propose the amendment, it died in Congress, and subsequent attempts to revive it in 1999 and 2006 achieved the same results.

8. In 1992, one of Bill Clinton's campaign promises was to completely overhaul the health care system and provide universal

health care for every American. During his first term, health care reform was a priority for his administration, but he faced pushback from the Republicans. He put Hillary Clinton in charge of the task force, but it failed to gain support, and the proposal died in Congress, despite Democrats having the larger percentage of members in both houses.

9. In 2000, George W. Bush promised to privatize Social Security, reduce government spending, and "change the tone" in the White House. He also promised to prevent sending troops all over the world when he said, "if we don't stop sending our troops around the world on nation-building missions, we will have serious problems down the road, and I am going to prevent that." However, under his administration, government spending shot up, partly due to the new wars American soldiers were fighting in Afghanistan and Iraq after the 9/11 attacks.

10. In 2008, Barack Obama promised to work to "close the partisan divide in Washington." However, for several reasons, by the time he left office in 2017, the partisan divide in Washington was wider than when he entered office in 2009.

11. In 2016, Donald Trump made several promises during his election campaign, including one to have Hillary Clinton imprisoned and to "build a wall" along the Mexican border with Mexico paying for it. He did none of these things in the four years that he was president.

All of these presidents had their administrations marred by the failure to meet up with the promises they made while campaigning. If they hadn't made them or had been successful in achieving them, it wouldn't have left a blemish on their time in office. If you are looking for a list of campaign promises not to make, this is a good place to start.

Chapter Thirteen

Invest In Good PR

"It is, therefore, necessary for the prince to have all the good qualities that I have described, but it is also necessary for him to pretend to have them." - Niccolò Machiavelli.

A s a politician, nothing can be more important to your career than your reputation. Machiavelli even says so himself:

1. *Nothing makes the prince more famous than his great achievements and exemplary gestures.*

While those great achievements and exemplary gestures could be about building and contributing to the community, they also contribute to building your honor, prestige, reputation, and glory.

That's the reason why during elections, candidates try to gain more credibility with voters by cozying up to well-liked, retired politicians. It is also the period where spin doctors weave the worst kind of smear campaign in the media to ruin the reputation of their opponents. If you are serious about your political career, it is important to invest in getting some good PR for yourself and your team.

2. *A prince should, above all else, strive in every action to be famous for being great and remarkable.*

When it comes to choosing who they feel is best to lead, people will consider both the character of the politician as well as their leadership capabilities. It pays to have an image that they can associate with the candidate - something that makes you more memorable.

Each time you step into the public eye, they will be on the lookout for the way you comport yourself, your speech, and the way you develop your narratives. Every eye, camera, and recorder will be on you, dissecting your every move until they find something to tear apart.

The presidential election between Hillary Clinton and Donald Trump is a good example of how letting spin doctors take your story beyond your control could damage your political chances. It is clear that Hillary Clinton suffered a lot of reputational damage due to several repetitional factors, including the email controversy. The opposing team pounced on that weakness and kept tugging until it left irreparable damage in Hillary's PR.

Although many people considered Hillary to be a very capable candidate, her reputation hung over her head like a shroud and hampered her ability to secure her position. They doubted her character, and that was her downfall. She worsened it by being evasive in her answers to questions about the emails, the data on her computers, her charity, and other areas. She was not able to strike confidence about her reputation in the hearts of the voters.

Public affection, human adoration, and voter support are very fickle. The reputation of a politician is one of the most fragile things on earth, and a simple mistake, an unguarded comment, a cheeky response to a question, or even silence when you should have said something could topple all of your hard work.

3. *I say that all human beings, when mentioned, especially princes due to their high status, are notable for their particular values that either bring them blame or praise. This is why people are known for being generous or miserly, generous or greedy, cruel or compassionate, unfaithful or loyal, soft and cowardly or daring and brave, friendly or proud, lascivious or chaste, sincere or cunning, easy or serious, religious or disbelieving, and so on.*

This quote from Machiavelli matches the message in the previous chapter - human beings get a reputation, whether good or bad, for a particular personality trait. This is especially obvious in popular figures like politicians. The way they can get identified by regular people is through their singular, noteworthy feats rather than the general way they behave.

Even though deep down we know that human beings are multifaceted (that is, they can be both good and bad, generous and miserly, believing and doubtful), we would rather create a perception of them through generalizations. If a politician makes the news for doing one or two noteworthy deeds, they get the reputation of being good.

4. *I know that some people will confess that it is praiseworthy for a prince to have all the above good qualities in him.*

It is good for a politician to stamp their name on something significant because that is the legacy that will be remembered in history. People will always remember a politician that has any of the above-mentioned good characters in a positive light.

5. *But our human nature does not allow us to have all of those perfect qualities. Therefore, the prince needs to be careful enough to avoid the reproach of those vices that would make him lose his state.*

However, we cannot always display all of these positive qualities. In fact, Machiavelli, with his usual pragmatism, notes that choosing to only display positive characters is an idealistic way of living when he said:

6. *Anyone who ignores the apparent reality for the imagination of what ought to be will sooner cause his own destruction rather than protection.*

The way that humans have to live in reality is quite different from the idealistic image that you may have in your head. There is no completely good person, so if you go around expecting people to be good to you because you are good to them, Machiavelli has this to say:

7. *A person who chooses to act completely moral will soon be destroyed among so many in the world who are not good.*

Politics is a cutthroat business. Everyone is on the lookout for ways to upstage you. Too much goodness on your part will bring nothing but destruction to you. The political world is filled with crafty people who will take advantage of your morality.

Just like choosing between being generous and miserly, you might have to choose between displaying more good characters that will bring you praise and bad ones that may bring you to censure.

327

8. *Hence, a prince who wants to survive must know how to do evil or not according to his need. So let's put aside the fantasies regarding the prince and discuss the realities.*

However, if you want to survive as a politician, you must learn how to switch between good and bad, according to your needs. That just might be the only thing that could save your career and give your community a chance to be better for it.

If it is necessary for you to be immoral, do it. If doing things that others consider wrong will bring about positive results in the long run, don't be afraid to do it. According to Machiavelli, there is no law that expects a politician to always act good - that is not a realistic expectation either. You must first weigh your circumstances and act in the best way that is profitable to your goals.

But then, if you are allowed to act badly, even though you know you will be judged harshly for it, how do you manage to maintain a good reputation, which Machiavelli also admits is important to politics, with the people? He answers that question with this next quote:

9. *It is, therefore, necessary for the prince to have all the good qualities that I have described, but it is also necessary for him to pretend to have them. I dare say this too, to have these qualities and to always exhibit them is dangerous. However, it is helpful for a prince to appear to have them – to appear to be benevolent, loyal, generous, religious, straightforward but flexible enough to take the display of the opposite of these qualities when needed.*

Since the way that other people perceive you is important to your political career, especially if your journey is just beginning, you can pay lip service to the idea of being good.

Machiavelli advises that even though you do not have any of the positive qualities that he describes, you should pretend to have them. Support a worthy cause if you have to; let your name be tied to positive things in the news, media, and on people's lips.

A modern example of a politician that invested in the best PR strategy is John Bel Edwards, the re-elected governor of Louisiana. In 2019, just before the Louisiana gubernatorial race, the incumbent governor launched a series of PR salvos that made him remain in the headlines and score free positive publicity with the media.

In Louisiana, all the candidates interested in the gubernatorial seat run for office simultaneously. So, Edwards' opponents included a combination of eight Democrats, Republicans, and third-party candidates. The pre-election polls placed Edwards, former U.S. Representative Ralph Abraham from the Republican party, and industrial CEO Eddie Rispone, also Republican, to be the likely winners.

Edwards' campaign and PR strategy included using his position as incumbent to capture the media's attention while simultaneously denying or diluting the quality of coverage his opponents got. As incumbent governor of the state, Edwards held the highest seat of power, so each time he spoke, all of Louisiana's news media had to listen. None of the other opponents had the same advantage to command the media as he could.

Understanding this and seeking to use this to his best advantage, Edwards planned a series of actions that would make him remain in the news for doing commendable things.

He held a press conference at the New Orleans Saints training facility to announce plans to renovate the Mercedes Benz Superdome for $450 million. In a state that has a large football culture, this was a huge development. He also promised to help the only NFL franchise in Louisiana extend its lease for another 30 years.

Apart from being a strategic move that would improve the social and cultural value of the state, extending the lease for the New Orleans Saints franchise was expected to have an economic impact of $1.3 billion in 2019. Thus ensuring that the continuity of the franchise reflected positively on both his position as the governor of the state, in terms of job performance, and his position as an election candidate, in terms of community and state service. He would also stage several photo ops with Saints' head coach, Sean Payton, and former quarterback, Drew Brees. As a former high school quarterback himself, he would run through athletic drills, sometimes even competing with Drew to the love of the Louisiana media. The people of Louisiana loved football, and he had not only successfully positioned himself with two of the most influential football figures as a part of his campaign PR.

These PR moves served two purposes for the Edwards campaign. One, it served as a piece of organic information that dominated several news cycles and kept him visible to the voters. Two, it suppressed similar press events from his major competitors and other opponents, as they did not receive as much significant press coverage.

However, the biggest and most defining move that kept the media buzzing about him for days and swayed public opinion in his favor was writing a letter to President Trump to request a Major Disaster Declaration, which would trigger federal funds to help deal with the unprecedented flooding of the Mississippi River.

By writing that letter, Edwards not only created a newsworthy act of a state governor conducting state business and fulfilling the duties of his office but also proved his readiness and ability to work with the Trump Administration. Edwards was an incumbent Democrat governor in a deeply conservative state, which placed him at opposite ends of the ideological chain with the major stakeholders in the state. Although most of their ideologies differed, by writing that public letter to a Republican president rather than using other methods - like a private phone call - he garnered a lot of media attention.

By using textbook crisis management and news management tactics, Edwards was able to create and manage a relationship with Republican voters and ensure he had their votes. By showing that he was willing to work with bi-partisan forces to fulfill his responsibilities, he showed himself as one of the most qualified candidates to become governor.

Edwards example is one that shows that having your name linked to positive acts, whether in the news or by word of mouth, is a strategy that can be used for effective PR comms and news management. He also shows that effectively sustained news presence can successfully sway public opinions towards you and your cause as a politician.

It does not matter if you genuinely support these causes or you take them on as a guide to clean up your image or justify your actions. The only thing that matters is the public perception of yourself. You don't have to be good; just act like you are.

Citing Ferdinand of Aragon, the King of Spain, as an example, Machiavelli explained how one could cover bad deeds under a cloak of respectability and acceptance.

10. *In addition, he always used religion as a justification for larger schemes. He applied cruel policies to push people out of the Moors kingdom. We cannot find a more admirable or rare example than that. Using the same excuse, he invaded Africa, waged war in Italy, and eventually attacked France.*

Therefore, his achievements and plans have always been great and kept the mind of his subjects in admiration and occupied with the outcome. He continued from war to war, leaving his subjects not enough time to think about opposing him.

Ferdinand grew his kingdom by conquering Islamic opponents and enlarging his empire; while acting in his own interest, he was able to cloak his behavior in respectability by pretending to others that he did it for the sake of his religion. So, people supported his pious cruelty as a necessary evil to bring more glory to the church.

Although Donald Trump may have spurred divided reactions to his promise to build a wall between the U.S. and Mexico in 2016, it gained him a lot of supporters. On the other hand, his democrat opponent, Hillary Clinton, in the same campaign made promises on immigration reform. However, rather than threatening to send immigrants back, she promised to offer law-abiding, hard-working immigrant families a path to citizenship. Her proposed immigration package would have liberalized future immigration.

When Donald Trump's detractors shut down his immigration ideas, arguing that building a wall and mass deportation of immigrants was unethical, racially inspired, and un-American, he decided to soften his stance and regroup so he wouldn't lose supporters.

He claimed that Mexico was sending their worst citizens to them and accused immigrants of being drug dealers, rapists, and drug dealers. In a televised speech, he claimed that every American was adversely affected by uncontrolled illegal immigration, and they were out of space to hold them to prevent them from joining the American population, so the wall would solve all their problems.

By spinning the media narrative to make it appear that he was putting Americans first and claiming that his policies would restore America to its previous glory, he was able to garner a lot of support for his anti-immigration stance.

He went on to chronicle a number of Americans that had been killed by illegal immigrants. He claimed that immigrant workers weighed down salaries and kept the American unemployment rates high, making it hard for Americans to earn a middle-class wage. He promised to create a hiatus where immigrant workers would not get jobs until employees had employed all available native-born Americans and legal immigrants first.

He cast Hillary as a candidate who cared more about protecting immigrant families than doing what was right to protect Americans first. He blamed his opponent, and Barack Obama, for the violence perpetrated by illegal immigrants against Americans because they supported visa overstays, sanctuary cities, amnesty, and the release of dangerous criminals. He also claimed that Hillary's promise to grant amnesty, Obamacare, Social Security, and Medicare to illegal immigrants would break the federal budget.

In his media interviews, he promised to put Americans first and protect them. He told the voters and everyone else who had special interests in the outcome of the elections that the debate of the U.S. immigration had only one purpose - to serve the well-being of the American people - and everything else was a very far second.

By the time he was done spinning the media narrative to paint his cause as good, he had already convinced the average white person (the largest population in the U.S.) that most of America's problems were due to illegal immigrants. He sealed the deal with a nicely wrapped bow by promising that America would not bear the expenses for building the wall because he would make Mexico pay for it. Even though opinions were still divided on his immigration stance, he had cloaked it in enough respectability to convince a large percentage of the population to support him. That, along with Hillary's shaky reputation, sealed the deal for him in the 2016 elections and ensured his victory.

Chapter Fourteen

Be Both Human and Beast

"If a prince is compelled to behave like a beast, he ought to choose the fox and the lion." - Niccolò Machiavelli.

Human relations require you to have complex personalities. There are times where you will need to be civil and times where you have to act on your baser instincts. According to Machiavelli, there is a time and place for both personalities.

1. *There are two ways to win - by the rule of law or by force. The first method is appropriate for humans, while the second is suitable for animals.*

Acting in a civil manner involves following the law and using it to settle your differences. It involves rational thinking and calm discussion - a method that sets human beings apart from animals. However, the law does not always favor us or work in our benefit. Machiavelli believes that in these instances there is another way to act - by force, which is the order of nature reserved for animals.

2. *However, because the first method is hardly ever effective, the second must also be used. It is, therefore, necessary for a prince to know how to use both the beast and the human ways.*

In situations where civility will not solve the issue to your benefit, Machiavelli proposes the need to behave in a more forceful manner to strongarm, frighten, and intimidate your people into doing things your way. It is good and reasonable to act compassionately, especially as a politician to the electorates, but sometimes being compassionate is not enough and you may need tougher measures to secure your position. These tough measures may require you to act differently and resort to an animalistic show of force.

3. *Therefore, it is essential for a prince to know how to use both natures, for one without the other is hardly ever enough. If a prince is compelled to behave like a beast, he ought to choose the fox and the lion.*

It is therefore important that you know how to switch between being a human and a beast, and more importantly when to do so. If you need the instincts of an animal to guide you, Machiavelli suggests choosing the lion and the fox as exemplary animalistic natures to mimic.

A lion is known for its boldness, strength, and courage. However, it is not very cunning or sly and may not know how to slip out of tight spots. On the other hand, a fox is very cunning and can weasel itself out of any tight situation, but it is not strong enough for a direct challenge.

The fox is not just wily enough to slip out of traps but also smart enough to spot them early on, so it doesn't snare it. A fox will see through deception and smell a plot from a distance.

A lion is not only brave and strong enough to face challenges head-on; it is also large and intimidating enough to scare off other predators. You will need both of these personalities to survive the chaotic environment of politics.

4. *As the lion cannot protect itself from traps, and the fox cannot defend itself against wolves. Therefore it is necessary to become a fox to sniff out the traps and a lion to fight off the wolves. Those who simply rely on the lion do not understand what they are doing.*

Machiavelli suggests that to survive the wilderness of politics, you can't be one without being the other. You will need both the cunningness of a fox and the strength of a lion - both deception and force combined. Where deception fails, brute force will work and vice versa.

It is erroneous to rely on the brute strength of the lion alone because unlike the fox, it is not shrewd and discerning. What the fox lacks in boldness and strength, it makes up for with its wiliness, spotting traps and deceptions easily and evading them. This is particularly important in diplomatic issues so you don't commit any errors that could spark bigger consequences.

Strength alone will not bring all your desired results. There will be times where you will need more subtle methods of accomplishing things. It is like that angry kid that always pummels anyone that offends him in the schoolyard - no matter how justified he is in his actions; he will just be seen as a bully. Some subtle tact should be applied in taking down your enemies.

Tone down your strength with cleverness, cultivate both behaviors, and use either of them when the situation calls for it. A leader that learns how to harness the power of both of these traits will become a formidable opponent, as the polar weaknesses of each beast can be managed by their polar strengths.

There is a common theme in all of Machiavelli's advice - there is no acceptable or unacceptable ethics, just as long as it is the right situation to display such behavior. As a leader, you will have to behave in ways that your situations dictate. If your situation calls for you to be bold, be bold. If it requires you to be cautious and wary, then be prudent enough to apply wariness and caution. If you have to be cruel, then ensure your cruelty is warranted. Your ethics should always be flexible and willing to change with your situation.

Most people believe in having rigid principles that won't falter irrespective of the situation they find themselves in. But Machiavelli believes that obstinate rigidity in a situation that calls for flexibility will only hurt you. Do not box yourself into doing something that will have a negative outcome on your plans, even though you have made promises to that effect.

5.   *Hence, a wise prince should not keep the faith when such a promise can be turned against him or when the reasons behind such a promise cease to exist. If humans were entirely good, then there would be no need for this rule, but since they are evil and will not keep their promises to you, you are also not bound to keep your promises to them.*

Basically, Machiavelli is saying that if it serves your purpose, it is okay to lie. As you can see from the previous examples of campaign

335

promises, most of them are either outright lies or an embellishment of the truth. They serve one purpose only - the people want to hear them, so politicians make the promises whether or not they can meet up with them. The promises usually revolve around reducing taxes or reducing government spending because that's what people want to hear. That's what gets you voted in. Nowhere in history has a person won an election by promising to raise taxes.

6. *However, Machiavelli is not saying that politicians should always make promises they cannot keep. What he means is that if after you make a promise and the premise for making the promise ceases to exist or that it could be your undoing, you shouldn't feel the slightest bit guilty about breaking your word.*

If you make a promise, you fully intend to keep but later reneged on it with good justification, that's not lying. This is a valid technique for survival in politics.

Machiavelli insists that if your situation finds it prudent for you to break your word, you can get away with doing it. He justifies this by saying if people were truly always good and kept their promises, then there would be no need for this rule. However, the reality is that most people will not keep their promises because they will chase their selfish interests first, then while you have to look out for both your best interests and those of the people you lead.

However, a prince ought to know the cleverness to disguise this behavior and be a good actor. Humans are so simple and, therefore, only concerned with present necessities, such that anyone who seeks to deceive will always find one person who will allow himself to be deceived.

However, people will not take too kindly to discovering that they have been hoodwinked or deceived. That sort of clever manipulation might not be seen as a strength, so be careful of how you present your wiliness. In a world where it is hard to trust anyone, you cannot afford to give yourself the reputation of a sly. So, if you can, hide your true intentions.

Do everything you can to remain in power, protect the people you lead, and ensure that the plans you have for them come to fruition. Be both cunning and bold.

An example of a politician that was so glib, he practically arm-twisted his opponents to win votes was Lyndon B. Johnson. One of his most notable feats won by arm twisting was an important vote he won from Senator Everett Dirksen.

In 1963, Lyndon Johnson became the President of the United States after John F. Kennedy was assassinated and inherited the Civil Rights bill from his predecessor. Kennedy had been trying to get the bill signed into law but couldn't quite get past partisan and segregationist Southern politicians who dominated Congress.

However, because Johnson had once been a player for that team, he knew the best way to play against the Southerners and beat them at their game. When he was a junior senator from Texas, Johnson had been part of the southern anti-Civil Rights bloc. But fast forward years later, in 1964, there he was, running for re-election in a Nation that expected the Civil Rights bill. But Johnson knew how to beat the Southerners at their game because he'd played it himself. As a junior senator from Texas, he'd been part of the anti-Civil Rights bloc. But in 1964, he was trying to get elected president of a nation that expected the enactment of a Civil Rights bill.

The Civil Rights bill was the object of the longest filibuster in the United States Senate history, designed to procrastinate or block the Senate from approving it. It took a whole 57 days.

Back then, one would require 67 votes to break a filibuster. As mentioned, all the Southern States were represented by Democrats who were opposed to civil rights, so even though they belonged to the same party, Johnson had to hope from those quarters. All hope lay in getting the 33 Republican senators to vote. To do that, he knew he had to cozy up to Dirksen, who was the Senate Minority Leader and win him over.

Dirksen had promised Johnson's predecessor to allow a floor vote on the bill, but when the bill got to the Senate, he stalled. Dirksen requested a few changes from Johnson that would have weakened fair employment sections and public accommodations in return, but he refused to make a compromise.

So Johnson approached Senator Hubert Humphrey of Minnesota, the bill's floor leader, and told him they all knew that the bill wouldn't pass until they got Dirksen on their side. So he told Humphrey that they were going to do everything they could to get him on their side.

As part of their crafty plan to get Dirksen on board, Humphrey went on Meet the Press and praised Dirksen's statesmanship. He said:

"He [Dirksen] is a man who thinks of his country before he thinks of his party. I sincerely believe that when Senator Dirksen finds himself in a situation where his decision, leadership, and influence would be required to get us the votes needed to pass this bill, he will not be found wanting."

There, they had managed to get Dirksen into a fine spot. If he couldn't get the Senate to sign the bill, Humphrey had created a target to collect all the blame. To seal the deal, Johnson reminded Dirksen that he not only led the Party of Lincoln but also represented Lincoln's home state. As the filibuster went on, several clergymen thronged into the Capitol, trying to lobby senators to vote for civil rights, until finally, after pressure from all ends, Dirksen gave in.

Johnson allowed him to make a few harmless amendments to the bill to make it look like he contributed to its creation. Dirksen would later tell reporters that he finally realized that it was time, and he could no longer be in the way of an idea whose time had come.

Dirksen agreed that it was time to call for cloture to end the filibuster. He called Senator Richard of Georgia and told him they had gone far enough; it was time to end it. Next, he placed a call to Johnson and promised to do all he could to get the bill signed and get the whole deal wrapped up.

The motion for the cloture was approved, and the votes were 71-29 in favor of signing the bill. Twenty-seven of those in favor were Republicans that threw their weight in because of Dirksen. The Civil Rights Act may just have completed the work begun by Abraham Lincoln, but it couldn't have passed the Senate if it didn't have the support of a Senator from Lincoln, and that couldn't have happened without the subtle maneuvering from Johnson. In a call with Dirksen, Johnson told him:

"You're worthy of the 'Land of Lincoln,' and the man from Illinois is going to pass the bill, and I'll see that you get proper attention and credit."

Build Political Alliances

"A prince is also respected when he is a true friend or an absolute enemy." - Niccolò Machiavelli.

The people you choose to align yourself with are equally as important as your opponents. Any politician that takes a firm stand on who their friends and enemies are is respected. Even when they lose, people will recognize that they made an attempt. Machiavelli was against neutrality and indecisiveness when it came to choosing who to align with. He said:

1. *In either case, it would always be beneficial for the prince to assist one of them to actively wage war. If the prince does not declare himself, he will fall prey to the conqueror. Then, the loser will be pleased and happy. As for the prince, there is no reason to ask for help, nor anything to protect or shelter him.*

When it is time to choose an ally to throw you back behind, Machiavelli suggests that you take a stand. Worrying about losing face because you chose the wrong ally will only be to your own disadvantage because neither winner nor the loser will respect you for deferring or remaining neutral.

2. *For whoever wins will not want people he doubts would help in difficult times, and the loser will not be willing to protect him because the prince was not willing to bring his troops to share his fate.*

That is because anyone who wins will not be willing to align themselves to a flaky person who may bail out on them in difficult times, and the loser will not be willing to be yoked with you because you will not hesitate to leave them to their fate.

Of course, if you are in a position of influence, people will lobby you for either your support or neutrality in key situations. To handle this situation, Machiavelli says:

3. *So it always happens that the people who are not your friend will ask for your neutrality, while your friends will beg you to hold your weapon by their side. The weak princes, in order to avoid the present danger, often go neutral and are often defeated. But when the prince bravely declares in favor of one side and if his side wins, even though the conqueror may be strong and have the prince at his mercy, he would still be indebted to the prince, and a friendship is established.*

You have nothing to lose by choosing to take a stand for someone or even supporting them. If the endeavor is successful, it will forever remain in your debts, and you can use it later to further other initiatives.

4. *Victories, after all, are never so clear that the winner must not show some regard, especially justice. But if one who the prince supports is defeated, the prince will be protected by them, and when it is possible, he may assist the prince, and they both become companions on a fortune that may come again.*

However, it is always better to be on the winning team rather than the losing one. This is because the winners get to choose the kind of treatment the losers get.

5. *When the two neighboring powers go to war, but the prince does not feel threatened by whoever wins, it is even of more importance for the prince to support one side. By so doing, the prince helps to sabotage one side by helping the other. With the prince's necessary help and interference, the winner will always be indebted to him.*

Machiavelli says that powerful alliances are created by appealing to the self-interest of a more influential and powerful politician. But when choosing who to side with, be careful with your choice. Whether they win or lose, people with more power can crush you, and an alliance with them may not always be in your best interest.

6. *However, it must be noted here that the prince should never ally himself with someone stronger than him to fight someone else unless absolutely necessary. As said before, if he wins, he becomes his prisoner. A prince must avoid, as much as he can, being in a position of indebtedness to anyone.*

Machiavelli further says that an alliance with people more powerful than you should only be brokered when it is absolutely necessary. Whether you win or lose, you will be the one indebted to them, and that is never a good position to bargain from.

Chapter Sixteen

Be Wary Of People Who Support You For Their Personal Gain

"The prince must always listen to advice, but only when he wants, not when others want it." – Niccolò Machiavelli.

One of the things you have to look out for is flatterers and silver-tongued sycophants who only flock around you for their personal gain. You know them - the ones who always have a ready compliment, who always have sweet words to butter you up and make you feel good. While you bask in their adoration, they are looking for ways to deceive and destroy you. Machiavelli has some choice words to say about them:

1. *I don't want to leave out an important matter because it is a difficult danger for the princes to watch out unless they are very careful and discerning. These are the flatterers that every court is filled.*

You see them in droves, hanging within the halls of government looking for an unsuspecting person to leech on to. They do not do this because they care about you or genuinely believe what they say, but to see how many personal benefits they can milk out of you by ingratiating themselves to you.

2. *Because people are so wrapped up in their own affairs or deceived within them, it is difficult to protect themselves from this danger. If they want to protect themselves, they risk being despised.*

The sad truth is that more often than not, it works. People fall victim to the deception because they are so wrapped up in their own heads.

They do not like being told they have made a mistake, so they would rather believe lies that call them infallible. The truth may hurt, but lies destroy.

3. *The only way to protect oneself from flattery is for people to understand that letting the prince know the truth is not offensive.*

If you do not make the people around you understand that it is okay for them to tell you the truth, even though you might not like it, you leave yourself vulnerable and open to flattery, lies, and deception.

4. *However, when everyone feels free to speak the truth, the prince's respect fades away. Therefore, a wise prince should hold a third method by choosing wise people in the country and giving only them the freedom to speak the truth. Even then, they can only speak the truth of the things the prince asks and not say anything else. But the prince should ask them about everything and listen to their presentation, and afterward, he can conclude himself.*

However, Machiavelli warns that allowing any and every one to speak to you in a blunt, free, and familiar manner breeds disrespect. When you limit the number of people that get to talk to you freely, it reduces the dangers of overfamiliarity. In addition, it reduces the opportunities they have to gang up against you to pursue their self-interests.

Choose a trusted person among the several paying you court and encourage them to be honest and open with you, but only at your request. And if you ask them to talk to you truthfully about something, listen to them but make your own conclusions after. If their recommendations do not tally with the plans you have, do not hesitate to discard them. But if you find wisdom in their speech, then take it.

5. *With these councilors, both individually and collectively, the prince must behave in such a way that each of them should know that the more freely they speak, the more they will be preferred. Outside of this group, the prince doesn't need to listen to anyone but pursue what has been settled and stick to his decision. Any prince who does otherwise will be buried in his career by flattery or often changes his mind because of different opinions and be laughed at.*

There is a popular saying that goes, "flattery gets you nowhere," but according to Machiavelli, that is not true because flattery does, indeed, get people somewhere. When it comes to climbing the social ladder, flattery gets people everywhere - including your good graces - and gains them favors. It is an important tool for personal advancement because people understand that you will need all the help and support you can get, especially as a newbie.

In 1869, President Ulysses Grant went from being a war hero to the president. From the moment he resumed office until his last day of office, his administration was under attack from users and supporters who were ready to take advantage of his naivety when it came to political issues.

The first of the beginning of his woes began when financiers who had wormed their way into his good graces tried to corner the gold market, which led to the 1869 gold panic. Then in 1872, it was discovered that some shareholders of the Union Pacific Railroad had been bribing lawmakers to win contracts for new rail lines. One of the lawmakers implicated in the scandal was Schuyler Colfax, Grant's vice president. Since that was a re-election year, he was later dropped from the presidential ticket.

Even with all these scandals, Grant won his re-election bid because he was revered as a beloved Civil War hero. So people overlooked the many corruption scandals that came with his administration. They blamed the corruption on Grant's disloyal friends whom he gave federal appointments.

However, he didn't learn his lessons in choosing better bedfellows and counsel.

He appointed another old friend, General John McDonald, as the supervisor for the Treasury Department's internal revenue operations. He got the job as a means to boost Republican efforts to re-elect the president. However, his presence there did more harm than good to Grant's political career.

McDonald created whiskey rings in different parts of the country to siphon funds from the federal tax of 70 cents per gallon on alcohol sales. This he did by underreporting alcohol sales, manipulating figures, and funneling the extra money to the Republican Party. After Grant's re-election in 1872, the whiskey rings became a full-blown criminal operation that had many government officials and whiskey distillers profiting. All of it without Grant's knowledge.

When a new Treasury Secretary, Benjamin Bristow, was chosen in mid-1874, he discovered that more than $4 million was missing in tax revenue in the two years that McDonald was head. He discovered coded telegram messages and unraveled evidence that proved the corruption went as deep as Grant's personal secretary, General Orville Babcock.

When Bristow took all of his accumulated evidence to President Grant, he refused to believe that people so close to him, people he trusted, could be capable of such nefarious acts. He had fought side-by-side with Babcock in the Civil War and genuinely believed he knew everything about his closest friend. Determined that there was more to the story and someone was playing something foul with the entire situation, he encouraged Bristow to keep digging and gathering more evidence. In his words, "if it can be avoided, let no guilty man escape."

To prove that there was no conflict of interest, he appointed the first special prosecutor in the U.S., Senator John B. Henderson, a Republican from Illinois and another Civil War veteran. He assembled a grand jury in St. Louis and began to indict and convict a large number of people involved in the scam. Among those sent to jail was McDonald.

To show there wasn't any conflict of interest, Grant appointed America's first special prosecutor. He was Republican Sen. John B. Henderson of Illinois, another Civil War veteran. Henderson convened a grand jury in St. Louis and soon began indicting and convicting scores of people. McDonald was among those who went to jail.

However, the moment the prosecutor started focusing on Babcock as well as other members of his family, Grant raised objections. Other Republicans also joined in the objections claiming there was a conspiracy to get to the president through his loved ones and friends.

In mid-December of 1875, Henderson was finally able to indict Babcock on charges of fraud against the American government. In his remarks to the court, he also hinted at interference and obstruction from the president. In anger, Grant ordered the Attorney General to fire Henderson, which he did on the basis that Henderson cast doubt on the president without any reason.

That proved to be a big misstep on the president's part as firing Henderson set off a public outcry, especially in democratic circles. People took to the streets to protest. One newspaper taunted Grant with his own words, saying he meant, "Let no guilty man escape unless he lives in the palace." When interviewed, Henderson told the New York Herald that he believed Grant's madness and thirst for revenge on hearing he had indicted his friend caused him to fire him.

Things were not looking good for the president, but instead of taking a step back to handle issues more diplomatically, he dug his foot in and blamed everyone for the mess, everyone except the people apparently responsible for it. He accused the press of being biased and fueling controversy. He tried to muzzle the press by asking the Attorney General to bring them before a grand jury to substantiate their claims. Grant was on a mission - one of self-destruction. At one point, he even tried to stop the prosecutors from giving key witnesses immunity for their testimony.

Grant had reached a state of full-blown hysteria and paranoia, complaining to anyone that would listen that the prosecution was targeting him and putting him on trial. Meanwhile, he adamantly defended his friend, Babcock, insisting that he was innocent. At a cabinet meeting, he declared that he would go down to St. Louis to testify at Babcock's trial, stunning everyone present. It was later agreed by cabinet members from both parties that the president should be questioned at the White House instead. In February 1876, Ulysses Grant became the first and only president of the United States to ever testify at a criminal trial.

The president's involvement in the case caused it to draw sensational attention, even rivaling O.J. Simpson's trial. Reporters came into the St. Louis courtroom from all over the country, waiting to hear the final verdict on the issue.

Babcock was eventually acquitted by the jury due to the president's testimony, to a large extent. However, he was forced to resign from his position in the White House. Of all the major targets probed for their involvement in the fraud, Babcock was the only one that walked away scot-free. The prosecutors were able to recover more than $3 million dollars from the stolen money and send over a hundred men to jail.

For the role he played in the outcome of the verdict, many Democratic newspapers called for Grant to be indicted for obstructing justice, but he was never punished for it.

The world of politics is very rife with duplicitous people looking for any means to benefit from you. Like Grant's story, even people you think you can trust with your life will not hesitate to use you for their personal gain if the opportunity calls for it. The problem is that they will more often than not drag you to your doom.

Grant was a war hero, but an excellent judge of character he was not. He was not equipped to spot these flatterers and users for who they were, and that made him an easy victim for unscrupulous men to take advantage of.

6. *Also, knowing that anyone, on any matter, has not told the prince the truth, he should let his anger be felt.*

The biggest mistake that Grant made was not standing aside to allow his closest counsel to be punished for lying and deceiving him. Instead, he chose to stand behind him, which could be interpreted as a reward for his bad behavior.

When you have selected the few people allowed to counsel you, warn them to avoid flattery or dissemination because you will not tolerate it. Otherwise, you will find yourself changing your plans to repeatedly fit the different whims of all your advisors.

Even worse than appearing to be a confused leader, flattery will cause you to make the wrong choices. When you get used to thinking all your decisions are fair and wise, when they are not, it may cause you to become autocratic and overconfident. You stop asking questions because you think everything is business as usual while everyone else laughs behind you for being foolish but keeps reassuring you that your decisions are wise to your face.

Machiavelli gave an example of a ruler, Maximilian, who almost never got anything done because of the differing opinions of his courtiers. He said:

7. *The emperor is a secret man - he does not communicate his plans to anyone, nor does he accept anyone's opinion. However, in putting them to practice, the plan is revealed and known. They are debated by those around the emperor; when they protest, he is immediately dissuaded from doing them. Therefore, the things he does today would be undone the next day without anyone understanding what he wanted to do, and no one can rely on his decisions.*

One of the downsides of flattery is the indecisiveness that follows. Maximilian was a man that kept his plans close to his chest, only revealing them when it was time for execution. Had he been one who followed through on his decisions, this would not be too much of a problem. However, Maximilian found it hard to follow through with his decision and didn't seek the advice of his counsel before he made plans.

Each time he brought forward a plan to be executed, his courtiers would argue in favor or against it depending on how much they stood to benefit from it, and at the end of the day, nobody would agree on a decision. They made a muddle of everything such that any plans that he started, he had to dump without anyone ever understanding what he hoped to achieve with said plans.

8. *So the prince must always listen to advice, but only when he wants, not when others want it. He must make it clear that he does not want advice unless asked. However, he must constantly ask questions and then be a patient listener about what he asks.*

To avoid unnecessary back and forth that will stall your project, always listen to advice. However, you should only listen to advice that you requested from people you trust and discourage unsolicited advice. And when you do get the advice you asked for, listen patiently and ask questions.

9. *There may be some who think that a prince can be wise not because of his own abilities but because he has good advisers around him. Such a belief is clearly false, for an unwise prince would never take good advice unless, by chance, he completely entrusted full control over to a*

brilliant and intelligent courtier. Indeed, in this case, the prince may be well governed, but it wouldn't be long, as such an eminent person would depose him within a short time.

When you create a select group of people you solicit advice from, do not make the mistake of thinking that every wise thing you do is a result of the council received. Wise counsel is as good as useless in the hands of a foolish person that cannot recognize the wisdom in it.

So while your advisors should be honest, capable, and competent, you also play an important role in how their advice turns out. If your advisors are truthful and competent, reward them for their efforts. However, be careful that you don't give away too much of your power to them or you may not regain it. When a power tussle comes, you will lose your leverage.

10. *If an inexperienced prince takes advice from many people, he always takes different advice, and he won't know how to handle it. Each advisor will think about his own interests and the prince will not know how to control or observe them. This is obvious since people always want to deceive the prince unless they are bound by a necessity to be honest.*

Like Grant, it is easy for newbies to the political world to fall into the trap of rewarding their friends, allies, and supporters with positions of authority when they resume office. Like Grant's situation, that will only spell disaster. Machiavelli warns that having too many advisors and not knowing who has your best interest at heart will make it hard for you to control them.

Too many people will fight to gain your trust and get in your good graces for their personal gain and, in so doing, will become flatterers and users rather than advisors and supporters.

11. *Hence, good counsel, from wherever it comes, is the result of the prince's wisdom. Not that the prince's wisdom comes from good advice.*

In conclusion, Machiavelli says that whether the quality of advisors you have and advice you receive is good or bad depends heavily on your skill and wisdom as a leader. The advice does not determine the quality of a leader's decision, but it is the leader's wisdom that makes a piece of advice good or bad.

Avoid Hatred

"A prince is scorned if he is considered to be fickle, weak, indecisive, wicked, or lowly." - Niccolò Machiavelli.

The first thing that you need to have at the back of your mind is that it is impossible to please everyone. Some people will just not be appeased, no matter what you do. However, if you cannot get everyone to like you, it is in your best interest that the reactions you get from them are not outright hatred. Machiavelli said:

1. *Now, because I have talked about the important characteristics that a prince must display, I would like to briefly discuss under the general topic the things that a prince should think about to avoid those things that would make him hated or despised. If he can play his part to the best of his ability, then he needs not fear any dangers of other criticisms.*

If you behave in all the manners that a leader is supposed to and try to the best of your abilities to ensure that you are successful in every decision to take, you don't need to bother yourself about criticisms. Your position will remain secure - unless you are caught doing something that allows you to be despised and hated.

2. *As I have said, what makes people the most resentful is the exploitation of the properties and women of his subjects. The prince must abstain from doing both of these things. When neither property nor honor is threatened, the majority of them will live happily. Then, the prince only has to contend with the ambitions of a few that he can easily control in many ways.*

When he discussed the different ways that a leader must act to gain cooperation from the citizens, Machiavelli mentioned that as long as you did not tamper with their properties, come after their loved ones, their honor, most people will have no problems with you. He listed that as a tactile line that must not be crossed under any circumstance.

Take care not to be caught diverting your citizen's finances for your personal gain. One way to make people hate you is to give yourself better benefits, a raise, or more perks than the common man, especially if you are working hard to get them to enjoy less. For example, cutting down costs in the budget, holding off on salary increases and benefits, etc. You should not be caught living lavishly while your people live in relative squalor and are worried about possible tax increments, inflation, and a fixed income. It is a thumb up the nose to people who already consider politicians to be more privileged and are already wary and envious of the benefits they enjoy.

Between 2013 and 2014, Ukraine experienced a series of violent protests that led to the ousting of the then-president Viktor Yanukovych. When Viktor won the elections in 2010, he was the people's messiah because they had been disillusioned by the Orange government that preceded his administration. He rode that wave to quick popularity among his citizens and would have remained the people's president had he done everything he could to avoid being held to contempt and hatred.

His first mistake came within weeks of being elected. When he chose members of his cabinet, instead of choosing members from both opposition parties to make up the seats, he filled them up with only headliners from his party. This sent a clear signal to everyone involved that his government would not be one of national reconciliation, defeating the purpose of electing him and disappointing those who switched from the Orange camp to vote for him. Thus, taking power and jobs from those who would have benefited from it.

Had he ended his mistake there, it probably would have been overlooked in light of his successful administration. In April 2010, he made another blunder by signing the Kharviv pact with Russia to allow the extension of the Russian lease on naval facilities in Crimea beyond 2017 to 2042 with an additional five-year renewal option in exchange for a multiyear discounted contract to supply Ukraine with Russian natural gas. The deal was widely criticized as a bad one that did not favor Ukraine at all and allowed Russia to gain control of Crimea.

Then he compounded it by signing a dubious constitution that ceded all power to himself in October. Within the space of 7-8 months, Viktor had gone from a democratically elected official to a dictator. It raised the alarm within circles that were more democratically minded. Had he had the foresight, he would have seen the pitfalls involved in becoming solely responsible for ruling a country.

The final straw that broke the camel's back was when he went back on the deal to sign the Ukraine-European Union Association Agreement that would allow Ukraine to join the EU and enjoy free trade, choosing instead to maintain ties and economic relations with Russia.

Viktor had set himself up because he proposed the deal and kept reassuring his citizens that it was as good as signed on his own end. He raised their hopes up as they saw it as an opportunity for both economic reforms and civilizational choice. An apt title because they were finally leaving to join the rest of civilization to progress. So when he went back on his promise, it was a big letdown to the people of Ukraine.

The Ukrainians were disappointed because they felt that Viktor had stolen an opportunity from them and took to the streets to protest in what became known as the Euromaidan movement.

On 24 November 2013, the police and the protesters began to clash. After a few days of protests, university students joined in the demonstrations en masse. Even with the snow and sub-zero temperature, Ukrainians were not discouraged - they had to get Viktor out of office.

In the early morning of November 30, government forces ramped up the violence against the protesters, which led to a surge in the number of protesters from between 50,000-200,000 in the preceding weeks to 400,000-800,000 on the 1st of December. The protests turned violent in response to government repression and police brutality that killed many and left others injured.

This went on for over a month. Several Western Ukrainian governor buildings and regional councils had been occupied by Euromaidan protesters. In several other cities, the protestors also tried to take over their local government buildings but were forced back by pro-government groups and the police.

Viktor tried to salvage the situation by having a meeting with key opposition leaders for constitutional changes and to restore certain players to Parliament. He also agreed to an early election by December. But the people were too far gone in their anger and hatred. On 21 February, an impeachment bill was introduced to Parliament.

When Viktor heard that protesters had taken over the country's capital, he fled to Eastern Ukraine, wherein in his absence Parliament voted 328-0 in favor of his impeachment and fixed a new election for May.

The only thing Viktor was interested in was enriching his own pockets from taxpayers' money. He and his family fled to Russia in February, leaving behind a trail of documents that showed how deep his thievery ran. By the time an investigation was concluded, it was discovered that Viktor and his cronies had stolen over $40 billion dollars in state assets. Three years after the tragic incident, Viktor was found guilty of treason and sentenced to 13 years in prison in absentia.

If Viktor had avoided being hated, he could easily have kept everything - the support of the people and his position.

3. *A prince is scorned if he is considered to be fickle, weak, indecisive, wicked, or lowly. All of these attributes should be avoided by the prince. In his actions, the prince should strive to show greatness, courage, bravery, and somberness. In his private dealings with his subjects, let him show that his orders are absolute. He must maintain his reputation in such a way that no one can hope to deceive or manipulate him.*

If your electorate sees you as being weak, fickle, indecisive, wicked, or lowly, you lose all credibility. As said before, appearances matter even if you don't have the same personality. Once contempt sets in, it acts like cancer, growing and spreading until it consumes everything in its path and is hard to control. It could begin with whispers from word of mouth, an angry post on social media, and it will spread like wildfire to people that are already susceptible.

You become despicable as a leader if you become an object for jokes in the media or among your opposition. This is a valid strategy to ruin the reputation of your opponent because nobody likes or respects a leader who is an object of public ridicule. However, as the recipient of this kind of behavior, it hurts your chances.

4. *For this reason, a prince only has two things to fear – an attack from within from his subjects and one from without from foreign forces. Against the latter, the prince is defended by being well-armed and having food allies, and if he has good arms, he will always have good allies. Things within will remain quiet if the things outside remain quiet, as long as it isn't disturbed by rebellion. Even if he is disturbed on the outside, if the prince has learned to prepare and act, as I said earlier, as long as he does not despair will be able to resist any attack.*

However, regarding his subjects, if there is an external disturbance, the prince also has to worry that his subjects are secretly plotting a rebellion. The prince can easily protect himself from this by avoiding hatred and contempt and by maintaining good relations with his subjects. This is important for him to achieve, as I have discussed above.

When it comes to threats to their positions, leaders only have two things to fear – internal rebellion from among their followers and an attack from their enemies. Of the two of them, rebellion from your followers is the biggest and deadliest threat, and Viktor's story is enough proof. They see your flaws, know your weak spots, and know the exact place to attack you to hurt you the most.

Even if he were to be attacked by external forces, as long as his people do not hate him, he would be able to quickly quell it with an effective team and enough resources. However, a rebellious electorate that has given up on you will be harder to control as you are there to serve their mandate. You cannot lead without their support.

Machiavelli does not mean that you need to be loved by everyone to remain secure in your position but try as much as you cannot trigger the ire or hatred of your citizens. Polite indifference and grudging respect are examples of emotions that you can trigger in your constituents that are not quite hatred or love. Even a leader that has to use cruelty can get away with being feared as long as he does not overdo it and cause the people to scorn him.

Complacency Is The Herald of Doom

"A prince should not have any other goal or thought nor choose anything else for his research, anything else but war and its rules and discipline."
– Niccolò Machiavelli.

Politics is a never-ending war cloaked in barely concealed civility. It is not enough for you to learn strategies to parry against your opponent and win, but also to remain prepared for war from any angle. You may not have to carry weapons into the battlefield, but you will constantly fight mental battles - in your community, on the council seat, sometimes, even with yourself, your ideals, and your weaknesses. The point is that losing focus even for one moment will leave you open and unguarded for attacks.

On remaining on your toes and staying one step ahead of the political game, Machiavelli had the following to say:

1. *A prince should not have any other goal or thought, nor choose anything else for his research, anything else but war and its rules and discipline. This is the only art that belongs to the ruler, and it enables those who weren't born princes to not only defend their status but also helps ordinary citizens rise to the princedom.*

There is no time to be idle. Even when you are not engaging in battle, you should be researching and learning everything that you can to improve yourself. Research on better tactics for battle, learn the rules of engagement in the political clime. Knowledge is indeed power. If you already hold office, knowledge can help you secure your position and remain in power longer, and if you aim to run for office, knowledge can help you climb steadily through ranks.

Any politician that misses the chance to learn the rules and apply self-improvement according to them is at risk of losing their reputation, status, or even more.

2. *It is common to see that when princes who think more of peace than of war lose their state. The reason why they lose their states is that they neglected this art. Along the same vein, the reason they expand their territory is from the mastery of this art.*

When you become complacent and relax because you think you have already gotten the position you always wanted, someone else hungrier and more prepared will snatch your seat right from under you. How conversant are you with the constitution? Do you know your procedural bylaw? Have you studied people that could be threats to you? Do you know enough about these things to catch your opponent off guard or deflect/counterattack when they try to catch you off guard? Do you have a mission or vision statement? What strategic plans do you have to work towards them? Do you have a code of conduct for yourself and your team? How do you sift through relevant and irrelevant procedures? Do you have safety nets and insurance put in place? Have you crafted your ground rules to reflect the legislation? The gag is that this is just the tip of the iceberg. There are so many other things you need to arm yourself with.

So you see, there is no reason why you should be idle and complacent as a politician. Every action you take should be intentional to bring you closer to your end goal. Each time your photo appears in the paper or on TV, there should be a motive behind it. Every speech you utter should have an intended target. You cannot afford to talk or act carelessly.

3. *Among the many evils which not having arms will bring you is that it causes you to be despised. This is one of the dangers that a prince must guard himself against.*

We have talked about the pitfalls of being despised, and one of ways to be despised is by being unarmed and unprepared. A politician should be ready to think on their feet and the only way to do it is arming yourself with enough ammunition beforehand.

4. *There is a big difference between the armed and unarmed. It would be unreasonable to expect one who is armed to willingly yield to one who is unarmed or that the unarmed man feels secure in the midst of armed servants. This is because while one person holds disdain towards the other, the other would be suspicious of them. Therefore, making it hard for them to work together.*

The general rule of thumb is that the most prepared player who understands the rules of the game controls the field and the outcome of the game. It would be unreasonable to expect the person who holds all the cards to yield to the other. What tools do you have around you that you can use to disarm your opponent? How will you keep yourself one step ahead of your opponents at all times?

Knowledge is one of the weapons that sets apart a successful politician from an unsuccessful one. The more knowledge you gain about the rules that apply to the game you are playing, the more ammunition you gather to fight your opponent on the field.

If you come on the field without adequate preparation and knowledge of these rules, others will spot that chink in your armor and if they know what you don't, they could use it to take advantage of your ignorance by scoring points that belittle you.

In 2010, Christine O'Donnell, the Republican nominee for the U.S. Senate in Delaware, was in a debate with her Democratic opponent, Chris Coons, before law professors and students at Widener University Law School. Christine criticized Chris' position that creationism should not be taught in public schools as it was a direct violation of the First Amendment by promoting religious doctrine.

Chris' argument was that creationism could be taught in parochial and private schools but insisted that religious doctrine had no place in public schools. She lashed out at Chris for not knowing anything about the constitution and challenged him to show her where in the constitution the church and state was separated. Chris, clearly the more prepared candidate of the two, responded that the First

Amendment stopped Congress from making laws respecting the establishment of religion or prohibiting its free exercise.

The moderator, noticing where this was heading, tried to move on but Christine dug her heels in and circled back to the topic and asked Chris incredulously, "are you telling me that the separation of church and state is in the First Amendment?", a gaffe that first caused the audience to gasp in stunned shock before they broke into laughter. It was laughable that a candidate seeking to be a lawmaker did not even know the Constitution!

It began to raise questions on whether or not she was fit for the role she was contesting. The voters must have agreed that she was unfit because she lost the election to Chris by a margin of 57% to 40%. The 2010 election was her third attempt in five years for the Delaware Senatorial seat.

From this exchange we can see that communication can be a weapon too. You need to know how and when to speak, the right things to say and not say. You also need to know how to align your argument to get your message across and switch the game, as well as when to deflect questions, shut up, and when to go off the record.

5. *Hence, a prince who does not understand the art of war, among other mentioned disadvantages, cannot be respected by his soldiers, nor can he rely on them. Therefore, a prince must never let the art of war leave his mind and, even in peace, ought to practice more than during the war. He can do this in two ways, by action or research.*

If Christine, on noticing that her opponent had the upper hand or realizing the wisdom in allowing the moderator to switch the topic, she would have escaped from the debate relatively unscathed. On the other hand, Chris Coons showed just how important preparation was. He was able to make his opponent look like an absolute fool without even trying hard.

Even worse than looking like a fool in the presence of your opponent is losing respect in front of your staff. Once they realize how easy you are to fool, they will take advantage of your ignorance to push things that will further their own agendas past you.

Machiavelli recommends that you learn all the relevant policies, laws, bylaws, and procedures, and know where to apply them so you know how and when to fight.

6. *In addition, it is advisable to practice as if in battle so that the body can endure and learn the nature of the natural terrain. The prince must understand the terrain of the mountains, valleys, plains and understand the nature of the rivers and marshes. He must learn about all of these terrains for careful analysis and planning. This knowledge may be useful in two ways. First, the prince learns to know his country and is able to defend it better. Then, with the knowledge and observations of the terrain in his country, the prince can easily understand any aspect that needs to be studied more.*

So, how hard are you studying? The internet is rich in resources that can help you prepare. You can also use it as a practice field before the main event begins. Go through blogs and social media pages, what are your colleagues talking about? Do you know anything about the subject matter? Can you share your thoughts on the subject with enough information to back your argument? If someone challenges you, can you flip it around and put them on the hot seat?

Christine is not the only person that has gone for office without knowledge of the Constitution as there are many who have come to the table unprepared without knowledge of their own political agenda and strategies, let alone policies and bylaws. Because they fail to do due diligence, they go off track, making motions contrary to already existing ones and stumble to answer relevant questions during debates.

This unpreparedness is a big red flag on how irresponsible, ineffective, and unsuitable a candidate is for a position. Voters can already tell that if they win, they will take the council on a merry chase that leads nowhere and wastes time and resources.

7. *But to exercise his brain, the prince should read the history and study the actions of famous people, see how they behaved in war, find out the causes of their victory or defeat in order to avoid the latter and achieve the former. Above all, the prince ought to follow what these famous men, who found someone who had been famous and praised*

before them to imitate, have done in the past and keep their achievements and actions in mind.

You can never be too informed about a subject. After you are done keeping up to date with current practices, Machiavelli suggests that you go back to history to read and study the actions of those that have walked this path before you and see how they behaved, how much influence their behaviors had on their victories or defeat so that you can recreate the former and avoid the latter.

Read up on your local history. Check out political events from the past. How did the news report these incidents? Pay particular attention to those as it will provide feelers for your course of action.

A politician with foresight will be able to forecast where their opponent is headed by observing their actions and the reports from news articles. That way, when they make their move, you are not left scrambling to catch up, but ready to parry them blow for blow.

A wise prince should observe some of such rules. He must never remain idle during peaceful times but increase his knowledge in such a way that he is always ready to respond in the face of adversity so that when his fortune changes and bad luck comes, he is always prepared to resist them.

How Not to Lose Your Office

"It will be a great contempt for those born as princes to lose their country for their lack of wisdom." - Niccolò Machiavelli.

I f it is your first time in an office, chances are that you will be closely monitored by the media and general public compared to an incumbent. With an incumbent, they already know what to expect - their flaws, their strengths, their quirks. But newcomers have to first prove themselves and so they become a mystery that must be observed.

1. *The actions of a new prince are observed more often than those of a hereditary prince.*

Apart from the natural aversion that people have towards new changes, the people need reassurance that you will do right by them. They want to know that they made the right choice in voting you in and once you have reassured them of that, you will have their full support and loyalty, even quicker than what the former incumbents enjoy.

2. *When the new prince is considered capable, he attracts more people, and they are more loyal than the ancient princes. This is because people are more attracted to the present than the past and when they find good in the present, they enjoy it and don't seek more. They will also strongly defend the prince if he does not harm them in other matters.*

Machiavelli insists that if you don't ruffle feathers, pass too many restrictive laws, raise taxes, or trample on their rights, most people will be content and that contentment with what you are doing in the present will make them not to seek comfort in the 'good old days.'

So one thing you can do to not lose your office is to make sure that as many people as possible are aware of how capable and good your administration has been. Shamelessly promote yourself as an exemplary character for good governance. Be in their faces. Let your name appear next to many good deeds on the news, social media, and even blogs.

3. *So it will be a great glory for the prince to have formed a new kingdom and made the country rich with good laws, good troops, good allies and good leadership. Likewise, it will be a great contempt for those born as princes to lose their country for their lack of wisdom.*

Incumbents have several advantages over new politicians, and it is disgraceful when these advantages are not enough to assure them of a win. It is a stain on their reputation that they will not be able to get rid of should they decide to run for another office. To the public, that is ample proof that they could not get people to support their campaign despite the headstart that they have.

4. *Hence, our princes should not blame fate for losing their power after years of possession but rather their own laziness. In peaceful times, they never thought that times could change (it's a common human weakness that in peace, no one thinks to prepare for a storm). When chaos came, they only thought of running away instead of protecting themselves. They hoped that the subjects, who were disgusted with the attitudes of the conquerors, would call them back. This, when other things fail, might be good, but it's a bad thing to ignore all the other factors to choose this course.*

Machiavelli says that any incumbent that loses their seat does so due to their own incompetence and not because they had a turn of luck. They grew complacent, lazy, preoccupied, and failed to change with the times. Not preparing yourself enough for the future challenges that will come with your position will quickly make you lose your seat to another more prepared for it.

How to Wield the Power of the Incumbent

"Unless affected by extraordinary or excessive things, all he only has to do is maintain himself in this state." - Niccolò Machiavelli.

The power of the incumbent is an effective tool that allows a politician who already holds an office to be reelected. Like the quote above implies, an incumbent does not have to do anything extraordinary to remain - no brave acts, zealous reforms, or principled stands - just simple inertia from the electorate.

As long as it does not negatively affect them, people are comfortable with not making any changes in a system that already somewhat benefits them. That is why people will continue to vote for incumbents years after, even though they have forgotten the reason they chose them in the first place or they have become ineffective in office.

1. *It is easier to preserve hereditary monarchy, especially when the people are already used to living with their prince's family, than new ones. This is because most people will prefer the stability of customs that they are accustomed to over the new policies of a new ruling family. All that the prince needs to do is preserve his predecessor's customs and carefully resolve conflicts as they arise.*

Machiavelli believes that it is easier to control an office you already hold. As long as you do not introduce too many changes and stick to the status quo, you should get along fine with the electorate. You don't need to create innovative ideas because they could either be a hit or miss. Just continue as you were.

He is saying that you shouldn't rock the boat by trying to be innovative as your ideas could either be a hit or miss, and that is risky.

2. *Unless affected by extraordinary or excessive things, all he only has to do is maintain himself in this state. This way, if he loses his throne, it is easier for the prince to get it back when his usurper encounters misfortune.*

Machiavelli says that the prudent way for incumbents to act is to only behave in ways that will maintain their position. That is, keeping the same reputation and not jolting the public too much. Barring any extraordinary event, an incumbent will not lose elections and can easily remain in power, even when they are only average or mediocre.

He also adds that even though an incumbent loses their seat, they have a very good chance of being reelected if their successor makes enough mistakes to lose the confidence of the electorates. A case of "a devil you know is better than an angel you don't know."

PART FOUR

Fighting With a Team

One - Leadership

"The general is the pillar of the nation. If the pillar is solid, the nation is strong. If the pillar is loose, the nation is weak."- Sun Tzu.

As a leader, you are the backbone of your political team. If you are weak, then your decisions and orders would be as well. This is why it is important to pay more attention to your opponent than their team. No matter how competent the team appears to be, the leader still has to give a final stamp of approval before they do anything. So if your opponent is weak, expect that everything that comes from that camp would be as well. If they are known to play dirty, everything that comes out of their camp would be too.

1. *We were faced with three challenges by which a leader can bring misfortune on his army:*

    a. *First is that if it is unclear for the troops to advance, but we keep them advancing, or we are not sure if the troops can back up, but we just tell them to back up. That's called tying up the troops.*

    b. *The second challenge is that if the position of the internal affairs of the troops is also unclear, by interfering with the military management, the officers and soldiers would be confused.*

    c. *Thirdly, if the military principle of adaptation to circumstances is unclear, but you interfere with the responsibility of commanders, the generals would have doubts in their minds.*

All of these allude to one thing - that the chain of command from leaders to followers is broken. Leadership without a proper chain of command will only bring misfortune to yourself and your followers.

When World War I began in August 1914, the British and French were caught in a bitter stalemate with the Germans on the Western Front, while the Germans were beating the Russians, allies of Britain and France, on the Eastern side. So the British formulated a new strategy to attack Gallipoli, a peninsula on the Dardanelles Strait which opened up to Constantinople, Turkey. Turkey was an ally of Germany, and if they could take Gallipoli, it would be easy to take Constantinople, and Turkey would have to withdraw from battle. With the bases, they would form in Turkey and the Balkans, they could also attack Germany from the Southeast and weaken its focus on the Western Front.

They had created a wonderful plan, but everything depended on the victory at Gallipoli. The plan was approved, and Sir Ian Hamilton was called in to lead the command. Winston Churchill and Hamilton believed the plan was foolproof and they had enough men to conquer the Turks easily. The only order Churchill left was to take Constantinople; he left Hamilton to work out the details.

Hamilton's plan was to land at three points - the southwestern tip of the Gallipoli peninsula, north, and the beaches. From the very moment that the troops landed, everything that could go wrong did. The maps they got were inaccurate and they had landed in the wrong places. The beach was too narrow for the troops to pass, and the Turks were surprisingly fighting back. After the first day of landing, a large percentage of the army could not join the fight because they couldn't pass the beach without being pinned by the Turks. Gallipoli, that should have been an easy win, was becoming a nightmare.

When it looked like the plan had failed, Churchill was able to convince the government to send more troops. Hamilton created a new plan where he would land soldiers in Suvla Bay - a vulnerable target with a large harbor and few defenses. Attacking from this end would force the Turks to split and break the stalemate. Hamilton placed the most senior Englishman available, Lt. Gen Sir Frederick Stopford, to command the Suvla operation, and under him, Major General

Frederick Hammersley would lead a division. Neither of these men was Hamilton's first choice, but he had to make do.

Hamilton's style of leadership was to tell his officers what they hoped to achieve with a battle and leave them to figure out how to go about it. Stopford made some changes to the landing plan, and Hamilton acquiesced. However, this time he made one request. Once the Turks heard about the attack on Suvla, they would rush to fight. He wanted the troop to advance to a range of hills called Tekke Tepe before the Turks, so they could dominate them.

The plan was simple enough but in order not to offend Stopford by interfering with his duties, he kept it as vague as possible and worse, did not stipulate a timeframe. However, his orders were vague enough that Stopford completely misinterpreted them. Instead of ordering his men to get to the hills as soon as possible, he told them to get there if possible.

When the troops landed ashore, Stopford's change in the landing plans muddled things up. They didn't know what positions to take and their objectives, and Stopford had remained on a boat to control the battlefield, so they couldn't reach him on time for confirmation. They wasted the whole day relaying messages back and forth the boat to work out the tangled mess of the plans.

Hamilton began to suspect things were not going according to plans, so the next morning, he went to investigate. On getting there, he realized that nobody had been able to do one thing right out of the plan they created for attack. Before they could rally together to fix the mistake, the Turks had already taken the Tekke Tepe hills and they lost their advantage.

Hamilton's plan was foolproof and would have worked but he forgot one important detail - the chain of command. A leadership with a broken chain of command will leave everyone confused and, in the confusion, your opponents might find opportunity to harass you, like Sun Tzu says below.

2. *If the troops were suspicious and bewildered, the vassal countries would have the opportunity to harass. This is called self-disordered troops and it is to lead others to victory.*

Hamilton's troops threw away the one chance they had at victory because they were confused and running around in circles, which gave their opponents enough time to regroup and attack. A leader's job is to ensure the team remains clear on their goals, mission, and vision, otherwise, everything descends into anarchy that the opponent can exploit.

No matter how advantageous your position is or how well-ordered your strategy is, if everyone on your team is not reading from the same page, you will lose that advantage - just as Hamilton did.

Choosing Your Team

"The first impression that one gets of a prince is by observing those around him." - Niccolò Machiavelli.

The first impression that anyone would have about you is your team. Before the public meets you to get to know you, they must have already had an interaction with members of your team. While you are the body, members of your team are the tentacles through which you have wider reach. In terms of how your team should represent you, Machiavelli had the following to say:

1. *The choice of personal staff is very important to the prince. Whether they are good or not depends on the prince's discrimination. The first impression that one gets of a prince is by observing those around him. If they are capable and loyal, the prince can be considered wise because he already knows how to recognize their abilities and keep them loyal. But when they were the opposite, people would unfavorably criticize the prince for the grave error that he made in choosing the wrong person.*

Just as the kind of counsel that you receive is an extension of your wisdom as a leader, the kind of people you choose to be part of your team shape your reputation as a leader. They are a direct and physical manifestation of your values and your sense of judgment. Everything they do is a direct reflection of yourself, so you have to be very careful when picking them.

If your team is capable and loyal, it adds prestige to your reputation but if they are the opposite, it is a big stain on your honor, and you will attract criticisms for making an error in judgment.

When choosing your councilors and other staff that will work closely with you, take the utmost care to make sure you have made the right choice. Make sure that the people representing you as delegates on several boards are equal to the task and able to pass on your exact message without deviating to further their own agenda. Even better, make sure that even when you are not present or monitoring them, they can effectively manage your decisions and wishes.

It, therefore, makes sense that your team should be made up of wise, capable, and smart people who can do their jobs without micromanagement from you. The lack of micromanagement will help them do their jobs better and encourage loyalty because you have given them a position of power, honor, and respect.

2. *The human mind has three types. The first one understands things by itself, the second has to listen to explanations to understand, and the third doesn't self-understand nor understand when it is explained. The first is the best, the second is good, and the third is useless.*

There are three types of people - those who are naturally smart, the ones that understand that others may be smarter and listen to them to learn, and those who are too stupid to realize they aren't smart or who cannot listen to understand when people smarter than they try to explain things.

As said, the first set of people are the best because they work instinctively without micromanagement. The second set of people are okay because they are willing to learn and, with time will be able to stand on their own. But the third set of people are absolutely useless to you. If you cannot attract the first set to join your team, then settle for the second. But by every means ignore the third set of people.

However, in typical Machiavelli manner, there are caveats:

3. *He had the judgment to know the good and the bad when it was said and done, and although he may not have the initiative himself, he could recognize the good and the bad in his employees. He praised the good and corrected the bad. Therefore, they could not hope to deceive him but were kept honest.*

The first caveat is to make sure that you can recognize both the good and bad people on your team so you can praise the good and condemn the bad. That way, you can tell that they are not sycophants, flatterers, or fools.

How can you then tell the difference between a genuine employee or a sycophant? Machiavelli lists it as his second caveat:

4. *When a prince sees an employee thinking more about his own interests than prince interests and searching for his own profits in everything, such a person never makes a good servant. The prince could never trust him either, because he who has the responsibility of another in his hands should never think of himself but always of the prince and never pay attention to matters that the prince does not care about.*

Be on the lookout for employees who are more self-serving than being concerned about your interests as a politician. You cannot trust them to have your best interests at heart because anyone that has been entrusted to manage your affairs should not be bothered about chasing causes that do not align with your goals.

Early morning of June 17, 1972, brought about one of the biggest scandals that shook the American political scene when several burglars were arrested as they tried to break into the Democratic National Committee office located in the Watergate complex in Washington, DC. However, these burglars were not your regular run-of-the-mill robbers as they were a part of Richard Nixon's re-election team and had been caught red-handed as they stole documents and wiretapped phones.

Before the Watergate break-in, the political scene in America was deeply divided, what with the United States' involvement in the Vietnam War. So, for President Richard M. Nixon to get better chances at re-election, they needed a more aggressive campaign strategy. The members of Nixon's campaign team called the Committee to Re-Elect the President (derisively called CREEP), decided that illegal espionage would be the tool they needed. So they broke into the Democratic National Committee's headquarters in Watergate to bug the office phones and steal copies of top-secret documents.

The installed phone taps did not work properly, so on that fateful morning, a group of five burglars went back to the building to fix the wiretap. As they were preparing to break into the offices, a security guard on duty noticed that someone had taped over many of the door locks on the building. He immediately raised the alarm and called the police, who arrived just in time to catch the burglars red-handed with the new wiretaps.

When the culprits were first arrested, nobody made the connection between them and Nixon's team, but when during the preliminary search, detectives found copies of the phone number for Nixon's re-election committee among their belongings, it began to raise suspicions. So an investigation was launched to get to the bottom of it.

Seeing how the blowback from the incident could hurt his career, Nixon gave a speech in August where he swore that none of his staff was involved in the break-in. Because Nixon was well-loved and famous, many of the electorates believed him, and he won his reelection in a landslide victory.

However, investigations proved that Nixon was not entirely truthful about his involvement in the affair. For example, a few days after the break-in, he had arranged to pay the burglars hundreds of thousands of dollars in hush money.

Discovering that he was caught, Nixon tried to bury the evidence that has been discovered. So he and his aides concocted a plan to make the CIA frustrate the FBI's progress on the case. To cover up a crime of espionage, Nixon committed an even bigger crime - abusing his power as the president to deliberately obstruct justice.

Seven co-conspirators in the espionage were rounded up and indicted on charges relating to the Watergate scandal. Nixon aides urged five of them to plead guilty and avoid trial, while the remaining two were sentenced to jail in January 1973.

The case had begun to attract the attention of several people (including Bob Woodward and Carl Bernstein, two reporters for the Washington Post, John J. Sirica, a trial judge, and a handful of members of the Senate investigating committee), who had begun to suspect that something bigger was in play.

Around the same time that some of the conspirators had begun to sweat under the heat of the cover-up, Woodward and Bernstein got an anonymous tip containing key information from a whistleblower called "Deep Throat."

They had finally broken through and gotten to a few of Nixon's aides, including the White House counsel John Dean, who testified about their involvement in the affair and the role the president had to play in it. They even testified that Nixon secretly taped all the meetings in the Oval Office, and if the prosecutors could lay hands on those tapes, they would have enough proof of the president's guilt.

Nixon tried to protect the tapes with his lawyers, arguing that his executive privilege allowed him to keep the contents of the tapes private. However, the Senate committee, Judge Sirica, and an independent prosecutor by the name of Archibald Cox were all determined to lay their hands on it.

On October 20, 1973, when Cox would not stop demanding the release of the tape, Nixon had him fired, which led several officials of the Justice Department to voluntarily resign in protest. This series of events became known as the Saturday Night Massacre. Eventually, Nixon gave in and surrendered some of the tapes.

By the beginning of 1974, all of the efforts to obstruct the investigation and the cover-up began to unravel. On March 1, a grand jury (appointed by a new special prosecutor) indicted seven of Nixon's former aides on several charges relating to the scandal. Not knowing if they could indict a sitting president, the jury named Nixon an "unindicted co-conspirator."

The Supreme Court ordered Nixon to submit all the tapes, and while he was still dragging his feet, the House Judiciary Committee voted in the agreement of his impeachment for abuse of power, criminal cover-up, obstruction of justice, and several other constitutional violations.

When Nixon finally released the tapes on August 5, it provided irrefutable proof of his involvement in the Watergate scandal. With impeachment looming on the horizon, Nixon decided to resign in disgrace on August 8.

When the Vice President was sworn in as president six weeks later, he pardoned Nixon for all the crimes he committed while in office. However, his aides were not so lucky as they were convicted for serious crimes and sent to federal prison.

John Mitchell, Nixon's Attorney General of the United States, served 19 months in jail for the part he played. The same applied to his Chief of Staff, H.R. Haldeman. John Ehrlichman spent 18 months in jail for attempting to cover up the break-in and the mastermind of the plot - G. Gordon Liddy, a former FBI agent -spent four and a half years in jail.

Although Nixon never openly admitted to any criminal actions, he acknowledged using poor judgment. It is obvious that his problems began when he chose the wrong group of people to work on his campaign team.

Chapter Twenty-Three

Organizing Your Team

"There has never been a new prince who has disarmed his subjects. On the contrary, whenever he has found them unarmed, he has always armed them. For when they are armed, those arms become yours." -
Niccolò Machiavelli.

One of the first things you should do when you get into the office is to gather your team. Find competent people who supported you in your campaign and reward them by giving them a place on your team. Because they will only enjoy their rewards when you remain in office, they will become your staunchest defender in the community. Machiavelli explains it better here:

1. *For when they are armed, those arms become yours; those who used to be mistrustful become loyal, and those who were loyal remain the same; from your subjects, they become your loyalists. Although not everyone can be armed, when those who you do arm benefit, the others can be dealt with more freely.*

Arms, in this case, are not military weapons but the power, privilege, authority, position, and status you reward your staff with. Giving a few people the power to represent you in places is a way to arm them.

The ones that you arm will appreciate it and be indebted to you. Even those who do not benefit from gaining positions will understand the importance of your choice. He further says:

2. *Although the treatments are different, they fully understand. Those who are armed become your supporters, and those who aren't armed,*

accepting that those who have more dangerous responsibilities should have the highest reward would excuse you.

Although the treatments are different, they understand and hope that in their continued support, you will also reward them with positions.

3. *On the contrary, when disarmed, the prince insults them by showing that he does not trust them, either out of cowardice or for want of loyalty. Both of these prejudices create hatred against the prince, and because he cannot be unarmed, he has to turn to the worthless mercenaries, as I have discussed.*

However, you have to note that once you give them positions, you cannot take them back, or it will cause them to lose face, and that will make an enemy out of your previous supporters - the worst kind to have.

4. *But when a prince occupies a new kingdom and adds it to his old one, it is necessary for him to disarm the newly conquered people, except those who helped the prince occupy the territory. These people, also, with time and opportunity, should be rendered weak and cowardly. Matters need to be managed in such a way that those who are armed in the state are only the prince's soldiers, who were raised in the old kingdom.*

So, where possible, put your own people in positions, especially sensitive ones, where they can watch your back and defend you if the need arises. Be on the lookout for committees, boards, even staff positions where you think having an inside person will serve you. However, this does not mean that you have to completely fill up the position with your supporters and neglect the others. But you can slowly sideline and weaken their influence over time so that only your strongest supporters have all the authority.

Reward and Punishment

"To keep his servants honest, a prince must reward, honor, enrich, be kind, share his glory, and care for them." - Niccolò Machiavelli.

For this chapter, we will revisit Ulysses Grant's story in chapter sixteen. Machiavelli insists that the right way to keep your staff honest is to reward, honor, enrich them, be kind, care for them, and share your glory with them.

Ulysse Grant did all of that with his friends from the Civil War when he gave them cushiony jobs in the government as a reward for their association with him, cared for, and enriched them. Yet, it was not enough to make them remain honest and blame-free.

Does that mean that Machiavelli's advice had no merit? No, because he had an additional clause that said:

1. *At the same time, he must show them that they cannot stand alone.*

According to Machiavelli, in enriching and catering for your staff, do not make the mistake of allowing them to think that they have enough power to operate on their own. This is obviously where Grant began to get it wrong.

He gave his staff too much leeway and space, and with the wings, he had allowed them to sprout, they flew straight into the sun, dragging him along with them.

It is good to delegate duties, as it proves to your staff that you trust and respect them. However, remember that giving your staff rank means you have bestowed on them the power associated with it. The moment you give them enough power to get their head drunk, they could turn and use that power against you.

2. *At the same time, he must show them that they cannot stand alone. So that receiving a lot of honors will not make them want more, much wealth does not make them desire more, and many burdens make them afraid of changes.*

Power is a heady thing. Once someone tastes it, especially one that never imagined they could ever get access to that kind of power, it becomes a drug they cannot do without. They will keep wanting more. So to avoid that kind of conspiracy, Machiavelli advised that you show your staff that without you, they would be nothing. Make them understand that their continued reward comes from the longevity of your position in power.

Everything that Babcock got he did because of his proximity to the president, but he didn't understand that. If he did, he would have realized how his actions were direct jeopardy to Grant's position and therefore, indirectly his.

3. *Once the relationship between the prince and the servants is kept at that level, they can trust each other. Otherwise, the end is always destructive, either for one or the other.*

Machiavelli insists that once you have found that spot where you have made your staff indebted to you, then you can trust them with your heart and vice versa. Otherwise, they will take you down when they spiral into self-destruction.

Managing Your Resources

"It is better for one to lose with his own army than to win the battle with auxiliary soldiers, as you cannot consider any victory won with them as being real." - Niccolò Machiavelli.

When Machiavelli discussed this subject in his book, he talked about soldiers in terms of war, but in the context of politics, your soldiers are the resources that will help you to fight and win against your opponents - finances, manpower, media, campaign, goodwill, etc. When it looks like your resources alone cannot help you win the battle over your opponents, the temptation to call in reinforcements from other people you consider allies is always there. However, Machiavelli expressly states that in that way lies the danger.

1. *The armies that a prince uses to protect his nation are either his own or mercenaries or auxiliary or mixed.*

There are four ways with which you can use the resources available to acquire a political position. You can either use yours alone, loan from several people who have no skin in the game (mercenaries), use your biggest political ally as a support system (auxiliary), or maintain a system that mixes all of them together. However, apart from using your own resources and abilities, the rest have limitations that Machiavelli has so kindly pointed out.

2. *The mercenaries and auxiliary forces are useless and dangerous. If a prince holds a nation that relies on these armies, then it is unstable and insecure because they are disunited, ambitious, indisciplined, unfaithful, courageous in the presence of friends, and cowardly in the*

presence of enemies. They are not afraid of God and are dishonest to people.

As he has stated, it is a dangerous thing to leave yourself at the mercy of others when it comes to resources because you cannot rely on them to always come through for you. At best, that makes your position unstable and precarious. At worst, that leaves you open for your opponent to tear apart completely.

If you have to bring in help from outside, it might be difficult to hold them united to your purpose and against your opponents. That is because people tend to be selfish and self-serving. They will always put their interests first, and if it so happens that your goals do not align with theirs, they have no qualms about throwing you under the bus completely.

3. *Destruction is postponed only as long as an attack is postponed, for in peace, they will plunder you, and in war, your enemy will. In fact, they have no other interest or reason for fighting other than a small stipend, which is not enough money to make them die for your cause. They are willing enough to be your soldiers while you are at peace, but if war comes, they either disappear or run from the enemy.*

Mercenaries are only in the game as long as they profit from it. Their loyalty goes to the highest bidder, so their support is very tenuous, volatile, and subject to change when someone with a better offer comes along. They do not have any skin in your political war, so they have nothing to lose if you lose or gain if you win, so long as you give them their compensation for helping you.

They are one of the weakest links you could have - at war, your opponents can exploit them to crumble your plans, and if you are at peace, they could be the ones exploiting you to their self-interest. When all seems to be going well, they will remain in your corner to back you up, but as soon as the first sign of trouble comes, they have no problems jumping ship and leaving you to drown in the brewing mess. They are not reliable at all.

4. *I want to further demonstrate the dangers of these soldiers. The mercenary captains are either capable men or not. If they are, one cannot trust them because they always aspire to their personal greatness,*

383

either by oppressing you, who is their master, or others against your will. But if the captain is incompetent, then you are destroyed in the usual way.

There are two ways by which the one who controls the resources you want to borrow can ruin you - by their competence and incompetence. If they are competent, they may begin to recognize opportunities that you are missing, or their greed can get in the way, and they will look for how to disenfranchise you to take your place. However, if they are incompetent, your ruin will come from the usual avenues.

Francesco Sforza served as a mercenary for Filippo Maria Visconti, Duke of Milan, and fought for and against him over a period of 20 years. But in that time, he started eyeing the seat of Milan, so he got betrothed to Filippo's only daughter and child, hoping to one day inherit the kingdom. However, his relationship with his would-be father-in-law was strenuous.

In 1434, Cosimo de Medici offered a large reward, including a seat in Florence to fight against Milan. Fighting for the Florentine-Venetian league against Milan, he won Verona in 1438 and defeated Milan in Anghiari in 1440. The next year, he married his fiancée during a period of uneasy truce. However, the truce did not last long, and he was soon fighting against his father-in-law again in 1443.

In 1447, the duke of Milan fell seriously ill while under threat of attack from a Venetian army, so he sent for his mercenary son-in-law to help. Before Francesco got to Milan, the duke died, and he found out that instead of willing the Duchy to him, his father-in-law had given it to Alfonso of Aragon, the King of Naples.

The Milanese took advantage of the confusion to rebel and proclaimed themselves a republic with Francesco as their captain-general. This sparked a three-pronged struggle between Venice, Francesco, and the Milanese republic. In 1449, Milan went behind Francesco to create a peace pact with Venice, and in response, he besieged the city and starved it into surrender. Therefore, in 1450, Francesco Sforza became the Duke of Milan after acting as a mercenary for years for the old one.

5. *I should have little difficulty proving this, for the destruction of Italy was caused but nothing else but relying on mercenaries for help for many years. Although they used to make some feats in the past and appeared brave among themselves, yet when enemy nations came, they showed us the truth about them.*

When the king of Naples, Ferdinard I offended Pope Innocent VIII by not paying his feudal dues to the papacy, he was excommunicated and banned from ruling Naples, and the Pope gave the Kingdom of Naples to Charles VIII, the grandson of the French King, Charles VII. This ushered in the French to Italy.

Just before the pope died, he made peace with Ferdinard and revoked the ban. However, the offer made to Charles VIII was still a bone of contention in Italy. There was also a third claim to the throne of Naples by Rene II, the Duke of Lorraine. The people of Naples had already offered the crown to Rene, but Charles VIII blocked it, saying he had more rights to the throne because his mother was closer than Rene's in the line of succession. In 1494, Ferdinand died and was succeeded by his son, Alfonso II.

That same year, Ludovico Sforza, who had been managing the Duchy of Milan, decided to claim it as his after showing a weak connection to the seat. However, Alfonso II challenged him over it because he also had claims to the throne. In the bid to get Alfonso out of his way, Ludovico encouraged Charles VIII to take Innocent's offer and claim the throne of Naples as his.

Charles VIII gathered an army of 25,000 soldiers, 8,000 of them being Swiss mercenaries, and blew through Italy to claim his seat. Thus, the first Italian war began, and it ushered in a slew of subsequent wars from other European countries seeking to take control of the divided Italian states.

However, Ludovico seeing how quickly Charles breezed through Italy and realizing his error in judging the French's power, became alarmed. Charles also had a claim to Milan, and he was afraid he wouldn't be satisfied with conquering only Naples. So he formed the League of Venice along with the emperor Maximilian I, the pope, and King Ferdinand II of Aragon to chase Charles out of Italy, and it worked.

However, the war already left behind its damage. The Italian states were weakened and left them vulnerable to the conflicting ambitions of both France and Spain. Charles' successor, Louis XII, seeing as he had some claim to both Milan and Naples, started plotting to invade the cities. The Venetians, having a short memory and not learning from their past mistakes, invited Louis XII to help them capture Lombardy on the premise that he would give them half of the Kingdom. King Louis invaded Lombardy, seized Milan, and quickly set his eyes on Naples.

Concerning the use of auxiliary armies, Machiavelli had the following to say:

6. *These soldiers can be helpful and good to their master, but it is a disadvantage to the one who asks for it. Because if they lose, the prince is ruined, and if they win, the prince becomes under their control.*

In the hands of your political allies, these resources may yield stellar results but accepting help and resources from them puts you at a great disadvantage. If they lose, you lose as well, but if they win, it places you under the control of your ally. They may want to use their help to cash in favors, some of which may be too costly for you to pay.

7. *Therefore, let those who have no ambitions to conquer use auxiliary troops, for they are much more dangerous than mercenaries. For them, your ruin is predetermined because they are all united and obey their commanders. But with the mercenaries, when they have won the battle, need more time and better opportunities to hurt you. They are unified, having been found and paid by you. Their commander is a third party installed by you, therefore, making it impossible for him to immediately have the authority to hurt you.*

Where the auxiliary soldiers become more dangerous to use than mercenaries is that they already have a functioning system and answer to one person that is not you. When you use the system of resources that your ally already set up, it is up to them to determine who they can spare to join your team, control the funds you receive, etc. - everyone is in their pocket. They can decide to sabotage you and will be successful because you do not have the resources to fight them back.

However, when you use several sources, it will take quite a lot of time for them to rally around a common cause for sabotaging you before they can act, buying you enough time to pull the plug on the plans. Either way, it is clear that using any of these methods is quite dangerous.

8. *A wise prince will, therefore, always avoid these types of soldiers and use his own army. It is better for one to lose with his own army than to win the battle with auxiliary or mercenary soldiers, as you cannot consider any victory won with them as being real.*

It is therefore advisable that you build your own system and effectively manage your resources, so you will not have to solicit help from others who will not hesitate to pull you down when the need arises.

CONCLUSION

Is there merit in converting the strategies in *The Law of War, The Prince,* and *The Five Spheres* into strategies for political warfare? Absolutely! You may not be able to draw the connections between them at first glance, but you can definitely see that the core essence of these strategies has been practiced in political circles from time immemorial.

There is a common theme behind these strategies, and that is flexibility. If you recall, from my introduction, I mentioned that society has tried to box us into acting according to predetermined structures to maintain some form of civil and fair order. But the reality is quite different. Life is chaos, and only those who are able to adapt to chaotic situations will thrive.

The world is not looking for more "good" people. We would benefit more from having capable people who are not afraid to do all it takes to bring the desired results that we can enjoy. Throughout history, there are stories of good people who, in their fair dealings, only made things worse than they should be.

In the line of battle, if you were to hand over responsibility for your life, would you choose a capable general or a good general? The problem with good people is that they always expect the rest of the world to be good as well. They will not account for the great evil that human beings are capable of.

On the other hand, capable leaders will take all of these into consideration and choose flexible means to deal with each situation according to how they merit. The world would benefit more from more capable leaders, and I hope that with this book, we can begin to work towards creating the movement.

INSIGHTS TO BETTER LIVING

Dive Into A Well-Being Lifestyle
With Lao Tzu

INTRODUCTION

The desires of man are insatiable such that when we create a goal and achieve it, we seek more, more money, influence, beauty, power, and the list goes on. It's no wonder the disharmony and imbalance we experience as individuals first, as a society, then as a nation, and lastly, the world at large. When we search deep within our hearts and critically get to the root of the violence and injustice we see in our environment, we can only come to one point, greed. Why do we seek more at the expense of others? Why is the Peace of our world threatened? Were we created for violence, famine, war, strife, and killings? Are natural disasters natural? Why does plastic surgery, feminism, racism, transgender, etc., seem to be the order of the day? These and many other questions have weighed the hearts of many of us.

In our search for happiness, freedom, wealth, and abundance, we forget that the things we seek must not conquer our inner Peace, Harmony, and Balance. The words Harmony, Balance, and Peace, if you notice, are repetitive. Peace is a state of tranquility, being free from thoughts and emotions that make you oppressed or restless. On the other hand, harmony is the ability to be united with yourself, being in togetherness with your personality, both good and evil, accepting your makeup. Finally, Balance is a state of equilibrium or stability. These highlighted words make up the foundation of Tao - The Way.

Earth, as we know it today, was not like this centuries ago. It was a scenic, picturesque, pleasant, and balanced place to live in. The energy (Qi) that flowed from its cardinal points brought Peace and abundance to humans and their inhabitants. What changed? The Earth or humans? The answer is quite glaring. We changed, and it affected the Earth's balance causing chaos and disrupting the flow of energy; hence, we experience natural (earthquakes, volcanic eruptions, hurricanes, etc.) and artificial disasters (global warming, desertification, oil spills, etc.).

The Way-Tao is a way of life that prioritizes Nature. Our oneness and balance with Nature will enlighten our spirits to see life's beauty and true essence. In this book, *"Insights To Better Living,"* we see a practical way to help us achieve the Harmony needed for our abundance while we journey through Earth.

As a famous quote goes, "where there is no law, there is no order." Laws, principles, codes of conduct, ethics, and punishments are put in place to govern our society effectively and put things in order. As humans, we have unique features that distinguish us from the other inhabitants of the Earth, such as our components of higher, complex thinking, problem-solving skills, will, and expressive nature. Therefore, about The Book of Ethics by Lao Tzu, which talks about the Way and virtues that should govern our culture and belief systems in poems, this book was developed as a guide to help you reflect and live your life at its maximum potential.

The book is divided into three parts: Part 1- The Body, Part 2 - The Spirit, and Part 3 - The Harmony of the Body and Spirit. The body is the reason we exist on Earth. Without the body, there is no functioning, no life; in fact, all we hope to achieve will be shadows. Another quote says, "Health is Wealth." Honestly, it is indeed. We know individuals or even individuals with unharnessed potentials, strong drive, will, passion, great ideas, fantastic problem-solving skills, to mention a few but, we are limited for factors like age, environment, diet and nutrition, physical well-being. When we have a deteriorating body, we become hindrances to ourselves and to others around us. Hence, the motivation for healthier living and hygiene. Taking care of your body is what you owe yourself to attain heights. You are responsible for what you eat and drink, and you also bear the consequences of the unhealthy lifestyle principles you live by. How do you perceive your body? How much worth have you accrued your body to be? Invest in your body, and it is the container that will get you before Kings and even make you one yourself.

Our spirit component is also vital in our quest for greatness and abundance. The state of our inner self and consciousness is discussed extensively in this book. Every mishap and violence happening in the world today was birthed from within. What is the state of your spirit? Have you learned to channel the flow of Nature's energy effectively? Why is our spirit essential? Out of the abundance of our hearts (spirit) yields the troubles of life. A lot of us do not pay attention to what or who we indeed are within. You can come to self-realization through meditation, yoga, and other healthy practices bolstered in the book.

Man is both body and spirit; both components are needed to be in Harmony with themselves. Harmony with our body components provides a balance that transcends to our environment, society, and our world at large. Every chapter of this book aims to spur us into a healthier and more natural way of living for our peace and world peace.

Going through every page and part of this book is an eye-opener that enlightens your spirit to live the right way. Never forget to be your number one motivation. You are the change the world needs. It has and will always begin with you. Be it and Earn it the Nature's Way.

PART I

The Body

Chapter One

The origin of the human body

In his book The Grand Design, physicist Stephen Hawking states that the laws of physics do not admit the possibility that the universe was created by God. If we reflect on the development of knowledge from the Renaissance to the present day, we can affirm that humanity is dismantling, relying on science, the entire set of religious beliefs about the world and nature, built or elaborated up to that historical moment. Modern science at the head of giants like Copernicus, Galileo, Kepler, Newton and closer to us, the entire generation of physicists at the beginning of the 20th century, has done nothing more than demonstrate that the universe is studied from itself, without need to resort to external forces. What Hawking does is reconfirm this current of thought.

The Catholic Church responded to these advances in the knowledge of nature with violence, burning alive (Giordano Bruno) or threatening to do so (Galileo), anyone who dared to disagree with its postulates of faith and its dogmatic beliefs. There is nothing so dangerous as the certainty of being in possession of the absolute truth. This belief has been the source of tragic human religious or political conflicts. Science, on the contrary, is not dogmatic, it proposes the openness and provisionality of knowledge.

This fact combines better with the flexibility present in the natural and social processes in which humans develop. The problem seems to be that unlike myth and religion which offer a vision of the whole and offer answers to all questions, science leaves a space of uncertainty since its answers are partial and feasible to reevaluate. With modernity, we then enter a world of true, verifiable but modifiable beliefs and we leave behind a world of false but coherent and total beliefs.

In any case, physics, despite its advances in the knowledge of the universe and the composition of matter, did not articulate with the human. The most forceful blow did not come then from this science, but from biology, from Darwin's theory about how species have evolved to give way to the many and wonderful diversity that is expressed before our eyes.

Darwin's theory thus becomes the greatest work of human thought by pointing out the mechanism by which all life on the planet has changed, has evolved in the course of time, how the offspring is modified from cumulative changes in time giving rise to some species giving rise to others, generating an ordered variability. Darwin dismantled an idea fixed in the minds of men and reinforced by religious thought, the immutability of species. Men and women thought that species were fixed, that they did not change, that they had been created once and for all by a creator. Darwin proposed change, the mechanism of natural selection that explains in a simple way, how some species can give rise to others. That is, we are all related. Marvelous!

Darwinian theory is completely sound and is accepted as fact today in the scientific community. There are discussions and debates but within the theory, not outside of it. It is a solid but open theory, not dogmatic. All the advances since the publication of Darwin's book have confirmed the fact of evolution. Paleontology and the fossil record, molecular biology and genome structure, comparative morphology, have offered empirical evidence about the evolutionary process.

Of course, religious ideas are part of our cultural heritage and are solid ideas in the minds of men, which permeate what we have been culturally. Religion and myth have helped us to endure the anguish generated by human consciousness. But religious ideas are only a possibility of our cognitive structure. The theory of evolution clashes head-on with the force of these ancient beliefs. But from 1543, the year of the publication of the book of Copernicus, the sun stopped rotating around the earth. And since 1859, the year of the publication of Darwin's book, the origin and diversity of species, including humans, ceased to have a creator. It is not easy to see and accept that there is no God, that we are simply one more species, like any other.

We should not fear seeing ourselves as is in the mirror. This blind and indifferent conception contains new ways of conceiving our lives. If we are able to recognize ourselves as a species, that therefore we are genomically related to distant and close species in the phylogeny, that we come from the natural world, whether we want to or not, we make a unity with that world, then a new ethic based in respect for nature so necessary in the face of predation practiced by current societies.

On the other hand, the idea of the absence of a creator, of a protective father, of a superior being to whom we can turn in moments of anxiety and anguish, generates psychological and corporeal distress. Thinking like this leads to a feeling of infinite loneliness. But that is precisely the human side of evolutionary theory. We are not dependent on anyone except ourselves. The course of humanity will be the sole responsibility of humanity itself. We are products of our own decisions. Like any species, we live on the edge, always on the edge, but extinction or survival will be the result of our own actions.

This awareness of loneliness, of who we really are, should lead us to recognize the value of human relationships. Perhaps we are alone as a species, but not as individuals since we count on others as support and traveling companions. That should be enough for us.

Scientific perspectives

The field of human evolution constitutes a multidisciplinary field of research, Paleoanthropology, highly controversial and in a constant state of boiling and change. In fact, the world related to our origins has revealed remarkable complexity and generated heated debates from the very moment that the theory of evolution was accepted by the scientific community.

Australopithecus afarensis

The subject is prone to multiple disagreements because it is an aspect of biological thought with a tendency to subjectivity, something that, on the other hand, is recognized today in practically all scientific work. But in addition, the interpretation of human origins has been overloaded with considerable gender bias. Let us clarify that with the term "gender" we refer not only to the biological differences between one sex and the other of the human species, but also to the social and cultural differences attributed to people based on their sex.

It is revealing to bear in mind that Paleanthropology is a recently created scientific discipline (early 20th century) and, practically until the 1970s, the vast majority of scholars dedicated to the subject were men. This situation has caused the interpretation of our evolutionary history to have been polarized by a notable androcentrism, that is, the identification of the masculine with the human in general. In this context, and despite the great variation in explanatory models proposed over the years, there has been a common denominator: giving the female sex a very insignificant role in such a significant process.

Homo Sapiens

Until just a few decades ago, scholars viewed women as simply passive participants in evolutionary change, and limited themselves to relegating them to the role of giving birth, feeding, and caring for their young. While, on the contrary, men were described as responsible for many of the innovations that define us as humans, for example, the emergence of bipedal gait, brain enlargement, tool-making, cooperative communication or symbolic representation.

Thus, it should not be surprising that research related to our evolution has, and still does, carry away the conventional sexist bias that has permeated the academic world and the models it produces for centuries. In reality, evolutionary studies have not moved in a vacuum, but immersed within the same line as the cultural history of the West. In fact, we all carry a "baggage": our gender matters, just as it matters who our teachers were, where we study, when we study, what our religion is, our cultural heritage, and so on. As the American biologist Ruth Hubbard has noted, among others: "There is no such thing: an objective, value-free science."

It can therefore be said that the androcentric bias that has weighed down studies on human evolution has been present since Darwin placed humanity within the evolutionary framework.

The recognized and admired father of the theory of evolution, following a tradition that came from ancient times, admitted without qualms, at least publicly, the superiority of man over woman as an indisputable characteristic of nature. We find it interesting to highlight the deep sexism that permeated Darwinian thought, one of the most influential in the history of biology.

Darwin's theory left women in the gutter of evolution

The Darwinian revolution, which changed so many things and swept away so many prejudices from the natural sciences, did not change the view held for centuries about the "natural" inferiority of women with respect to men. The only notable change in this regard was that hierarchical differences between the human sexes, previously attributed to the god or gods, were now attributed to science.

Although many have blamed the English naturalist for the evolutionary underestimation of the female sex, many experts today claim that it was mainly some of his exalted followers - "more Darwinists than Darwin" - who defended such marginalization most emphatically.

However, The Origin of Man, the book in which Darwin devoted more space to women, was a clear reflection of its author's attempt to turn this ancient prejudice into "scientific truth": women "by nature" are inferior to men. The scientist affirmed that many of the typical faculties of the female sex (intuition, rapid perception and perhaps also those of imitation) "are proper and characteristic of inferior races, and therefore correspond to a past and lower state of culture."

In contrast to these feminine characteristics, she emphasized that "the man developed superior mental faculties, such as observation, reason, invention or imagination" that, finally, made him superior to women in all areas. Darwin concluded: "in body and spirit man is more powerful than woman."

To explain male supremacy, the famous Briton, and most of his in-numerable followers, resorted to the different functions that the two sexes of the human species fulfilled. Since the natural function of men was to support and protect women and their young, they had to fight for survival in dangerous activities that required great intelligence. This obligation of care and supply was the engine that led them to develop great courage, aggressiveness and energy.

Nature, on the other hand, made less demands on women since, being their only activity procreation and nurturing, their role was purely physical. They hardly fought, their food supply to the group was secondary, they did not have to solve new situations or face risks, challenges, etc. The reproduction and care of the offspring required only passive and domestic maternal qualities.

Supported by this reasoning, Darwin argued that the value of a woman lay in her reproductive organs. And, since neither the development of a child in the womb, nor delivery or milk production depended on the female ability to think, they did not require that their brains and minds evolve at a speed equal to that of males.

Male activity

Darwinian reasoning further held that men in general had acquired the ability to think first; as this trait was crucial for survival it then passed to women, which allowed them to evolve as well. In other words, thanks to the fact that girls and boys inherit the characters in an equivalent way, the evolution ran evenly for both sexes. In this sense, the naturalist reflected: "if it were not for the law of equality in the transmission of inheritance, the physical and intellectual difference that separates us from women would still be greater than it is."

Only when referring to reproduction, in Chapter IV of The Origin of Man, Darwin attributed to women an important evolutionary role. According to the scientist, in most species the members of one sex, usually the male, compete with each other for access to mating with the other sex. But, he also considered that female predilections for accepting a mate had an influence: the chosen males achieved greater reproductive success compared to those who were not chosen.

In this regard, he wrote: «In courtship, of the two sexes, the male is the most active member. The female, on the other hand, with very rare exceptions, is less impatient than the male... she [although] shy and passive, in general exercises some choice and accepts a male preferring him over others.

It is evident that the core of the Darwinian thesis contained a contradiction: the female sex carries out the sexual choice but at the same time its attitude is one of great passivity. This is a paradox that was hardly discussed when the book came out. Rather to the contrary, it was overlooked. In fact, efforts were concentrated on underlining the subordinate role in which the great scientist had placed women.

Finally, it is interesting to insist that The Origin of Man (1871) generated an avalanche of discussions and endless replies among the scientific community and in society in general, both at the time it was published and later.

However, with regard to the situation of women, saving the last decades, there have been almost no controversies that reached the general public, but rather a tacit majority acceptance of Darwinian theses. In reality, it should not surprise us too much since these theses hardly changed the dominant conceptions and no one felt, at least openly, offended or surprised by the sexist content of the work of such a famous author.

Today, although considerably less widespread than in the past, androcentrism still persists. And this is not a marginal abnormality. As the American essayist Adrienne Rich has so well pointed out: "objectivity is the name given in patriarchal society to male subjectivity."

Religious perspectives

The religious perspective about the origin of man is the belief of a divine creation is responsible for the life and the universe, contrary to scientific consensus that supports a natural means of evolution.

Since evolutionary phenomena have been described in astronomy, geology and biology, creationists (those who believe in religious part of human origin) have maintained controversy in this regard, because the scientific explanation of these phenomena is not compatible with their interpretation of religious texts. The debate raises important political issues, in particular in matters of education, scientific research, freedom of opinion and beliefs.

Creationist currents show a great diversity, from those who support fixism by developing a theory of theistic nature ("Jeune-Terre creationism" and "Vieille-Terre") to those with more deistic positions who embrace the transformist theory (hypothesis of the intelligent design and directed panspermia).

The "Creationism Young-Earth reads the Bible or the Koran as scientific and historical books, conveying the belief that the story of the creation of the universe, as provided by religious texts, gives a literally accurate description of origin of the Universe. This literal interpretation of texts like Genesis is based on the conviction that these texts were "dictated by God" as absolute, definitive and indisputable truths (the case of certain Protestant churches, the majority in the Bible Belt of the United States). This current of thought is generally associated with the rejection of any idea of biological and geological evolution.

Most monotheistic religious traditions (Judaism, Christianity and Islam) postulate the creation of the world by a supreme God. The fundamentalist reading is refused by the majority of current Christian Churches, which favor a hermeneutical reading.

For Catholics, the creation of the universe by God is not in itself opposed to evolution: creation is above all the relationship between creatures and a Creator, their first principle.

Creationism is not, however, restricted to currents that interpret religious texts literally, but also includes Old-Earth creationism which admits that the universe is well over 6000 years; the partisans of intelligent design, of currents which admit aspects of the theory of evolution but exclude man from it; theistic evolution which admits that the evolution of species takes place but that it is directed or influenced by divinities or a Creator who would give birth to the universe, to the living and to the mechanisms allowing them then to evolve by them.

According to creationism, everything starts from God. The stance of creationism suggests certain philosophical dilemmas: How did the world came to be? Is it even possible to create something from nothing?

There is a metaphysical principle that "nothing comes out of no-where." If the universe, which encompasses everything that exists, had an origin, it would have arisen out of nowhere, nullifying the aforementioned principle. To overcome this contradiction, it would be necessary to accept that the universe always existed. For creationism, that existence is given by God, who is eternal and has always existed.

As aforesaid, creationism is often claimed to be opposed to the theory of evolution proposed by Charles Darwin. This scientist explained that species, including humans, are derived from others. This would therefore assume that God did not create man out of nothing. For creationists, on the other hand, each species is the fruit of an act of divine creation.

A part of the Christian creationists assure that our planet is young, so young that it does not reach 10,000 years old; more specifically, they usually point out that it was created by the god Yahweh 6000 years ago, as described in the Ussher-Lightfoot Calendar. In other words, this ideology does not take into account scientifically based theories of the emergence of the universe and the Earth.

Many Protestant churches in North America support the Young Earth vision: Statistically, this is the theory that is respected by approximately 47% of North Americans, and about 10% of Christian universities teach it in their classrooms. Some Christian organizations, such as the Creation Research Institute and the Creation Research Society, also believe in this ideology.

To find the age of our planet mentioned above, which does not exceed six thousand years, the followers of this branch of creationism rely on deductions and calculations based on the ages of the characters in the Bible, as mentioned in Genesis and Other books. Young Earth creationism is divided into three views:

- The one that rejects the theory of the evolution of species categorically, as well as any indication of evolution of planet Earth, according to geological studies. This is the most common form of ideology;

- The one that is subtitled "ambiguous", which contemplates the possibility that all living beings except human beings have evolved;

- The so-called "of a rapid evolution", according to which the god Yahweh carried out the creation in a few days, so that the evolution did take place but it occurred in just one week.

In the field of literature, finally, creationism is the name of a poetic movement that emerged in the early twentieth century, postulating the absolute autonomy of the poem. According to this movement, the poem does not reflect the appearance of nature, but rather follows its internal logic and impulses.

Chapter Two

The union of the human body and mind

L ife is a matrix - the ancient Greek thinker Plato, made this idea clear in the allegory of the cave: There are people chained in a cave and only see images of the real world - as shadows that a fire casts into the cave from outside. What we perceive with our senses is only a flawed copy of a perfect world that exists independently of space and time. A sphere is round, this truth always applies, regardless of whether all seemingly round objects have dents and corners under the microscope.

Reality is thus divided into two parts ("dualism"): into an eternally immaterial "world of ideas" and a physically perishable "world of senses". While the latter can deceive us as in the allegory of the cave, infallible knowledge lies in the world of ideas, where the idea of a sphere or of the "beautiful in itself" exists objectively. We only get there from the cave through our thinking - because our spirit lives in the immortal soul, which is temporarily trapped in the body, but actually comes from the world of ideas. If we use our reason, the soul can remember the ideas and thus also recognize what is good and just. But the body also plays a central role in Plato's educational ideal.

Through sport, we learn to control our body with its desires and thus also train our soul. But the body also plays a central role in Plato's educational ideal.

According to Aristotle, there is no thinking without a body;

Aristotle wants to turn the philosophy of his teacher Plato upside down on its feet. For him, the essence of things is not in the ideas, but in the things themselves. Without the football and all the apparently round objects, we would not come up with the idea of rounding things off. So the idea reflects what the senses perceive.

With this, Aristotle rehabilitates sensory perception - and introduces an immortal soul through the back door. For Aristotle, as for Plato, this is a universal principle that breathes life into the body, but is itself immaterial. A part of the soul, the "active spirit", is even immortal - if only as a kind of cosmic principle that breaks free from every individuality after human death. Because here Aristotle is again a materialist - and empiricist: thoughts are only filled with content through perception.

You can think without a body, Descartes believes;

The French René Descartes was a notorious skeptic. Because not only the senses deceive us, but also our intellect, for example when we dream, Descartes questioned everything. What remained was the doubt - and the thinking: "I think, therefore I am." So thinking is also possible without a body, because the world breaks down into two independent substances: the soul as the immaterial inner world of free thinking ("res cogitans") As well as the physical ("res extensa"), which as pure matter follows natural laws.

Contrary to ancient beliefs, however, the soul does not need it for life. Perception and movement are mechanical - with which (unreasonable) animals become "machines". But the human being is a double being with body and immortal soul. The aim is to give the reasonable mind control over the weak body. But how do mind and body actually interact? Because Descartes asked himself this question, he is considered the father of the "body-soul problem" - which he was only able to solve in an unsatisfactory manner. To substantiate the mutual influence of body and mind, he claimed that the soul sits in the middle of the brain in the pineal gland.

For Marx, property and power relations shape our ideals;

For the famous critic of capitalism Karl Marx, thinking depends on the economy. "It is not the consciousness of people that determines their being, but their social being that determines their consciousness." In "dialectical materialism" being and consciousness are indeed in a kind of interaction, but ultimately social and individual beliefs depend above all on it economic, historical and social conditions.

Ownership and power relations thus significantly shape our ideals of beauty as well as ideas of justice or freedom. Because in capitalism, this often serves to maintain power structures instead of the well-being of the people, Marx also speaks of "false consciousness". But the world is not determined: a change in conditions is possible.

There is agreement that the body has influence over the mind;

In 1979, the American neurophysiologist Benjamin Libet caused a sensation with an experiment. Subjects should raise their hands at a freely chosen time. The measurement of the brain activity showed that the unconscious neural impulse to move was present before the conscious decision.

Are the human mind and consciousness materialistically reducible to nerve activities? This would reduce our free will and also the jurisprudence based on the question of guilt is absurdum.

Other scientists are more cautious because the experiment has a weak point: the test subjects already knew what action to take, and an active decision was no longer necessary.

In another experiment recently, the researcher John-Dylan Haynes showed that that our consciousness can affect unconscious decisions. In any case, the debate continues to this day, especially philosophers disagree with neuroscientists.

They doubt that complex rational decisions can be explained in the same way as simply raising one's arm. What the brain researchers remind us in any case is the influence of the body on our mind.

The body is punished and trimmed by the powerful, says Foucault;

The French philosopher Michel Foucault sees the body determined by social power structures - and disciplined by those in power. The

Church preaches abstinence and fidelity and makes human sexuality the subject of religious laws and discussions.

In the Middle Ages and under absolutism, confessions were extracted under torture and physical torture was a widespread punishment. The destruction of the body of a delinquent was also a popular discipline. In the 18th and 19th centuries, the obvious brutality increasingly faded from discipline, and according to Foucault, the body is now made more subtle in public institutions, in prisons, but also in schools, orphanages, clinics and in the military.

In this way, power structures are internalized by the individual. The aim is, as it were, their submission and the increase in economic usefulness. "The human body enters a machine of power that penetrates, dissects and reassembles it. In this way, the discipline fabricates subjugated and trained bodies, docile and passive bodies." For Foucault, the body is the surface on which power is inscribed.

Spivak sees the female body as exploited in capitalism;

For Gayatri Spivak, a co-founder of the post-colonial theory, who sees the current balance of power as a continuation of colonial structures of rule and strives to overcome them, the female body in countries in the global south is the scene of patriarchal supremacy and sufferers of global inequality.

Transnational corporations realize their profits on the backs of the workers in the low-wage countries. In the context of unrestrained capitalism, women become objects of exploitation, without the possibility of political participation or self-representation - because, if at all, others are talking about them.

According to Spivak, this is also to be understood as a criticism of the hegemonic tradition of many supposed liberation discourses by Western intellectuals.

Butler believes that the body and mind are subject to cultural norms;

According to contemporary philosopher Judith Butler, physical reality is also shaped by how we talk about something. As soon as the midwife says: "This is a boy", many allegedly follow typical male attributions. As early as the 1970s, feminists took up the distinction between biological (sex) and social sex (gender), which came from psychoanalysis and sociology, to point out the oppression of women and the fact that gender roles are socially constructed.

Butler, being a feminist, rejects the Descartes-related dualism between supposedly unchangeable nature (sex) and culture (gender) - ultimately between body and mind. This maintains the separation between "man" and "woman" and the associated power relations.

Ending the debate about body and mind interaction;

This has always been a problem that keeps human beings arguing all the time. That is: Does the body control the mind or the mind control the body? The philosophers participating in the debate have their own opinions, which can be roughly divided into two viewpoints: materialism and idealism.

The mind and body are not two incompatible aspects. Both the mind and the body are part of our life, and both are expressions of life. We should understand their relationship on the basis of seeing life as a whole.

Foreseeing one's own actions in advance is the most critical role of the soul. Knowing this, we can realize: how the mind controls the body - the mind sets the direction of the next action for the body.

If we don't have a direction to work hard, but only receive some scattered movement signals, it is useless. Since the mind can determine the direction of our actions, it occupies a pivotal position in life. At the same time, the mind is also affected by the body, the body is the executor of the action, and the mind can only exercise commanding powers within the scope of the body's abilities. For example, if the mind wants the body to run to the moon in the sky, it is nonsense unless it can overcome the limitations of the human body.

The horse and the horse rider are a vivid metaphor. The horse rider can direct the horse to go, but he cannot specify the details precisely. It cannot be forced. It can only be guided. In the end, it will be decided by the horse.

Mankind's ability to foresee the future will definitely develop in the long term, and mankind will work hard for the goals set by itself in order to consolidate the important position of mankind in the environment.

By studying the meaning contained in the various expressions of the individual, find a suitable way to understand the object, and compare his goals with the goals of other people.

In most cases, the mind affects the body. When a person thinks about something in his head, he will work hard on the matter, and finally give feedback to the body.

Chapter Three

The components of the human body

Endowed with gesture and speech, the human body is distinguished from that of animals by a whole series of physical characteristics, the inventory of which has undoubtedly not finished being drawn up: true bipedalism, liberation of the hand, capacity cranial.

Whether the differences are accentuated or blurred depending on the animal species to which he is compared, he nonetheless remains a singular being, and requires, as such, a specific approach. Inert or alive, all other bodies appear as objects placed in space, *partes extra partes*, in an exteriority and a distance conducive to cognitive reflection.

The human body, as composed of flesh and bones, can certainly be analyzed as a being in itself, but this mode of apprehension ignores its particularity and its incomparable character to other bodies. To truly understand him and to grasp something other than his remains, you have to change people and go from the third to the first.

So then, what are the components that makes up the body?

The brain: The seat of desires and emotions

The brain is made up of three major parts: the neocortex, the limbic system, and the reptilian system. The latter represents the primary brain, responsible for instincts (survival, flight…). The limbic system is the center of emotions and memory. The neocortex represents the center of higher cognitive functions and thus concerns, for example, strategy, spatial and long-term reasoning, perception, conscious thought or even language. The latter, the neocortex or "new brain", developed from the limbic system in the evolutionary history of the human brain, which could explain the crucial role of emotions on the functioning of the brain and especially of thought.

Until a few years ago, the location of emotions in the brain was localized by the scientific community exclusively to the limbic system. It was established that emotions run a single systematic genetic circuit. But advances in research have made it possible to discover that the areas of the brain causing emotion are multiple. As the neuropsychologist Aroa Gomez Marin tells us: "We know that the different emotions are not the result of the activation of a single cerebral structure: but that they are the result of the activation of a circuit of determined connections that allow communication between different areas of the brain."

Other theories agree on this point: the areas affected by emotions in our brain are numerous. They further argue that there would be no genetically established circuits in our brains. The circuits responsible for the appearance of emotions would, on the contrary, be the result exclusively of the learning process: through our experiences or through language.

In terms of functioning, there is an important emotional circuit to know in order to understand the power of emotions in our brain. Joseph LeDoux, American neurologist, was the first to show the central role of the amygdala in the emotional circuit of our brain. This small organ explains that man is able to act following an emotion even before his thought system has been able to make a decision. "Anatomically, the system that governs emotions can act independently of the neocortex. Certain reactions and certain emotional memories can be formed without the slightest intervention of consciousness, of cognition," describes Joseph LeDoux.

When the brain receives sensory signals, two pathways are taken in parallel by the information received. Take the example of an emotional reaction of fear following a visual signal: that of the appearance of a tarantula in our field of vision (do you feel the shiver run through your arms and your back at this thought?). Let's get back to how our brains work:

The visual signal leaves the retina during the vision of this tarantula to go to the thalamus.

The thalamus is then responsible for transmitting information, according to the language of our brain, to the visual cortex.

The visual cortex is ultimately responsible for analyzing the received signal to find the necessary response.

If the appropriate solution is of an emotional nature, the signal will again be transmitted from the neocortex to the amygdala, located in the limbic system and therefore at the center of emotional controls.

But in parallel with this path, part of the signal is sent by a single synapse, by the thalamus directly to the amygdala, and can thus generate an emotional response very quickly. This fast track nevertheless remains primitive and detached from any cognitive analysis. It is thus completed a posteriori by the path taken by the neocortex, which can establish a more elaborate and adequate plan of action.

Emotions can thus be triggered without the slightest intervention of thought and gain the upper hand over reason for a given time, before the cognitive system has been able to analyze the information rationally. If this operation has saved lives many times in human history, it can also be the source of an inappropriate reaction in our daily lives.

The role of the amygdala in emotional memory should not be overlooked. This instance of our modus operandi is an essential guide in our choices. Indeed, Antonio Damasio has studied the role of the amygdala in decision making. He studied personal or professional choices, small or very important. His studies have shown that emotions and feelings are essential when making rational decisions. They are warnings to guide our choices in the right direction, the one where reason can be best used thanks to the emotional memory stored throughout our life.

Two forms of intelligence, therefore, inhabit our mind, our brain: intellectual intelligence and emotional intelligence. Intellectual intelligence has long been considered the only intelligence, but as An-tonio Damasio says: after the paradigm of intellectual intelligence, the new objective is to link reason and emotions to better decide!

The blood: The familial bond

The natural bond of parents with their children and also that of the latter between them has always been considered "blood". It has the psychological value of an identity affinity of ways of being, the con-firmation of which is sought in the physical and character similarity. The natural bond, of which we now know the genetic constitution, is the foundation of a relationship that is claimed to be defined from the start, in its own right.

In reality, the particularity of the bond between parents and children and between siblings is built, for better or for worse, through their relationships never detached from the environment outside the fam-ily.

The difference in the parents' relationship with their adopted chil-dren compared to that with their natural children can be significant only for the more complicated mutual investment, which there can be, certainly not for irrelevant biological reasons. The blood bond is a relatively recognized belief that supports the defensive and mis-leading need to separate the value of family relationships from their actual erotic/affective quality.

The only blood bond that has a relational meaning corresponds to the fact that we meet the world for the first time through close con-tact with the maternal body, after having lodged within it. The blood of this body fed us. By virtue of this exceptional common psychoc-orporeal experience, the mother invests us in an exceptional way as soon as we are born (and waiting for this to happen). A special rec-ognition to which we respond in an equally special way.

The blood bond with the mother, to which Jewish law associates the right of citizenship, would lead to our annexation to a maternal uni-verse closed to otherness and entertaining a "hit and run" relation-ship with the world, if it were not animated from the law of desire, the law of equal differences of desiring subjects. The equality of dif-ferences requires the structuring presence of the erotic relationship between the parents which assigns a function of equalizing redistribution of the currents of desire within the family to the father: the one who does not come from the womb of the mother and does not have a blood bond with her nor with the children.

The responsibility of parents towards their children that gives them greater blame if they harm them. This does not change in anything due to the fact that they have adopted them instead of procreating them. They are committed to taking good care of them because they are human beings whose destiny is heavily dependent on their dedication. This care, which they can be called to account for, will not bring it to fruition because it is part of their natural prerogative, which does not really bind them, but because they are capable of loving while respecting the particularity of the loved object. On this level, each child is adopted: he is not treated by his parents as his own extension, but is recognized and accepted in his difference and loved by taking care of it.

The law of blood contradicts the principle of universal brotherhood which ignores natural bonds and is based on the equal exchange between our different declinations of the common human matter. It violates the foundation of justice, it is an unjust law.

The limbs: Tools for creation

"The hand is the man himself." - Anaxagoras

Anaxagoras affirms that man is the most intelligent of animals thanks to having hands; so it is reasonable to say that he got the hands because he is the smartest.

Hands are in fact an instrument, and nature, as an intelligent person would do, always attributes each of them to those who can use them; since it is more convenient to give flutes to someone who is already a flutist than to attribute the art of the flute to someone who owns flutes.

Nature attributes the lesser to the greater and more important, not the noblest and the greater to the lesser. So if this is the best way, and nature in the field of possibilities realizes the best one, then it is not that man is the most intelligent thanks to his hands, but he has hands thanks to being the most intelligent of animals.

Simply put, the most intelligent must be the one who properly knows how to use the greatest number of tools; now the hand seems to constitute not one but several instruments: in a certain sense it is an instrument in charge of other instruments.

Therefore, to him who is able to master the greatest number of techniques, nature has given, with his hand, the instrument capable of using the greatest number of other instruments.

As for those who maintain that man is not well constituted, indeed worse than all other animals (they say in fact that he has no protection for his feet, he is naked and without combat weapons), their speech is incorrect. The other animals have only one means of defense, and they are not allowed to replace it with another, on the contrary they must sleep and do anything else while always keeping, so to speak, their shoes on their feet, that is, without putting down the armor they have on their body nor can they change the weapon that has befallen them.

Man, on the other hand, is granted many means of defense, and he can always change them, also adopting the weapon he wants and when he wants it. In fact, the hand can become a claw, hoof, horn, or even a spear, sword and any other weapon or tool: all this can be because everything can grasp and hold.

The shape of the hand was also designed by nature in this sense. It can be articulated and divided into several parts, because the capacity for cohesion is also implicit in the division, while the first is not implicit in the second. And it is possible to use it as a single organ, two or many.

Aristotle has this to say in his book – "The Parts of Animals"

"It is not because he has hands that man is the most intelligent of beings, but because he is the most intelligent of beings that he has hands. Indeed, the most intelligent being is the one who is able to use the greatest number of tools well: the hand does indeed seem to be not one tool, but several. Because it is, so to speak, a tool that takes the place of others. It is therefore

to the being capable of acquiring the greatest number of techniques that nature has given by far the most useful tool, the hand.

Also those who say that man is not well constituted and that he is the least well shared among animals (because they say he is without shoes, he is naked and has no weapons to fight) are in error. Because the other animals each have only one means of defense and it is not possible for them to change it for another, but they are forced, so to speak, to keep their shoes on to sleep and to do anything, what else, and should never put down the armor they have around their body or change the weapon they have been shared. Man, on the contrary, has many means of defense, and he is always free to change them and even have the weapon he wants when he wants. For the hand becomes a claw, hoof, horn or lance or sword or any other weapon or tool. She can be all of that, because she is able to grab everything and hold everything."

Intelligence is the faculty of inventing means to achieve an end. Suffice to say that his approach is always to manufacture tools. The invention, the manufacture, the use of tools are therefore all elements of the first approach specific to intelligence. For Aristotle, nature is wise: it would be foolish to give a tool to someone who does not have the intelligence to use it. To man, because he is the most intelligent being in nature, nature has given an organ which he is able to use: the hand, not as a tool, but as a multiplicity of tools.

Modern anthropology proves Aristotle and his finalism wrong. But the image of the hand, the tool of tools, remains beautiful and strong.

The tongue: The vehicle for propagating ideas

The tongue is one of the essential members of the human body. It is precisely because of the existence of the tongue that we can taste the taste of various foods and know what is sour, what is sweet, what is bitter, and what is spicy. Therefore, for the tongue, the most important role is to be able to sense taste. Of course, our human tongue also has other functions, which can be specifically manifested in the following aspect; speaking.

The role of auxiliary speaking

We should all know that human beings cannot only speak without their vocal cords, but also an important organ, the tongue. The tongue is a heavy-duty organ that assists in pronunciation. Without the tongue, we humans cannot speak or pronounce at all.

Humans have the vital need to relate. These relationships in the social context are possible thanks to communication, which implies entering into relationships with others and an exchange of views, since we are alternately emitters and receivers.

Communicating is, then, expressing or manifesting to others our thoughts, desires and our interpretations of things and the world. All this, however, is not possible without language, since it is through it that communication relationships are established.

Now, what then is language? Well, in a broad and even metaphorical sense, people often speak of the "language" of flowers, stars, hills, and so on. Animals that live in a community also have very subtle communication procedures, as in the case of bees and ants. However, all this is not language in the strict sense.

Language becomes a unique and exclusively human activity, which allows us to communicate and relate to our fellow human beings through the expression and understanding of messages. In other words, language is the ability that everyone has to communicate with others using oral, written or other signs.

This concept of language, as it can be understood, has a broader significance than the production of articulated sounds that make up words and phrases.

- There is language through symbols such as traffic signs, military signs, etc.

- There is body language such as mimicry and gestures.

- There is language expressed through linguistic codes, which is the most important means of human communication, which is called oral language or speech.

It is this latter form of language that is addressed in this book. It becomes a personal act in which the speaker emits a message using the signs and rules that he needs at a given moment.

Language, then, is a very important quality of the human being thanks to which it communicates, knows its past, can analyze, interpret and understand its present and, consequently, project itself into the future as an individual and as a social being.

Why is speaking important?

To highlight its importance, it should be noted first of all that human beings live immersed in a veritable verbal ocean, in a world or an eminently competitive social reality, where the word, especially that expressed verbally, is a decisive factor that constitutes the bridge, the noose, the weapon, the important means or instrument of union or disunity; of understanding or misunderstanding; of success, recognition or indifference; of failure, frustration or marginalization among human beings. In other words, speech becomes a vital process that enables communication with others, increasing the opportunity to live better in a society like the current one.

Thus, all human beings need verbal language to express our needs, thoughts, feelings and emotions; We even need it to solve the most basic things in our life: hunger, thirst, shelter, work. We also need it to acquire knowledge, to abstract and project ourselves symbolically and truly in time and space, as well as to communicate and adapt to the environment.

We can do all this thanks to verbal language; But when there are defects in this quality, a series of problems are generated that can limit and marginalize us socially.

Having said that, it is important to understand that the tongue is an essential instrumental aspect for the life of relationship. Without it, man is a socially mutilated being, without the ability to project himself symbolically. It is also considered as a fundamental aspect for the development of intelligence and for all cognitive activity related to life. However, it is good to point out that this quality does not refer to a purely "mechanical" fact, nor to something that is acquired or given in a natural way, such as learning to walk, but rather it is something much more complex, and that behind of all this is the fact of feeling and thinking well, having a personality and being a man.

The child and the power of language

Since birth, the child lives in an eminently verbal context, where people, radio, television and a thousand and one other forms of interrelation establish verbal bridges with him; that is, the child at birth passes from the "amniotic bath" of the mother's womb to the "verbal bath" of the social environment, which becomes the conditioning factor for the acquisition and development of language.

This social environment with its manifestations of language, not only surrounds the child but also makes him or her receive and assimilate it directly, since the child is spoken to from the first day of birth together with the physical demonstrations of affection: hugs, kisses, caresses and tender words almost sung.

This influence of the sociolinguistic environment makes the child, at first, associate verbalizations with situations of human contact and feelings of well-being, constituting a strong incentive for the acquisition of language. Later, as you progress, you become aware of its instrumental value for the demands and requests related to your needs.

The child, around the eighth month of birth, discovers that certain types of vocalizations manage to attract adults around him (call function), which begins to explode. In this we can see the beginning of a vocal communication relationship that later became the core of all verbal activity.

In the second year of life, the child discovers the power of the word, particularly the "name." He realizes that just by naming objects or actions adults obey him, either by bringing the objects closer to him or by performing the actions. In addition, he also obtains verbal answers on the topic he proposes, which is enriching and facilitating his linguistic development. Later the child will use this quality as a means of "controlling" and "directing" the actions of others and, later, of himself.

Thus, at different stages of acquisition there are different motivations to keep going. However, the deep roots of these motivations must be traced in affective relationships within the family, since without this support language either does not develop to its full potential, or it atrophies. Hence, the affective family climate and the opportunities provided by parents for the child to practice language are basic conditions for the establishment, development or subsistence of this quality.

Thus, thanks to tongue, the child is overcoming the here and now; You can draw on knowledge from experience to solve current problems and plan for the future.

The tongue also enables you to interact more fully with other people and share your individual world of fantasies, beliefs, hopes, and regrets.

In this way, human beings have been using the tongue to create huge and complex civilizations, and they continue to use it to promote scientific and technological progress. Unquestionably, language, speech, is one of the instruments of enormous importance and power.

The language and the psychological adjustment of the child

When the acquisition of speech is done within an environment of security, love and understanding; When this learning takes place in a family environment without tension, with mature and happy parents, all obstacles are simple and easily overcome by the child, reaching the different stages of development in an expected period that may vary, but with a certain graduation in that acquisition.

Thus, children who come from balanced homes, in which their parents provide them with love, security, stimulation and understanding, are generally happy children who express themselves normally, confident of themselves and with a wide disposition for relationships with others, the rest. This also means that they have the best possibilities to develop harmonically and integrally, adapting adequately to their sociolinguistic environment.

Instead, let's imagine the origin of those children or young people who feel disabled or affected in this quality that most humanizes us, it is quite likely that they come from inadequate or poorly formed homes, where the parents were not interested or worried about stimulating and helping them in the acquisition of speech, this being,

THE GAME CHANGERS SERIES

sometimes or most of the time, the cause of the speech defect or disorder, and these, by not expressing themselves normally, are the target of ironies, rejection, of "pity" or "compassion", going through tensions and frustrations that negatively affect the development of their personality and social adjustment.

Therefore, the adequate development of language in children enables the harmonious development of their personality, constituting a valuable instrument or means for learning and social integration. But, when there are defects, the child tends to present developmental maladjustments, generating certain behavioral-mental reactions such as shyness, feelings of inferiority, isolation and frustrations that, in short, lead to unhappiness.

What happens when there are defects in the tongue?

This question leads us to question ourselves in an extreme way, what would happen if we could not talk with our partner, children or other people? What would happen if they were accusing you of being a terrorist and you could not say that it was not true? And if you were sick, what if you couldn't say what hurts or how you feel?

All these questions make us aware of how important and essential the tongue is in the lives of human beings. It is with it that we can communicate, inform ourselves, read and understand, work and learn everything related to our life. However, when there are defects or disorders in this quality, there are serious interferences and limitations in the development and psychological adjustment of the affected person to their social environment.

This is the case, for example, of stutterers, for whom the defect not only constitutes an impediment to speech, but also to their lives, since it prevents them from following their educational and vocational aspirations and their development and social reciprocity.

To better understand and assess the consequences of a speech defect, let's look at the case of a 23-year-old young man who came to a psychological consultation due to his stuttering.

He states the following:

"(In a restaurant ...) ... I wanted a coffee and a tasty cake that was displayed on the counter, but I asked for a tea and a bread ... because I knew that if I tried to say those others Words would stutter a lot and I didn't want the lady who was attending me to feel sorry for me ... I hate bread alone ...

Since I was a child I isolated myself from my schoolmates for fear that they would make fun of me ... I have no friends who consider me ..., I have never had a girlfriend because of my defect."

In this story we can realize that the defect is not only a speech impediment, but is also a serious limitation for his development in life, since this prevents him from freely expressing what he wants, inducing frustration and social isolation.

This painful situation is rarely understood by normal people. Daily activities, such as answering the phone, asking or answering, talking to any other person, etc., constitute for subjects with this defect a source of deep concern, restlessness and tension, even becoming a true "nightmare". For them, everything goes well as long as they do not speak, but it is enough for them to know that they have to talk so that everything falls apart, tension and "panic" surface, blocking all aspects of their personality, hiding as a result of this in tics and tricks. I do not know if you know the story of the bullfighter named Belmonte, who was a stutterer, he preferred to face the worst of the bulls, the most ferocious miura.

According to these references, can we still doubt the importance of speaking well? Not really! Speaking well and with a good voice is the best quality that a person can have in a world like the one we live in. This allows him to communicate, feel active and useful to his peers; that is, to be much more human, since you can think, say what you feel and think, understand and help others using language.

The tongue and verbal language functions

Language fulfills a number of important functions in the life of human beings:

a. Communicative function: The primary function of language is communication. Human beings have a vital need to relate and this is possible thanks to language.

b. In this communication process, speech constitutes the decisive instrument of communication and social interrelation.

c. Cognitive function: Language also has a cognitive function; that is, it is a powerful instrument for learning and abstraction. Thanks to language we can project ourselves from the concrete to the abstract, from the proximal to the distal.

d. With the position of this quality, a human can elaborate his first elementary abstractions and concepts, with which he will understand and dominate his environment.

But, when there is a defect with the tongue, the person involved will have difficulties to abstract and, as such, it becomes a handicap for active performance and other cognitive activities.

a. Instrumental function to satisfy immediate needs: Verbal language allows to satisfy immediate needs such as hunger, thirst, shelter and is the most dietary and effective means to ask for help or assistance in situations of risk or danger. Without this quality we would perish.

b. Personal function: Man, through verbal language, can express his opinions, feelings, motivations, personal points of view and aspirations, sharing feelings, ideals and fantasies with others.

c. Informative function: The tongue allows us to obtain information about what is happening around us and in the world in which we live, contributing to the solution of problems, anticipating and adapting to changes. In this way, the tongue allows us to live more satisfactorily.

d. Adaptive function: The verbal language or speech allows the individual to adapt adequately and competently to the social environment. That is, it facilitates the adjustment and self-realization of the person, which translates psychologically into well-being or discomfort. The discomfort occurs precisely because of speech defects, constituting a limitation for life, as occurs with those affected by stuttering.

e. Regulatory function of behavior: Language has an important function as a regulator of the individual's behavior through internal language and, also, a "controlling" function on the behavior of others, through external language. This allows the child, like the adult, to establish and maintain social relationships.

These are, among others, the most important functions of tongue and verbal languages, characterized by being a valuable instrument of communication and thought.

Chapter Four

Antagonists of the human body

In medicine, when we refer to everything that is disease, war terms are depopulated: we talk about "fighting" the problem, "fighting" against the pathology, using the "therapeutic paraphernalia" in an exhausting "battle" for health. Here then is that Medicine becomes the strategy of "conquering" that primary and undisputed good which is health.

A misleading metaphor

In this war perspective, however, the body is no longer perceived as part of the patient, but becomes a battlefield, where doctor and disease collide, while the interested subject becomes a helpless spectator able only to witness what is a conflict decisive for his fate.

To understand how this perception came about, the reflection of Norman Doidge, psychiatrist winner of important literary prizes for his best seller "The infinite brain", illustrates how this vision is partly the result of the discoveries of the twentieth century, which led to the absolute centrality of the brain in the performance of many functions.

The discovery of his control of the body has led to the belief that everything happens in the brain, to the point of considering it almost as an entity in its own right with respect to the body. Consequently, the body would be nothing more than a mere appendage of the brain, a simple executor of it and the structure within which it is stored.

A one-to-one relationship

Such a conception of the human body is limiting and does not allow us to grasp the profound relationship that distinguishes the link between the brain and the rest of the organism: there is a continuous and one-to-one communication, guaranteed by the dense network of neurons present within the whole organism. This ensures that the exchange of information between inside and outside is constant and that body and mind are able to influence each other. The discoveries of recent years, precisely with regard to the neuronal networks distributed in the body, have led to the identification of networks that are so dense and organized that they can be defined as "brains."

In this regard, see:

The gut: our second brain sensitive to emotions the heart: our third brain with a powerful electromagnetic field. In this way the perception of the human body as a mere effector loses its thickness: the intertwining with the nervous system is so dense that it makes no sense to try to separate them.

A step back to move forward

Hippocrates believed that the body was the most important medicine. It was believed, in fact, that the body had its own therapeutic abilities and, as a patient and doctor, acting according to nature, was to elicit them, thus guaranteeing healing. The Hippocratic perception of medicine was holistic and was human-centered.

Paraphrasing Medicus, a film that conveys a different perception of the Doctor than today, the principle is that one should not take care of the disease, but of the person who has the disease. This is the key to hoping for the best results.

This is the message also conveyed by better known masterpieces such as Patch Adams:

"If you cure a disease, you win or lose, if you treat a person, I guarantee you that in that case, you will win whatever outcome the therapy has" and "The point is that to become doctors, we must treat the patient as well the illness. We have to dive into people, navigate the sea of humanity."

So, if we take care of the person in his entirety, we understand how his organism - the body - is an integral part that cannot be ignored: it is a very sophisticated machine, which works incessantly to guarantee each of us the best possible level of well-being.

Precisely from the knowledge of its responses to different conditions (knowledge still far away in its totality) an optimal approach to the disease can be born when we talk about the human body, we are dealing with its laws which often do not correspond to that rationally one could think intuitively.

Moreover, the recent scientific discoveries are helping us to understand the incredible potential of the human body, first of all neuroplasticity, or the ability that the brain possesses to modify its own structure and functioning in response to mental activity and experience. And perhaps the most peculiar aspect of the efforts of neurology is how more and more doctors (and Dr. Norman Doidge returns to be illuminating in this regard), to make the most of the potential of neuroplasticity, are seeking a marriage between Western neuroscience and practices of oriental medicine - knowledge that has always placed at its center the joint action of energy and mind in healing.

At that point, one wonders if looking back is really a going back or if sometimes it is essential to turn around and become aware of past traditions in order to hope for better progress. One certainty remains: man, and the body he inhabits, remains the fulcrum of every medicine that aims at the well-being and health of man himself. The body, in this case, becomes an ally. Ally, because it is the first tool that each of us has at his disposal to get to know each other: educating oneself to listen to one's body can become a crucial aspect in the path of daily health.

What it really means to listen to your body? It is a path of knowledge, and like every path it presents a certain gradualness. It is important to get to know each other in everyday life, to learn to decipher the simplest sensations and then understand what is happening. Learning to know when you are full is the key, for example, to avoid overeating and avoid unnecessary stomach pain and - in the long run - weight gain.

Learning to feel when thirsty allows you to drink more frequently and stay hydrated. Knowing when your body is tired can become the tool for going to bed earlier in the evening rather than abusing coffee. What seem like trifles can become a valid help in everyday life and in solving those problems that are secondary to an inappropriate conduct that often imposes itself on us. Big results can be achieved in small steps. And that same knowledge of one's own body can be crucial in managing the disease, as no one can know the tricks to improve one's well-being as the person concerned. This is what it means to have your body as an ally: from respect for it comes the respect for one's person.

Germs/Diseases

Viruses, bacteria, pathogens, microbes… The tendency is quickly to amalgamate. Our hands carry 80% of infections. Our body does not have one, but three types of enemies. Diseases are caused either by viruses, bacteria or fungi. Enemies, who feed and reproduce differently.

Germs are present everywhere in our environment. Germs are the cause of most illnesses and infections. They are invisible to the naked eye. Viruses and bacteria attach themselves to surfaces and are dependent on exterior movement for their own movements. Fungi can be volatile and "catch" in the air. The lifespan of germs depends on their own nature, but also on the environment in which they are found.

A friction, a handshake, a touch, are enough to move germs from one place to another and from one body to another. Like all living things, germs need an environment conducive to their survival. As a priority, they therefore seek to attach themselves to surfaces on which they will find food and conditions that suit them (humidity, temperature, etc.).

Carrying a germ on you does not necessarily make you sick. We can very well have bacteria on our hands, without them generating an infection in our body. But, we can still transmit them to those around us by direct or indirect contact. An infection may start in a person even though it did not start in the person who passed the germ to them.

The three types of germs

Bacteria are microorganisms. That is to say that they are living beings which are made up of one or more cells. For example, some ear infections, tonsillitis and diarrhea are caused by bacteria.

Fungi are also microorganisms, made up of one to several cells. Their way of multiplying is particular. They release their spores into the environment (air, water, surfaces). These spores can reproduce autonomously (asexual reproduction), or they may need contact with a similar spore to become a new fungus (sexual reproduction). Itching of the scalp, feet or mucous membranes can be caused by fungi.

A third type of germ is the cause of many diseases. These are viruses. Nasopharyngitis, influenza and most tonsillitis are caused by viruses. These entities are not microorganisms, they are not made up of cells. Not having their own mechanism for producing energy like a bacterial cell does, they are dependent on the outside. Thus, viruses can only live and reproduce inside the cells of a living being (man, animals, plants or micro-organisms). They are constantly trying to colonize cells to feed and multiply.

What happens when the body attacks itself?

Tiredness, difficulty sitting up, swollen limbs and bleeding, these are some of the many and varied symptoms that may be announcing the suffering of different autoimmune diseases, when the body's defenses become their attackers. Due to the low specificity of its symptoms, the diagnosis involves difficulties and can be delayed: a compelling reason to go to the doctor at the slightest suspicion. In these diseases, early diagnosis is crucial to avoid irreparable damage, even in young people.

Autoimmune diseases are those disorders that consist of making defenses (or immunity) against ourselves (hence the prefix "auto"), so that our immune system stops working as a pure defensive system - and harmless to the human body and becomes your enemy. This means that, instead of making defenses against pathogenic microorganisms that invade the body, they make antibodies that are directed against the cells of our own body and damage them.

The list of autoimmune diseases is extensive; more than 100 have already been identified. These include known diseases such as fibromyalgia, multiple sclerosis, celiac disease or Crohn's disease. But also others, which are perhaps less well known by the population, such as pernicious anemia, rheumatoid arthritis, Behçet's disease, antiphospholipid syndrome, Sjögren's syndrome, scleroderma, vitiligo, different types of vasculitis, inflammatory myopathies or myasthenia gravis. Some diseases affect a single organ, such as diabetes mellitustype 1 or juvenile diabetes, while others affect several of them (multi-organ or systemic), such as systemic lupus erythematosus (SLE).

Chapter Five

Humans

You have them too, like everyone else. It is a nuisance to make them protagonists, but in this entry it touches: Who are your adversaries and what to do with them?

Let's see if the little pleasant time that we are going to spend thinking about who opposes your interests is of any use and that you are happy. Because that's just the figure of the enemy. The upset begins.

Your 'antagonist' is someone who opposes your interests, either because it collides with theirs or because they have something personal against you. He hates you.

The enemy wants your bad, in contrast to the friend, who is who feels good when you are well.

We may not all have friends. But enemies, yes. Of those we always have.

Why say this?

Because, to be friends with someone, you need to build the relationship (from respect and trust), share interests or hobbies ... In short, work on it. Friendship is very beautiful, but it is a relationship that must be taken care of. If you don't take care of it, you can lose it.

It's easier with enemies. You don't have to do anything to have them.

Sometimes a person takes it with you and you are fatal to them without eating or drinking it. He finds out that you are from a football team other than his and he already has bad will on you.

Other times, in the fight for his own interest, he finds you in the middle ... And he takes you ahead or crushes you, as he sees fit. You have something you want. Or he sees you as a threat that separates him from his goal.

A real threat. Or a threat that is only in your head.

The possibilities are many. But no effort is required on your part either. One day you wake up and you see the destruction that he has done to you, the very nice one. And maybe then you find out that he was your enemy. But then, there are other chances that you don't have a bigger enemy than yourself?

Self

In many of our experiences, we have felt abused and humiliated, and we think we got past that when it is not that simple.

Over time, this abuse disappears, but we start to exercise it against ourselves without really being aware of it.

This is where we need to realize how we really are. People with low self-esteem, full of insecurities, frustrations, fears, guilt ...

If you find it very difficult to value yourself, accept yourself, and recognize that you are capable of achieving everything that others have already achieved and achieved, you are surely becoming your own enemy.

You can choose to be your enemy or not

Your worst enemy is not other people, but what is on your mind. How is it possible? How can we become our own enemy?

All the criticisms that you can receive, the humiliations, the opinions, the judgments that you must make on yourself... All of this, you can accept them or not.

This decision-making power is within you. Do you think you deserve it, really? Do you agree with what others are saying?

Taking on something just to be accepted by others only fuels low self-esteem and that inner enemy.

It is obvious that being surrounded by diverse opinions makes you doubt who you really are. So, it is necessary to distance yourself from these people in order to be able to reflect on who you really are. Once you know it, you can face these opinions and judgments much more confidently.

How to stop being your own enemy?

1. Accept yourself and be sure of who you really are.

2. Question any negative messages that come to you.

3. Learn to make mistakes.

Don't try to please everyone.

It's hard to stop being your own enemy, but it's within reach. You need to be confident in who you are and not let others dictate your conduct.

You have to start seeing mistakes not as burdens or shame, but as experiences that can be learned and then done better.

Everyone is wrong, but you feel humiliated. Know that there is no learning without errors. We learn more from mistakes than we think.

Who are you?

This is a very simple question, but it is difficult to answer. Do you know who you really are? If so, why do other people's criticism affect you so much?

You need to learn not to compare yourself to others, to be confident in yourself, and not to get carried away by what others may say. You are unique, extraordinary and irreplaceable, with flaws but also with qualities.

Trust, believe in yourself, and don't allow yourself to be how others want you to be. Being yourself will help you achieve the happiness we all dream of.

Your decisions are the ones that will mark your life from today. Who will decide in your life? You or the others?

Be a little selfish with yourself and stay away from what people say. Your life is yours, you alone decide how to live it.

Think that the confidence you have in yourself will allow you to move forward, to test, to experiment. If you don't trust yourself, insecurities will arise.

Ask yourself where you are heading your life. Want to be so perfect that you can't do it anymore? Perfection is by no means the right answer.

Be natural, try to improve yourself, make mistakes, learn and live the way you want. Free yourself from everything that is said to you, which blocks you and paralyzes you. Be free from all of this and move on. Never allow yourself to be your own enemy.

Okay. Now you know this and you're obviously prepared not to be your own enemy. Still, there might be a problem. Someone, or people might just hate you more.

Others

"The man is a wolf for the other man", affirmed the philosopher Thomas Hobbes to remember the tendency of the human beings to fight the one against the other.

Of course, the wolfish gaze of the gentleman sitting across from me in the airport boarding area bites. "Get away, flock of sheep," he seems to say in his wordless language. Perhaps he is having a bad day or he is one of those aggressive toxic guys who circulate with his loaded hostility submachine gun, which is certain, is that the man in question has decided that his frustration at the flight delay is his neighbor's fault. He dislikes everyone!

Has it happened to you that, sometimes, you get up on the wrong footing and everything bothers you? Have you ever perceived that others are superficial and stupid? Have you felt like a weirdo for hating humanity? Do you want "to stop the world that to allow you to get off"? If you have answered yes to any of these questions, do not worry, the most likely explanation is that you are a victim of stress, fatigue or the feeling of not being understood.

"To fall badly or well" is an attitude that serves to regulate the proximity that we are willing to allow to other human beings. It is something intuitive, a sensation based on details as minute as the clothes they wear, how they speak or sustained by prejudices as serious as their gender, their skin color or their creed. The brain warns from the depths of the limbic system: the amygdala is activated because someone gives it a bad feeling.

Negativist Bias

This hatred of humanity is consolidated thanks to the power of the tongue. There are ways of getting hooked on negative thoughts that make us approach others in an unconstructive way.

By virtue of the so-called negativity bias, negative expressions grab the mind's attention and produce an immediate emotional response while positive ones don't have it so easily. A simple "okay" doesn't generate much enthusiasm, while "it's wrong" hits us right away.

Christine Liebrecht, from the University of Tilburg, and her team published their research on this linguistic gap in the 'Giornal of Language and Social Psychology'. In the study, the subjects exchanged opinions about a restaurant. Those who thought the food was good weighed less than those who criticized it because it was bad. Surely the finding does not surprise you, just read the comments of others on any social network, in general, negative words make a greater impression than positive ones.

These hostile comments towards humanity serve to quickly charge us with reasons and justify the rejection of people that we do not want to overlook under any circumstances.

When we consider that the problems come from others, we end up disliked by everything they do. For highly dependent personalities, temporary negativity towards others is the only way to allow themselves time and space: while the anger lasts, they can stay away.

Mirror Effect

The problem arises when judging our peers as unworthy people lasts too long and becomes a habit. In these situations, the fact that you dislike others can hide the fear of being rejected and, as a compensation mechanism, you previously reject yourself.

Sigmund Freud referred to this behavior as "the expression of the defense mechanism of projection": you avoid feeling emotional discomfort in yourself and you put yourself on another person (you project yourself).

Our own emotion comes to be seen as something belonging to the other. In short, hating someone means hating in their image something that we have ourselves (positive emotions are also projected as in falling in love).

Jacques Lacan was a French psychoanalyst who spoke of the mirror stage, a stage that occurs in children between six and eighteen months. These infants, seeing themselves in the mirror for the first time complete, feel joy. This is the moment of the formation of the ego of the subject.

What Lacan highlights is that the recognition of one's own mirror image occurs with the help of and in relation to another similar one. From that moment on we get to know each other through relationships with others that thus become our mirrors (and we mirror of our fellow men). Therefore, when we meet someone we really do not like, we must ask ourselves what this person has to do with me, what bothers me so much and why, before assuming that the world is against us.

Envy and Resentment

Sometimes it is the rancor and resentment that do not heal and persist in the present that make others lazy, superficial, insensitive, ignorant or careless and by judging them in such a way we have a free hand to unload on them our bad vibes.

Others, we cannot allow ourselves to do the same as that person or, we simply want what the other has and that unleashes anger and frustration. Instead of acknowledging the unhealthy envy and transforming it into an appreciation or a proactive emotion, we tend to generate a negative feeling towards which we believe makes us feel bad.

When you dislike everyone, think about these aspects because perhaps you are putting your own ghosts and fears in others in facing life, or perhaps, you hope that someone will rescue you and take care of you as when you were a child.

Human beings need others and it is true that sometimes beyond our state we can run into difficult, selfish or narcissistic personalities, but the important thing in these cases is that we can manage our emotions without clouding our judgment.

Chapter Six

Death: The destination of the human body

Death is too exact; all the reasons are on its side. Mysterious for our instincts, it is drawn, before our reflection, limpid, without prestige and without the false attractions of the unknown."

- EM Cioran, Breviary of Rot.

Every passing day, man is growing to become more complicated than this world, his world and he are in a constant differentiation and tangle. Its biological constitution and the variability of its environment have led to development and physiological and neurological transformations with immeasurable levels of complexity. Such complexity weaves a network over all spheres and areas of man from which nothing escapes.

Under this pathos, death has become more complicated, it is no longer a simple event, as our Neanderthal ancestors thought (Morin 2000: 113-115), now it is something that is embedded in the very consciousness and bio-ontological constitution of man. There is a recognition of mortality and transcendence, in whatever form. That is, the life of man, from the moment in which he became conscious - true original sin, has revolved around death, even to the point of affirming, as Heidegger tells us, that being-is-for-the-death (Heidegger 1987: 276).

In this sense, we can say together with Camus, that all the fundamental and serious problems of Philosophy and Anthropology they refer to death. Every philosophical (and anthropological) attempt to find meaning in life and man falls back on a reflection on death (Camus 1996: 9).

The following work tries to give some insights on the different transfigurations of death that have occurred to this day. Death continues to be a constitutive phenomenon of our reality, although it is banalized and seen as the simple end of a life, like a breakdown or a disease, just as our consumer societies do. However, the consequences of "living," death and interpreting it under the logic of consumerism and hegemonic commercialism are self-destructive, pernicious and in many cases, irreversible.

Death has been reduced to a scientific fact, a simple positive fact subject to observation and experimentation. These representations of death are intrinsic to the subjective movements of societies, our post-industrial era radiates and confers particular signs and meanings to death. Death becomes the representation of the machine that does not work, that is damaged, becomes the limit and fails of the production and re-production of the human being, of social systems and of the great economic machinery.

The last anthropological limit of human existence

"If I kill myself, it will not be to destroy myself but to rebuild myself." - A. Artaud, Van Gogh: the suicide by society.

Throughout history, death has been present in one way or another in man's thought, either as an event of social, religious, political, etc. (Evans-Pritchard 1973), as a record in memory as an abstraction or as a philosophical or scientific reflection.

In Anthropology, these different ways of thinking about death converge, together with the different sciences of man. In this sense, death, being a multidimensional phenomenon inherent to man, is studied from an anthropological perspective. That is, every phenomenon is studied from its fundamental unit, and man is this fundamental unit. In order to understand what we are, we have to study death, and in order to understand death, we have to study man. Death, then, appears to us as a "subject-object" of study, pathos by which humanity has traced its existence.

Anthropology claims to be the most ambitious science par excellence, it wants to embrace man from all his angles, seeing him from an infinity of raw materials; but like any ambitious project, it fell short. Knowledge, science, anthropology, cannot go beyond our life, our senses, our language, our world, and only through this combination of elements can we form any system of thought or representation. Death is presented as that limit from which we cannot escape. We cannot know, know, much less explain, what is there after death. Ancestral, biblical question, prehistoric, that continues and will continue to reverberate in our heads, fluttering chaotically like a butterfly in the back of our minds. Perhaps it will be selfish death that does not want to reveal the secrets of life to us, or complex life that does not want us to know the secrets of death. However, death inscribed in life, but also overflowing it, expanding as rapidly as time. Death encoded in man (Morin 1999), part of the primordial component that sustains, bases and forms life. Endless fundamental cycle from which all cycles start.

Death is the great project; it is the totalizing end. In death the consciousness of man ends, dissolving into the unknown. Death is, in part, metaphysical, but it is also an event, randomness, focus, accident, death is Hegelian, but it is also Nietzschean; it is dialectical and eternal return at the same time. It is the zero point of our world, it is the moment that we cannot grasp, of which Ernst Bloch speaks. Death is the infinite horizon that escapes us at every moment, synthesized disorder and order, a dislocated fragment that is diluted in history, in life, in our being.

Death is presented to us as biological, but also as cultural, it is empirical data, but also symbolic, it is the most human trait (Morin 1999: 13), MORIN would say. We are the only living beings on earth who reflect on death, and not just death, but usefulness of life, itself.

Although this is more important - our own death is the next step that leads us to a new maturity, knowing that we are dying and that others are also going to die. No animal has the ability to make its own death conscious, it only dies, there is no death for animals, but that instinct, which, like us, is biogenetically established: the survival instinct. The animal is not aware that it is dying moment by moment, that each day that passes inevitably approaches, that at any moment it can unexpectedly break into our life, ironic? or can life also break into death?

Life bursts into death at all times, in the constant eternal return of the instant and the unrepeatable creative act; thus, some die so that others can live. In ancient times, the dead were those who had life, preceptors, advisers and guides of the living. Dead or alive, man serves and will serve life.

"Man not only mythically appropriates the law of death-resurrection to find his own immortality, but also strives to magically use the life-engendering force that constitutes death, for his own vital purposes." (Morin 1999: 121)

The death that gives us life, makes us aware of our finitude, of our ephemeral and transitory state, maintains and delimits existence, death distinguishes us, without it we are nothing or nobody. The main characteristic is that of being human: our dignity. In this sense, all subjectivity is traversed by death, as well as all objective limitations of human practice.

Since man became aware of this phenomenon, the great myths appeared, the majestic legends that gave life to hominid history. Death is, duplication, the image of the other. The dead, in prehistoric societies, possess food, weapons, clothes, desires, thoughts, motivations; the dead are doubles of the living and vice versa. Death is rebirth, an endless cycle, as in the Christian and Buddhist religions, although each of them interprets death-rebirth differently, even in a contradictory way.

It is evident that we do not know about death, we only know about our attitude towards it. We only know about pains, agonies, processes, phases, stages, not of death itself, but of dying; absolute death, sudden death, apparent death, what difference does it make, we don't know anything. So, agony is the medical, psychological, sociological condition of people who are in the final phase of a disease or severe trauma, it is the last moment of existence. We know what happens just before it bursts into consciousness and vanishes everything. We only know the biological data immanent to the material body.

In this way, we must see death in its complete nakedness, decontaminated from us, unmasked; we have to take away that "personality", or rather, stop conceiving it as a person (mask). A mask built by society and the superego. We must stop seeing it outside of us, and see it inside, not as that ghost, double, spirit or soul that reflects our own being, but as a reality, as a constituent element of us and our world.

This mask arises from the impossibility of making the experience of one's own death conscious, therefore, consciousness will have to adopt a representation of death given by the society in which the subject is inserted. In this sense, we only know our death thanks to the death of others since death annihilates the means and the senses that human beings have to verify their existence. For consciousness, death is the last anthropological limit of existence.

The great German poet Rainer Maria Rilke underlines the advantages of appropriating death, becoming familiar with it, which does not mean becoming obsessed with it. In reality, anonymous death, which the consumer society cultivates, only leads to anonymous, depersonalized, dehumanized life. It is a great alienation to never think about death, live as if it does not exist, or only think about it in terms of life insurance, which is actually death insurance. Some seek in vain to hide their fear in fun, flight and escapism.

According to Rilke, if we are afraid of death it is because we have not known how to cultivate the death that each one of us carries within. Humanizing death is understanding and living its meaning. The question about the meaning of death arises urgently and inescapably. By presenting death as the last and the end of life, it gives it its ultimate meaning and purpose.

Every human being has to take on a great task, take charge of his life, and learn to live. Death prompts us to live a more authentic existence: accept our finitude, appreciate our itinerant condition, relativize the accumulation of goods and social functions, disqualify selfishness and the desire for profit, not to waste time, but to enjoy the seriousness of life - present moment and task. We seek to explore the face of death and discover what it teaches us with its silence and silence. The celebration of the Day of the Dead helps us to remember, to bring to our hearts, the memory of our loved ones.

Many ancient and modern thinkers point out that philosophy, the love of wisdom, has among its main functions learning or teaching how to die. Deep down, learning to die is learning to live, which implies giving life a purpose, a direction and a meaning, which goes beyond the instinct for self-preservation and cultivates the instinct for self-improvement.

Man does not limit his performance to satisfying basic survival needs, but rather seeks to confer value and meaning on his life and death. Even in moments when life seems to lose its meaning, in times of crisis and decadence, anxiety, restlessness and anguish appear as paradoxical witnesses that the search for meaning, value and the demand for an end and an order, they never disappear from the human mind and heart.

In fact, death is an event that raises legitimate questions about the being and the work of man. Death is not just a big question mark that encompasses all of life, but a reality that raises many unknowns.

Apparently, it is convenient to consider the framework of the human condition, its itinerant vocation, since death is on the way. But what is death? Is it something specific, or rather an ingredient of life? His face is enigmatic, but also multifaceted: death is something distant and close, friend and foe, natural and unnatural, and it performs a critical function for man and for society.

We must bear in mind our mortal condition, as travelers, as passing through this world, pilgrim beings who always glimpse death on the horizon, which helps us to walk wisely on earth.

The Spanish poet Jorge Manrique uses the metaphor of the river: "our lives are the rivers / that go to the sea / that is dying". The rivers are for Pascal, roads that walk. The essence of the river is not to stagnate, always flow, always run, precipitously in the rapids, calmly in the backwaters, but always, continuously, constantly, advance.

Is it possible to have a rest, as the Roman epitaph suggests: Stop, walker! Stop in space, not in time, the itinerant condition always leads us to move forward. In any case, the human being does not have permanent residence here, nor is he on this earth as at home, "to be is to be on the road": not to be dormant, always to move forward, to be attentive and vigilant to the signs of the road and the risks that it implies.

For the pilgrim, it would be absurd if the path led to nothingness, if it led to annihilation. The goal, the end, the culmination of the path would not be the what is expected, it would be meaningless. It is important to be in search of an end, beyond which it is not worth prolonging the journey. Be open to novelty and the sense of the invisible. The goal, however, illuminates the entire path: hope shines in the chiaroscuro of faith.

Chapter Seven

The Way And The Human Body

The Way gives birth to one
One gives birth to two
Two gives birth to three
Three gives birth to the universe
Everything that carries negative holds positive
Combined, they are in harmony
The human hates orphans, widow, and useless ones
But the king sees himself as that
Therefore, his thoughts increase but also decrease
And then his thoughts decrease but also increase
The words that others and I promote are
"Violent man has brutal death!"
That is the main point I recommend.
Chapter 42 – The Book of Ethics

We see the numbers one, two, and three recurring in the poem above, which are easily relatable to everyone. However, in this poem, one, two, and three are not in a numerical context. According to the Way - one implies the universe, two- Yin and Yang, and three- the Heavens. Earth and its Inhabitants (people) who multiply all things, comprising of Yin and Yang, which produces Harmony. Our world is full of harmony, the fruits of Yin and Yang.

Since one is recognized as the universe, it is sensible to make this correlation. First, with a question, what does this Taoism have to do with the body? The Way - Tao is not practiced without an aim, and the reason why the Way is existent will no longer be possible if the body is absent.

Without the body, harmony, balance, yin, and yang, and other fundamentals, which are discussed in the subsequent chapters will not be achievable. The Way seeks to reconstruct the body to the earliest energy (Qi) felt and enjoyed at creation (free flow), so that the body is no longer a means to an end but the end itself. The body becomes the Universe (One).

Stanza four of the poem in Chapter 42 - The Book of Ethics says, "Three gives birth to the Universe." Do you see the connection? Three is the earth and its inhabitants (You). It means You give birth to the universe. This makes sense because only the You-niverse can birth the universe. It is a fact that the Way centers on the body; therefore, it should be treated with utmost priority to harmonize the world. The body is a transporter of feelings, thoughts, actions, representation, and expression of a practice, religion, ideology, school of thought.

According to Tao, the body is underrated when perceived as a physical container that houses other components or a spirit-material (flesh) component. It is revered as a means of journeying into Immortality, which you must understand maximum function. The body's symbolism is not just bringing various practices, meanings, and observations together but, most importantly, it gives full expressions to these perspectives. Through the diverse connotations, the body is put up to its full potential and is maximized by the practice, harnessing, and cultivation of The Way.

Nature is quiet
Strong wind does not blow the whole morning
Heavy rain does not fall all-day
Why? Heaven and earth!
If heaven and earth can't do it
How can humans do it?

THE GAME CHANGERS SERIES

One with the Way
Then becomes one with the Way
One with Virtue
Then becomes one with Virtue
One who loses the Way and the Virtue
Then becomes one with loss
When one is one with the Way
The Way welcomes one
When one is together with the Virtue
The Virtue is always there
When one is together with loss
The loss also follows one
One who is disbelieved
It should not be believed.
Chapter 23 - The Book of Ethics

Nature is a fundamental of Tao, and it preaches returning to the source, which means different things, particularly returning to the original body - emotional energy and good health. We lose our golden/original body as we grow and evolve due to stress, trauma, depression, bad eating habits, and the likes. The Way is after a system to reverse the deterioration of the body to flow with nature and function from its original state freely.

The origin of the human body; Science or religion?

The religious perspective about man's origin is the belief that divine creation is responsible for life and the universe, contrary to scientific consensus that supports a natural means of evolution.

Since evolutionary phenomena have been described in astronomy, geology, and biology, creationists (those who believe in the religious part of human origin) have maintained controversy in this regard, because the scientific explanation of these phenomena is not compatible with their interpretation of religious texts. The debate raises important political issues, in particular in matters of education, scientific research, freedom of opinion, and beliefs.

447

Creationist currents show great diversity, from those who support fixism by developing a theory of theistic nature ("Jeune-Terre creationism" and "Vieille-Terre") to those with more deistic positions who embrace the transformist theory (hypothesis of the intelligent design and directed panspermia).

The Creationism Young-Earth reads the Bible or the Koran as scientific and historical books, conveying the belief that the story of the creation of the universe, as provided by religious texts, gives a literally accurate description of the origin of the Universe. This literal interpretation of texts like Genesis is based on the conviction that these texts were "dictated by God" as absolute, definitive, and indisputable truths (the case of certain Protestant churches, the majority in the Bible Belt of the United States). This current of thought is generally associated with the rejection of any idea of biological and geological evolution.

Most monotheistic religious traditions (Judaism, Christianity, and Islam) postulate the creation of the world by a supreme God. The fundamentalist reading is refused by the majority of current Christian Churches, which favor a hermeneutical reading.

For Catholics, the creation of the universe by God is not in itself opposed to evolution: creation is above all the relationship between creatures and a Creator, their first principle.

Creationism is not, however, restricted to currents that interpret religious texts literally, but also includes Old-Earth creationism which admits that the universe is well over 6000 years; the partisans of intelligent design, of currents which admit aspects of the theory of evolution but exclude a man from it; theistic evolution which admits that the evolution of species takes place but that it is directed or influenced by divinities or a Creator who would give birth to the universe, to the living and to the mechanisms allowing them then to evolve by them.

According to creationism, everything starts from God. The stance of creationism suggests certain philosophical dilemmas: How did the world come to be? How is it possible for something to be created out of nothing?

There is a metaphysical principle that states, "nothing comes out of nowhere." Therefore, if the universe, which encompasses everything that exists, had an origin, it would have arisen out of nowhere, nullifying the aforementioned principle. To overcome this contradiction, we would need to accept that the universe always existed. For creationism, this means that existence is given by God, who is eternal and has always existed.

As earlier said, creationism is often claimed to be opposed to Charles Darwin's theory of evolution. This scientist explained that all species, including humans, are derived from other species. This would therefore assume that man wasn't created out of nothing. On the other hand, creationists believe that each species is the fruit of an act of divine creation.

Taoist (Dao) perspective of the body

The human body is defined based on three terms:

One, ti/body meaning the physique; Two, xing/form means to form or being; Three, Shen/person implying the whole human; material and non-material. The body is a complicated term in Taoism due to its various contexts:

- The body and state: they are two microcosms related to each other and the macrocosm. The concept of microcosm-macrocosm states that humans are microcosms (smaller universe) which corresponds significantly to the macrocosm (large universe).

The big country seems to be located in low land
That is the gathering place of all species
The mother of all things
Females prevail over males due to their stillness
Take stillness as a low place
Therefore, if a big country is humble with a small country
Then it will conquer the small country
If a small country is modest with a big country
Then it will be protected by the big country
So staying below to get it

Or staying below to be protected
A big country wants to accommodate many people
The small country needs many people to accommodate
Each side gets what they want
So, the big country should learn to be humble.
Chapter 61 – The Book of Ethics

- The body and cosmos: this is based on the supernatural form of Laozi known as Laojun, the supreme Lord of Tao, including its Virtue. In the Scriptures, Transformation of Laozi and Opening of Heaven, the man, Laozi, is seen at the creation of the cosmos and reappearing throughout life in various bodily forms. Cosmos is taken to be his body.

- The body as a home for gods, celestial bodies, and spirits: in the book Laozi zhongjing, the description of deities who live in different body parts was explained as one supreme being in forms (Taoiyi). These deities perform a balance function in the viscera: liver, kidneys, lungs, spleen, and heart. In addition, they are the abode of unseen forces. The Heshang gong describes the hun soul as Yang, po soul as yin, essence as jing, spirit as Shen, with you residing in the five viscera.

Five colors make people's eyes blind
Five sounds make people's ears buzz
Five flavors make people's tongue lose taste
Chasing hunting horses makes people go crazy
Rare and precious possessions make one degrade
Sage prays for a full stomach
And yet there's nothing spectacular
Therefore, leave this and get that.
Chapter 12 – The Book of Ethics

- The body as a mountain and landscape: The five's: planets, sacred mountains, and viscera are related to wudi zhenfu (five emperors) in the Wushang biyao (Supreme Secret Essentials Book).

By keeping body and soul together
Is it possible to keep them apart?
Pay attention to breathe
To be soft
Can one become an infant?
With spiritual cleansing
Can the stain be gone?
Love people and rule country
The heaven gate opens and closes
Through everything
Can't we do anything?
We are born and raised
Instructions without possessions
Made without merit
Instruction without ruling
Such is the root of the Way.
Chapter 10 - The Book of Ethics

- The body related to Internal Alchemy: the major constituents of the internal state (breath, essence, spirit, shen). The focus is not the bodily form rather the loci (pivotal points) where energy is channeled from five points to achieve balance.

The Taoist View on Gender

Male-Female balance, otherwise known as yin and Yang, was formed in the 6th century by Lao Tzu, the Taoist scholar in Tao De Jing. His classical work was the stepping stone for respecting women. Several philosophies and ideologies allow the female to be discriminated against, ignored, or subjected.

Until just a few decades ago, scholars viewed women as simply passive participants in evolutionary change and limited themselves to relegating them to the role of giving birth, feeding, and caring for their young. While, on the contrary, men were described as responsible for many of the innovations that define us as humans, for exam-

451

ple, the emergence of bipedal gait, brain enlargement, tool-making, cooperative communication, or symbolic representation.

Thus, it should not be surprising that research related to our evolution has, and still does, carry away the conventional sexist bias that has permeated the academic world and the models it produces for centuries.

However, in Taoism, women are dignified and given a chance to express themselves by being independent. In the history of Tao, Wu Chengzhen is the first female master who applauded Yi Ching, the Chinese Classic on Gender equality. The awesomeness of balance, equality of yin and Yang (water and fire, good and bad, male and female, etc.) is elaborated, which were then in Chinese history, the best thing to happen in her words. According to Tao De Jing, the female body is related to the potency of Tao, illustrated as a divine gate bearing lives, a valley, and a power source.

Know the male and keep the female,
Making streams for people.
Making streams for people,
Virtue does not leave
Return to the childhood
Know the light and keep the dark,
Be an example for the world.
Be an example for the world,
Virtue does not leave
Return to infinite
Know the honour and keep the humiliation,
Make a cave for the world.
Make a cave for the world,
Virtue is full
Return to the rustic
Rustic is not divided
Sage uses it to provoke hundreds of officials
So, the great spell is not undercut.

Chapter 28 - The Book of Ethics

The yin (female) is concluded to be equivalent to the yang in both strength and Importance. We have to accept yin to understand Yang. They also ate interdependently and related to reproduction, and only in this is the oneness of the element achieved. Every individual has a touch of masculinity and femininity. The Way encourages the understanding and cultivation of yin to the extent of Yang.

The union of the human body and mind

This has always been a problem that keeps human beings arguing all the time. That is: Does the body control the mind or does the mind control the body? The philosophers participating in the debate have their own opinions, which can be roughly divided into two viewpoints: materialism and idealism.

The mind and body are not two incompatible aspects. Both the mind and the body are part of our life, and both are expressions of life. We should understand their relationship on the basis of seeing life as a whole.

Foreseeing one's own actions in advance is the most critical role of the soul. Knowing this, we can realize: how the mind controls the body - the mind sets the direction of the next action for the body.

If we don't have a direction to work hard, but only receive some scattered movement signals, it is useless. Since the mind can determine the direction of our actions, it occupies a pivotal position in life. At the same time, the mind is also affected by the body, the body is the executor of the action, and the mind can only exercise commanding powers within the scope of the body's abilities. For example, if the mind wants the body to run to the moon in the sky, it is nonsense unless it can overcome the limitations of the human body.

The horse and the horse rider is a good example. The horse rider can direct the horse to go, but he cannot specify the details precisely. It cannot be forced. It can only be guided. In the end, it will be decided by the horse.

Mankind's ability to foresee the future will definitely develop in the long term, and mankind will work hard for the goals set by itself in order to consolidate the important position of mankind in the environment.

By studying the meaning contained in the various expressions of the individual, find a suitable way to understand the object, and compare his goals with the goals of other people.

In most cases, the mind affects the body. When a person thinks about something in his head, he will work hard on the matter, and finally, give feedback to the body.

Everything has origin
At the beginning of everything is the mother of all
By keeping the mother, one knows the child
By knowing the child, one keeps the mother
Therefore, one should not be in danger for a lifetime
Close-lipped, breath held
Life is full
Open-lipped, always busy
Life is futile
Seeing hidden is bright
Hold strength is strong
Use Virtue to return to the Way
Do not let the body be in trouble
Thus, the Way is eternal.
Chapter 52 - The Book of Ethics

Chapter Eight

The Taoist View on Death

People are not afraid of death
Why use death to scare?
If it makes people always afraid
And if every criminal is caught and killed
So, who is left?
Killing is carried out by the executioner
Replace that person
Like replacing a woodcutter
Which rarely cuts hands?
Chapter 74 - The Book of Ethics

The Way explains how things are done naturally; the way plants grow, the way we breathe, the way water flows, etc. Transformation happens consistently in both humans and nature; hence, when individuals have insight into the natural way things occur, they will find it simple to accept pain, sorrow, grief, or joy and be unaffected by it. With understanding, the surge of emotions can be subdued. For instance, a family is preparing for an evening outing when a heavy downpour of rain begins. The children will naturally be unhappy and probably cry because they would be unable to go out while the parents having understanding do not get mad but see it as a natural cause. Zhuangzi, the ancient philosopher, stopped mourning when his wife died because he realized that it was a part of the change. Just as seasons come and go, death is such; the springtime, summer, the autumn, and winter. Hence, to mourn is going against the law of nature and acting oblivious. In the cycle of change and the Earth, life and death are embedded therein. We live to die and die to live. This is nature's way; plants grow, animals consume them (herbivores), other animals consume them (carnivores), man kills them, and we also die and are taken into the Earth where microbes feast on, making the soil fertile. The inability of a man to unbound himself from his classification of life and existence is why Grief is experienced; the dead and the living are alike. Death is inevitable, Man must die, yet his essence is permanent.

The theory of Zhuangzi is in line with Tao Te Ching (Daode-Jing). Man is to exist as a member of Nature worth other parts of and within Nature. It is only in freedom that he understands the Tao. Freedom from:

- Man's ideologies and intellectual bias.

- Emotional surge (insight into the way life is).

- Barriers are due to natural occurrences.

When we see death as transformation, not disappearance, we appreciate life better and see death as a drive.

The Concept of Death

We all remain a part of the Tao. We live as a constituent of Tao and die as a constituent of Tao.

- Based on yin-Yang theory, the transformation from being (existing) to not being (not existing) is death; change from Yang to yin. Nature sees no variation in life and death. Instead, a harmonization for balance is to be obtained. Death should be viewed as the same.

- We are taught to accept all things as essentials, whether good or bad. Death is part of the forces of eternity. Life and Death complement the Way.

The Concept of Afterlife

Newborn humans are pliable
When they are dead, they are stiff
Newly born trees are soft
When they are finished, they are complex and dry
So stiff and rigid represent death
Pliable and softness mean life
Strong and violent is the dead
Hard trees are cut
So hard and strong should be put under
Pliable and softness should be put above.
Chapter 76 – The Book of Ethics

1. Life after death is indifferent; the same as it was while you were on Earth. They are One.

2. Whatever you believed in before death is what is Incorporated. Do you believe in God or gods? You will be a part of them in your Afterlife.

Usually, the memories of our dead linger, and some persons may add that to their rituals to invoke and pay homage to their ancestry and memories, for example, the Qingming festival.

Chapter Nine

A Lifestyle For A Longer Life

The role of the body in spiritual enlightenment, longevity, balance, and harmony is indispensable. There is no way out without the body. The earlier you understand this and take the necessary action in preserving and maintaining your physique according to Nature's Way, the better you'd achieve.

> *A skilled plant is difficult to eradicate*
> *A skilled grasp is difficult to slip*
> *Virtue will be honored from generation to generation*
> *By fixing Virtue in oneself, Virtue will be real*
> *By fixing Virtue in the house, Virtue will have redundancy*
> *By fixing Virtue in the village, Virtue will grow*
> *By fixing Virtue in the country, Virtue will be in abundance*
> *By fixing Virtue in the world, Virtue will be everywhere*
> *So, by oneself that considers others*
> *By one's house that considers other houses*
> *By one's village that considers other villages*
> *By one's nation that considers other nations*
> *By one's people that consider other people*
> *How do we know what people are? Thanks for that!*
> *Chapter 54 – The Book of Ethics*

Taoism does not see the body differently from the spirit because it believes that our actions create a spiritual impact.

• Purity -The body is kept in purity for the purpose of maintaining spiritual well-being. Purity is attained by avoiding specific kinds of nutritional choices and physical activity. Attributes that should be avoided are dishonesty, immorality, pride, etc.

- Meditation - It is a mandatory practice, and essential for achieving stillness, mindfulness, and boosting mental health.

- Breathing - Engaging in the various breath practices like qigong helps Taoist receive ch'i (energy).

- The flow of Energy - Ch'i can be generated, achieved, and fully harnessed by the right exercises, nutrition, and meditative practice.

- Martial arts - Original Taoist exercises like Tai Chi are encouraged.

- Diet -Not all crops and meat sources are permitted for consumption.

Improving body posture and food digestion

Taoist standing routine

Centuries ago, inside the Mount of China, the Taoist Monks attained a healthy life through posture and spine maintenance, a healthy and balanced diet, physical fitness routine coupled with martial arts prowess. Their show of balance and energy together with these features is known as Tensegrity.

Tensegrity

The term was formulated by Buckminster Fuller while working on his Geodesic Dome in the 1940's. This dome functions by joining and maintaining the balance between its components tension and compression in contrast to a work that will stack its components upon themselves leading to the whole weight carried by the bottom.

This is applicable to the way we make our bodies function. It is in both manners either dumping the majority of one's weight on some joints or allowing an even distribution of the weight across all parts. The choice is yours.

Your body is a Tensegrity medium that maintains the spine for the functioning of other body systems.

Tensegrity and Birth

When a child is born, the muscles are still being developed. Think back to when you put your finger in a baby's hand and the reaction; tightening his hand around your finger with a subtle force caused by muscle and soft tissue movements (tensile), transmitted into the phalanges (compression) resulting in the tightening of the baby's hand.

Naturally, the muscular and skeletal systems work more effectively as the child grows older. Tensility moves up, down, sideways, to all parts and the body becomes stronger to walk, run, carry things and graduate to even more demanding activities. This push and pull is an avenue for the body to be massaged. Through this movement, the visceral organs like the liver, gastrointestinal organs, etc. are being exercised. When we make tensegrity the basis of our movement, our body systems particularly digestive and excretion will function maximally.

Why do we not experience tensegrity?

Sadly, many of us do not maintain this tensegrity and in a matter of time, our bodies move to stack. Hence, the lower limbs and back take responsibility for carrying a major part of the body's weight and keeping the torso against tipping the pelvis (hips). Initially, the lower back and pelvic region are strong. However, due to (lack of use-synonym) the lower part of the abdomen gets weak.

After a period, the region from the navel, through the body's midsection, to the spinal cord, and the hip floor gets exhausted and (tight-synonym) leading to the Colon's inability to move and affecting excretion. The weakness of the colon is caused by friction in the lower limbs, abdomen, and pelvis. When challenges with excretion surface, it is no doubt that absorption will be affected.

What is the way out?

Our solution lies in returning to baby-like functioning. Make use of Nature's Way and blessing to our body; Tensegrity. The energy from the lower limbs (legs) to the abdomen has to be harnessed and grown. Block training is an easy method of understanding and grooming tensegrity founded by John Bracy (Master).

To strengthen your muscles, bring your body into alignment, and boost your digestive system, follow this Taoist standing routine for 300 seconds only!

1. Purchase a cinder block or a 6 inches thick wood (wood higher than the ground for you to stand with both feet shoulder apart).

2. Get on the block. Ensure your feet are straight (check if your second toe is straight) and relax your shoulders.

3. Quickly check the alignment of your body by ensuring your ears over shoulders, shoulders above hip, and hip above the ankle. Your knees should be slightly bent. Prevent your heels from bearing the weight.

4. Your jaw should be relaxed by allowing your teeth to touch, and not clenching them. The tip of your tongue should rest on your oral roof.

5. Locate a point to light a candle on the wall or space 6 feet from you and focus on it.

Standing for a period of 5-10 minutes daily is advisable for a start till you can increase. It may seem like you're doing nothing. In fact, you are working hard because inactive muscles are being used.

Shaky legs are common during the exercise and after it. Muscle soreness is also normal. Your denatured core muscles are being trained. Surfers seem to avoid denaturing because their muscles are pushed to ride the waves.

Block training is an activity that helps an individual attain balance and prevents the possibility of stressing the body leading to losing tensegrity. The legs are being strengthened together with the abdominal muscles and pelvis. In addition to enhancing balance and eliminating body tension, it boosts unison in the body systems.

In caring for others and worshiping god
There is nothing like restraint

Restraint begins with giving up one's will
This belongs to Virtue gained from experience
If you store a lot of Virtue, nothing can be undone
If there is nothing one can't undo, then there's no restraint
If there is no restraint, then one can cure the country
Knowing the root of country treatment is long-lasting
That is called deeply-rooted, durable descent
That is the Way to live long and see throughout.
Chapter 59 - The Book of Ethics

The purpose of Taoism is to boost the well-being and longevity of individuals. Diet has a major role in this mission. The ancestors of Taoism have endorsed and thoroughly scrutinized the Taoist diet. Though diet differs across generations, a meal of grains, vegetables, meat, and fruits is constant while water and tea are beverages. The pillar of Chinese culture is Taoism. According to the Chinese word for food, Yin Shi (beverages/food), they complement one another. The major prominent lineages are:

The Zheng Yi Dao lineage: allowed to eat anything except a few.

The Quan Zhen Dao: strict nutritional rules (no meat and alcohol).

Meals

1. Selecting ingredients

A basic meal should include about 70% grains, 30% is a mixture of vegetables, fruits, and meat. Grains contain Yang energy which Taoists believe to supply nutrients and boost vitality.

The Quan Zhen forbids garlic, chives, coriander, etc. from cooking since it affects the flow of energy and Harmony.

The Zhen Yi allows all things without restriction but advises cooked food over raw.

Ingredients must be mature and ripe without artificial enhancers.

2. Vegetables over meat

Instead of meat, which is eaten in small quantities, vegetables are preferred. The meat encouraged for consumption is fresh and quality. These animals are prohibited for all who practice Taoism:

- Buffalo - are selfless and hard-working animals that consume grass and secrete milk. So, they are respected and seen as sacred.

- Mullet - this fish is sacrificial, exhibits genuine love and respect for its mother since the babies offer themselves to be eaten by their mother.

- Crane - faithful to one partner throughout their lifetime.

- Dig - loyal and of great help to man.

3. A little flavored and balanced meal

The harmony between your body and spirit is attainable when you also pay attention to diet. The five significant flavors from the Earth's element are connected to diet in Tao:

- Excess sour hurts spleen, Sourness for Wood

- Excess sweetness hurts kidney, Sweetness for the Earth

- Excess bitter hurts lung, Bitterness for Fire

- Excess spice hurts liver, Spiciness for Metal

- Excess salt hurts heart, Saltiness for Water

Balance in the Way cuts across all aspects of life. There should be no need for a flavor to overshadow another in a meal. All tastes should be in the right proportion for harmony.

Food like whole grains, vegetables (consumed steamed or fried), and a small proportion of meat is the ideal diet for Taoists. Fishes like salmon with high Yin components should be avoided while others are eaten once a week, red and blue hearts are prohibited, and games are consumed in moderate forms.

What do you eat?

To enjoy longevity, eating wisely is non-negotiable. Make sure to consume natural foods to boost your body's balance and functioning for optimum results. Healthy food should be consumed to preserve our bodies.

What is healthy food?

These are animals, minerals, and plants consumed or externally used on the body to hinder and provide healing for ailments by restoring the energy flow and making quality nutrients available for body (cells and tissues) regeneration.

Disobedience to nature's provision causes Bing; abnormal health in man. Diseases have been categorized into Air, Water, and Blood Dis-ease. This helps to understand the causes of these problems and tackle them at once.

4. The ideal medicine is food

The effect of food on our minds and physique is great. A lot of us eat thrice daily yet, we make the wrong food choices and end up consuming toxins. After a prolonged period, it accumulates and causes health challenges. Taoist advocates know how to use meals and herbs in balancing and providing nourishment to the body and mind to the extent that the body becomes light and our consciousness expands. Taoists treat diseases with the food eaten daily, for instance, Yang deficiency is cured using mutton soup, Chinese angelica, and ginger; endemic goiter is cured with seaweed medicinal wine while night blindness is cured pork liver.

5. Don't fill your stomach

It implies two things: eat till about 80% satisfaction. Do not fill your stomach. Also, avoid or eat little meat/oily food. Tai Ping Jing states that eating enough is vital. These days, most of us pay attention to the energy we get from food regardless of the energy our body will require to break down the meal. When the food is complex, it will take more energy to break down. Overloading our stomach with food keeps it active in doing work. This will shorten your lifespan and a belly filled till it's brim will hinder the flow of energy. Eating less makes your heart open and doing otherwise invites diseases.

Guidelines for the major meals of the day

We are advised to eat based on the energy shift from yin-yang daily, that is, having a proper and full course breakfast but less when noon-time is past. Dinner should even be less than lunch because as the body's yang reduces, digestion does likewise.

Drink when thirsty; Eat when hungry. You are what you eat, digest, and cannot digest. When there is food in your system and you eat, it is as good as useless. Your body cannot make use of it because it is blocked. It either gets excreted or remains as toxic substances in the body. Drinking water when you are not thirsty leaves much work for your kidneys and may not be expelled. Eating late-night meals is bad rather, get a healthy snack and do not fill your stomach. It is easier to get a good night's sleep with your body at rest.

6. Pay attention to your body

It is better for you to pay attention to your body than its senses or nutritional advice. Lao Tzu urges us to know what our body needs both intrinsically and extrinsically. The fact that it looks attractive, tastes amazing, or is advised by the doctor does not mean it is good for you. What is good for the goose may not be good for the gander.

How to treat your body to aid digestion:

- Let your mood be happy when you eat: play some good tunes as you eat for your spleen and digestive process. Fix your mind on chewing, talk less, or do not at all.

- When you are served a meal of different temperatures, begin with the hot meal, next is warm, last the cold meal.

- After each meal, make sure to rinse or brush your mouth.

    » Mouth washing with tea removes bacteria and freshens breath.

    » Mouth wash with warm water is preferable after a hot meal.

    » Mouth wash with cold water for a cold meal.

- Massaging the stomach to take out bad energy from food consumed is popular among Taoists. Digestion is aided by massages and walks. However, serious physical activities are not allowed after meals.

Drinks

A major part of our body is formed by water. Taking healthy and living water is important to health. Water is not just in the volume or mineral constituents instead; it is the amount of life contained in it. Taoist believes in live water because it is easily absorbed by the water. Unfortunately, we do not have access to live water hence, tap or bottled water is more consumed except citizens of Switzerland and Norway. Water from natural sources like; rivers, springs, mountains, lakes should be taken if possible (it has more life/essence compared to bottled water).

Drinking about 8 cups or more of water daily is not something Taoist believe in. Find the right quantity your body needs and make that the standard for you. Average consumption of teas is preferable to living water. Why? It purifies the mind and is an accurate antidote for the body. A little bit of alcohol is permitted in some Taoist ancestry; it supports the flow of energy, herbal absorption, skin nourishment, and blood circulation. Consuming large quantities of alcohol destroys the kidneys and liver since they function as detoxification.

Bigu/Pigu Fasting

The Shen Nong Bible is also a Taoist classic which states that individuals who consume grains are full of wisdom hence, the Qi will make them live forever.

Bi: not to eat, Gu: grains translated no to grains. Taoists hold a belief that consuming grains hinder them from getting enlightened. It is a process of switching off the body's Yang and turning on the Yin. The brain functions uniquely at that state, the physical and spiritual energy are well harnessed, stress is reduced, there is a greater sense of enlightenment and connection. Bigu is in two forms:

- Abstaining from food and consuming Qi (Qigong professionals)

- Taking herbal mixtures without grain consumption

Bigu is a means of detoxification highly esteemed by Taoists.

On a final note, maintaining diets is a personal goal and business. There is no food that is bad or good. Just as advised by Taoists, know yourself and create the standard you would follow. No two persons are the same and Tao also taught that it is good we accept ourselves. Do not feel discouraged if one person has been keeping up with his dietary changes or yielding results. Go at your pace because your immunity and body metabolic level differ from others; some are fast, others slow. These summarized habitual patterns should be at the tip of your fingers:

1. Have a natural attitude and flow with nature

2. Eat proper and balanced energy meals

3. Focus on your body's language

4. Keep fit, exercise regularly

5. Have a positive outlook

6. Engage in a spiritual activity

7. Practice!

A healthy body and total wellness cannot be achievable if we do not consciously work at it, and there's no better time to start than now. As long as you're flowing with nature, you are good on the Way.

PART II
THE SPIRIT

Chapter One

What is the human spirit?

The word spirit comes from the Latin spiritus (derived from spirare, "to blow") which means "breath, air." It could also mean "to inspire" (lat. Inspirare) and "to expire" (lat. Expirare). "Spirit," or spiritus, is also the translation of the Greek pneuma and the Hebrew ruach.

The word "spirit" could be given to anything that is very subtle and very active, so we find it in expressions of the old chemistry like spirit of wine (alcohol) or spirit of salt (hydrochloric acid).

The spirit can also refer to the principle of life or to the individual soul. We no longer meet this use, taken up by Leibniz, except in theological or even mystical discourses.

"Reasonable spirits or souls" are "images of the Divinity, or of the very Author of nature; so that the Spirits are able to enter into a kind of Society with God."

In contemporary philosophical language, "spirit" can be opposed to different notions:

- Opposed to matter, with a distinction between thought and the object of thought, matter; with analogies with subjective/objective or uniqueness/multitude in certain relationships;

- Opposed to nature for example in the freedom/necessity distinction;

- Opposed to the flesh and the instinct of animal life, we find here a meaning close to that of Reason:

"The flesh desires contrary to those of the spirit, and the spirit desires contrary to those of the flesh."

The Spirit in the religions

• *Spirit in Christianity*

In his first epistle to the Thessalonians , Paul of Tarsus prays that our "whole being, spirit, soul and body" will be kept blameless at the Coming of the Lord (1Th 5:23).

The Catholic Church teaches that the distinction between soul and spirit does not introduce a duality into the soul. In the 9th century, during the Fourth Council of Constantinople in 869, there was a controversy over the relationship between soul and body. The 11th canon of this council affirmed the uniqueness of the soul.

It is the 9th century that the distinction is formalized between the soul and spirit. The spirit being traditionally associated with the thought and the soul with the feeling, it was previously considered that man could have a multiple nature (body, soul and spirit). The Christianity asserted the contrary, the unity of the human person (a body and soul) by denying the existence of the spirit, because it coincides with the soul:

"The unity of soul and body is so deep that one must regard the soul as the form of the body; that is to say, it is thanks to the spiritual soul that the body made up of matter is a human and living body; mind and matter, in man, are not two natures united, but rather their union forms a single nature."

The Roman Catholic Church therefore sought to deepen the meaning of the terms, which was not without controversy between the Church of Rome and the Churches of the East. In the catechism of the Catholic Church, the notion of soul is attached to an individual (unity of the human person and of the soul), while the spirit is also considered from a collective angle:

"The sacred heritage of faith (depositum fidei), contained in Holy Tradition and in Sacred Scripture, was entrusted by the apostles to the whole Church. By attaching themselves to Him, the whole holy people united to their pastors remain assiduously faithful to the teaching of the apostles and to fraternal communion, to the breaking of bread and to prayers, so that, in the maintenance, the practice and the confession of the faith transmitted, settled between pastors and faithful, a singular unity of spirit."

This is particularly well revealed in the introduction to the encyclical Fides et ratio:

"Faith and reason are like the two wings which allow the human spirit to rise towards the contemplation of the truth. It is God who put in the heart of man the desire to know the truth and, in the end, to know Him himself so that, knowing Him and loving Him, he can attain the full truth about himself."

The word "spirit", with a lower case (therefore that of man), appears very often in this encyclical, while the word "soul" appears only five times.

The word Spirit written with a capital letter, or appearing in the names Spirit of truth, Spirit of adoption… (always with a capital letter) designates the Holy Spirit.

- *The spirit in the Kabbalah*

Jewish mysticism, from the 11th century, believes that man has, besides the physical body, many souls. The Jewish neo-Platonists Abraham ibn Ezra (c. 1150) and Abraham bar Hiyya Hanassi distinguish three parts: nêfesh, ru'ah, neshamah; kabbalists add hayyah, yehidah. The five names of the soul are, in ascending order: the nêfesh ("vitality", "bodily double"), the ru'ah ("breath", the "personality", the anima), the neshamah ("the divine perfume", "higher soul", "divine spark", "spiritus"), the hayyah ("Divine life", equivalent of Buddhi) and the yehidah ("union", "oneness", indivisible principle of individuality). If we group together in an acronym the initials of each of these terms, we obtain the word naran-hai, ("Living Fire"). This is the doctrine of the Kabbalist Isaac Louria, around 1570, at Safed.

- *The spirit in Buddhism*

The Buddhism denies the existence of the soul (considers as an illusion) and emphasizes the interdependence between the deep body and mind. The individual is considered there as a set of aggregates, the first of which is the body, accompanied by four other concepts that can be linked to the notion of spirit: sensations, perceptions, volitional formations and consciousness.

These aggregates are impermanent and interdependent processes, not immutable objects. The mind is linked to the body and becomes truly independent of it only in the sublimated states of meditation which are the dhyānas in view of nirvāna.

The mind is considered, not as a "ghost in the machine" of the body, but as a sixth sense (manas) in addition to the five senses usually recognized. Buddhism is neither spiritualist nor materialist: the mind is not an eternal entity, but it is not an epiphenomenon of matter either. The brain is only a kind of "terminal" which operates the interface between the mind (immaterial) and the world of the five senses (material). Experiences of altered states of consciousness, common in advanced meditators, seem to confirm this view.

Ajahn Brahm explains:

"The sixth sense, the mind, is independent of the other five senses. In particular, it is independent of the brain. If there was a brain transplant between you and me, you took my brain and I took yours, I would still be Ajahn Brahm and you would still be you."

The Dalai Lama expresses a similar opinion:

"The highest level [of consciousness] escapes material support. Consciousness is independent of physical particles."

The fundamental functioning of the mind and its conditioning in saṃsāra are described by the causal chain of conditioned co-production. Some schools, like the Cittamātra school, teach an unconscious aspect of the mind, Ālayavijñāna.

The spirit in philosophies

• *Classical Western Philosophy*

In the 17th century, Descartes separates the body from the mind (he identifies the soul) in a dualism: the body is an extended substance and is the mechanical (hence the theory of animal-machine) while the soul is a thinking substance. When passive, the mind is intellect; as an asset, it is will. The unity of the two remains a thorny problem, and Descartes sees the pineal gland as the place of communication between the two.

More simply, Descartes breaks down the mind into three components: thought, imagination and memory.

Conversely, the proponents of philosophical materialism refuse the existence of an immaterial principle and the mind is conceived as the manifestation of physiological phenomena governed by the laws of physics: "the brain secretes thought as the liver secretes bile " (Pierre-Jean-Georges Cabanis, 1802).

Philosophy of contemporary spirit

The generalization of the monistic naturalistic paradigm in the sciences of the mind, known today as the cognitive sciences, often leads today to putting between the brain and the mind the same type of relationship as between the material ("Hardware") and software ("software") in IT.

This thesis known as the brain-computer metaphor also knows its adversaries, those who refuse to see in the mind only an epiphenomenon of neurobiology, opposing the optimism of those for whom, the field of "this which remains to be explained in the functioning of the mind" is finished and is shrinking from year to year.

Spiritualist philosophy

The spiritualism is defined as a spiritual philosophy and grant an essential place to the concept of mind. For this doctrine, the spirit is the intelligent principle of the universe, whose true nature remains to be discovered.

In the sense of the spiritualist doctrine, the Spirits are the intelligent beings of creation, which inhabit the universe outside the material world, and which constitute the invisible world. They are not beings of a particular creation, but the souls of those who have lived on earth or in other spheres, and who have left their bodily envelope.

The spirit in the sciences

By etymology, psychology is the science of the mind. But faced with the religious and mystical connotations of the word, scientific discourse has preferred to use more neutral terms such as those of mental faculties or processes or even psyche (especially in approaches inspired by psychoanalysis) or cognition. In contemporary cognitive science, the term cognition does not only refer to the faculties of knowledge and intelligence (of thought) but to all the psychological processes at work in the human (and non-human) mind, including perception, motivation, decision or emotions.

Indeed, it is found in 1983 used in the translation of the book of the philosopher Jerry Fodor, The Modularity of Mind and in the following expressions:

The philosophy of mind, the branch of contemporary philosophy which focuses on the problems of the concepts of mind, mental states, consciousness, etc.

The theory of mind is this psychological faculty in a very small number of animal species, or, according to some researchers, specific to humans that allows an individual to understand the mental states (beliefs and intentions) another individual.

The "Society of the Mind" is the title of a book by Marvin Minsky in which he proposes to analyze human cognition as a holistic phenomenon, emerging from the interaction of a very large number of agents themselves unintelligent.

The notion of ecology of the mind was developed by anthropologist Gregory Bateson in his book Ecology of the Mind and can be compared with that of ecology of consciousness by neuropsychologist Gerald Edelman.

Chapter Two

The role of the spirit in the (physical) world

The term spirit can be applied, according to the oldest interpretations, to living beings in general (plants and animals) as its constitutive principle. According to some interpretations, such as Aristotle's, the soul would incorporate the vital principle or internal essence of each of these living beings, thanks to which they have a certain identity, which cannot be explained from the material reality of its parts.

The term is also used in a more particular sense if it refers to human beings; in this second case, according to many religious and philosophical traditions, the soul would be the spiritual component of human beings.

In the course of history, the concept of the spirit goes through various attempts at explanation: from the dualism of philosophical idealism and gnosis to the existentialist interpretation of a whole with two specific aspects that are: the material and the immaterial.

For the Christian religion, man consists of three parts that are: body (the physical), soul (related to the emotional) and spirit (related to the spiritual). According to the Christian tradition, the spirit is one of the aspects of the human being that unifies him as an individual and "launches" him into activities that go beyond the material. Thanks to the soul, the human being has free instincts, feelings, emotions, thoughts and decisions, and can return to himself (self-consciousness).

Although it is not very frequent, the term "soul" can also be used referring to any human being as a whole, ignoring the religious or philosophical meaning, as in the expressions "there is not even a soul" or "city of 40,000 souls."

The soul in western philosophy

•   *Greek philosophy*

Plato considered the spirit as the most important dimension of the human being. Sometimes he speaks of her as if she were imprisoned in a body, although this idea is borrowed from Orphism.

According to the Timaeus, the spirit was composed of the identical and the diverse, a substance that the demiurge used to create the cosmic soul and the other stars; Furthermore, the lower gods created two mortal spirit: the passionate, which resides in the thorax, and the appetitive, which resides in the abdomen. Above both would be the rational soul, which would find its place in the head.

Something similar is narrated in the Phaedrus, where the myth of the winged horses is exposed: the charioteer is the rational spirit, the white horse represents the passionate part and the black the part of the appetites (always rebellious). The charioteer's task is to keep the black horse at the same gallop as the white. In the Phaedo, the spirit is seen as a substance that seeks to detach itself from the limits and conflicts that arise from its union with the body, and that will be able to live fully after the moment of death; This dialogue offers various arguments that seek to prove her immortality.

Aristotle defined the Psyche as "a specific form of a natural body that potentially has life, (From Anima, 412 a20)." He also understands it as "the essence of such a type of body" (412b10). The form or essence is what makes an entity what it is. By this we understand that the soul is what defines a natural body. For example, if the ear were an animal, its spirit would be listening and its matter the ear's own organ. An ear that did not have the function of hearing would be an ear only for words. In this case, the spirit configures matter in an organized natural body.

Thus a substantial unit (composed of matter and form) is formed. Spirit and body are not separable in the living being.

The spirit is also defined by the Stagirite as "the first entelechy of a natural body that potentially has life" (412a26). This indicates that the spirit is entelechy or the first act of the living body and soul and body are united simultaneously. But since the spirit is the act, it can be said that it has priority over the body. It is first not in time, but in importance. It is the first action from which the faculties and powers of the living being arise.

Aristotle points out, finally, that there could be operations of the soul that did not depend on anybody.

The dualistic vision that emerges from Platonism distorts reality and the consequences come to a disregard for physical realities, the human body and sexuality, among other things. The spirit is imagined as something independent, part of the divine and of the good, like a white sheet stuck in a poor material envelope from which it is urgent to free itself.

However, Aristotelian monism allows us to understand the human being as a unit made up of body and soul, giving the body just value by not understanding it as the prison of the soul (as Plato did), but as an essential part of what man is.

Thomas Aquinas

With Thomas Aquinas, anthropological reflection (explanation of what the human being is) takes a more realistic turn. Drawing on Aristotle more than Plato, Thomas Aquinas speaks of principles, no longer of opposite realities. For Aristotle, all beings in the physical world have matter (which is pure indeterminacy) and a substantial form (which is the determinative principle).

These two realities are inseparable, so they have no independent existence. We would say that these are two "aspects" of the same reality. Thomas Aquinas describes the human being as material on the one hand (his body) and not material on the other (his spirit). The human being is immersed in the material and obeys its basic laws of space and time. At the same time, it shows that it is not material at all, being able to go beyond space and time with its reason: planning the future or arranging the arrangements on an existing space in its daily life.

Example: I can prepare an agenda for tomorrow and conceptualize what the dining room of the house will be like without having to be present in that dining room.

Spirit and body become co-principles in the explanation of what the human being is like. The human being is fully bodily but has something of his own that allows him to go beyond the bodily: his spiritual soul. However, it is the soul that has the being in the first place, while the body exists as united to the soul.

Later western thought

Western thought fell on the dualism between body and spirit:

Descartes defines soul as a thinking thing as opposed to an "exten-sive" thing (res cogitans versus res Amplia).

a. Baruch Spinoza speaks of the soul as an attribute and mode of the divine substance.

b. Leibniz calls it a monad closed in on itself.

c. Theodor Lessing, as infinite aspiration.

d. Kant describes it as the impossibility of learning the absolute.

e. Fichte, how to know and action.

f. Hegel says that the soul is the self-development of the idea.

g. Friedrich Schelling defines it as a mystical power.

h. Nietzsche, invention and imaginary entity of the common peo-ple, that helps to strengthen the beliefs of the existence of a god or, more specifically, of "God".

i. Freud, as the difference between the "I" and the "super-me".

j. Jaspers defines it as "existentiality".

k. Ernst Bloch, as the original realization of the future.

In the Judeo-Christian tradition

According to the Judeo-Christian religious tradition, the spirit is the main identifying quality of movement in living matter, making it non-moving (inert) to moving, independent of the displacement of others.

According to the biblical records, in Genesis (Genesis 1: 20-28) it says:

20, God said: "Let the waters be filled with a multitude of living beings and let birds fly over the earth, through the firmament of the sky."

21, God created the great sea monsters, the various kinds of living beings that fill the waters by gliding in them, and all species of animals with wings. And God saw that this was good.

22, Then he blessed them, saying: "Be fruitful and multiply; fill the waters of the seas and let the birds multiply on the earth.

23, Thus there was an evening and a morning: this was the fifth day.

24, God said, "May the earth produce all kinds of living things: cattle, reptiles, and wild animals of all kinds." And so it happened.

25, God made the various kinds of animals of the field, the various kinds of cattle, and all the reptiles of the earth, whatever their species. And God saw that this was good.

26, God said, "Let us make man in our image, after our likeness; and that the fish of the sea and the birds of the sky, the cattle, the beasts of the earth and all the animals that crawl on the ground are subject to it.

27, And God created man in his image; He created him in the image of God, He created them male and female.

28, And he blessed them, saying: "Be fruitful, multiply, fill the earth and subdue it; dominate the fish of the sea, the birds of the sky and all the living beings that move on the earth.

The term also appears in the anthropological vision of numerous cultural and religious groups. In the modern era, the term "soul" is used more frequently in religious contexts

The spirit, in Christian theology

Christian theology, mainly German Protestant theology, is inspired by Idealism (current based on ideas) and comes to conceive of the soul as only "subjectivity". This same Idealism influences through Descartes the thought of some Catholic currents. Indeed, Descartes, by stating "I think, therefore I am", encloses philosophical reflection in the world of ideas. He is considered the father of idealism.

The philosophers cited in the previous paragraph are, for the most part, "idealistic" philosophers.

The philosophical realism gave birth to both the empiricism and the Marxism as existentialist philosophy (existentialism) and Christian existentialism (Gabriel Marcel, personalism of Mounier).

In the Bible

In the Bible, the word "soul" is given as a translation of the Hebrew word (ne '• phesch [נֶפֶשׁ]) and the Greek word (psy • khe'). From the use of the word in the Bible, it is clear that the soul is the person or animal itself referred to by the term, or the life that the person or animal enjoys.

The rúaj, which is "wind", "spirit" in Hebrew, in relation to anthropology is the 'breath [of life]', breath of the divinity itself: when Yahweh breathed on man his breath of life (Genesis 2: 7), it became a living being. Man lives while Yahweh does not withdraw his reach, (Job 27.3). The term strongly marks the relationship between creature and creator, her absolute dependence on Him.

The Ruach receives other meanings in the Bible according to the contexts. The nephesh (נֶפֶשׁ) means "throat", "jaws" (2 Samuel 16:14), "one who breathes" (Job 41:13, 20, 21). Néfesch comes from a root that means "to breathe", and in a literal sense it could be translated as "a respirator."

Exactly the same Hebrew expression that is used for the animal creation, namely, néfesch jaiyah (living soul), is applied to Adam when it is said that after God formed man from the dust of the ground and blew into his nostrils the breath of life, "man became a living soul" (Ge 2:7).

In the instructions that God gave to man after creating him, he used the term "nefesch" again to refer to the animal creation: in which there is life as a soul [literally, in which there is a living soul (nephesh)] "(Genesis 1:30).

Sometimes the word né • fesch is used to express the desire of the individual, which fulfills him and then pushes him to achieve his goal. Proverbs 13:2 says of those who treat treacherously that 'their very soul is violence,' that is, they are staunch supporters of violence, and actually become violence personified - so it has to do with interaction as well. between the mind and active personality of an individual, "life" (1 Samuel 26:21).

Also, the Genesis 9: 4 record says that the blood is Alma and Leviticus 17:11 says that the blood is the soul, because each living cell that makes up the blood is capable of moving in itself, differentiating animal beings from plants, which do not have blood or cells related to it; the blood, whose cellular movement allows the convolution of respiration, shows its distinctive characteristic of Animal Life. The word néfesch (שׁפנ) appears a total of 754 times in the Hebrew Scriptures (Genesis to Malachi) and its Greek equivalent psykhḗ (ψυχή) 105 times in the Greek Scriptures(Matthew to Revelation) and is never associated with the immortality that some religious, philosophical or other currents give it. But most notably, there are hundreds of biblical texts that associate it with death; in fact, there are 13 texts where it is mentioned as «dead néfesch» (dead soul).

Also, they do not have to do psykhḗ (ψυχή) and the Latin word anima (words that are related to the Spanish term «animal," making the expression « rational animal « logical for the human being) with the word spirit (gr. pneuma).

So, the spirit is defined by inseparable interaction of three movements in living matter that make it up: Mind/Heart (conscious-unconscious psychological principle of the Self [pneumatic movement]), Blood (principle of the animal or carnal body [lymphatic movement]) and Life (principle of activity-habit [dynamic movement]).

Without these three, the soul is dead. From this interpretation arises the importance of valuing both the human spirit and that of a beast. Strengthening the ethical evaluation from the most sensitive part of the soul (mind/ heart) until the toughest part of it (life).

The basár (flesh) is a concept that is not opposed to rúaj (breath) but they are juxtaposed. An acceptable translation would be "my person", which can be touched, experienced. When Paul says: "Your bodies are the temple of the Spirit (in gr. Pneuma) ... (1 Cor 6,19)" or "You are the temple ... (1 Cor, 3-17)" he highlights the aspect experienceable of the concept.

The Catholic Magisterium

The dogmatic definitions of the Magisterium of the Catholic Church deal mainly with the relationships between soul and body. The main:

The man has a spirit

• The spirit exists in each man as individually distinct and is immortal in this individual diversity.

• The spirit is a corporeal form by itself.

From Pope John XXII:

a. The spirit can have the full vision of God, only after death. The spirit is created and infused immediately by God at the moment of conception.
b. The spirit does not belong to the divine substance.
c. The spirit does not lead a pre-corporeal existence.
d. The spirit does not have a material origin.
e. She constitutes the vital principle of man.
f. It is superior to the body.

g. Your spirituality can be demonstrated.

The Second Vatican Council goes beyond the soul-body scheme and speaks of the person. "Man is one body and soul, and in his interiority transcends all things ..."

Pope John Paul II in a Sunday locution, published in L'Osservatore Romano (01/14/1990), said that "animals possess a vital breath received from God", quoting Psalms 103 and 104, being recognized, therefore, the 'sensitive soul' (Greek 'pneuma', breath, air), without forgetting that the word 'animal' comes from the Latin 'anima' (spirit). "Animals have a spirit and human beings must love and feel solidarity with our younger brothers."

Iconography

The early Christians represented in their monuments the human soul free from the shackles of the flesh and addressing the heavenly homeland by means of the following symbolic figures:

a. A horse running as if to get the prize in the circus games.
b. A ship sailing with unfolded sails towards a lighthouse or arriving at the port.
c. A lamb or a sheep alone or restored to the flock by the Good Shepherd.
d. A dove sometimes flying, sometimes next to an empty glass, an image of the body abandoned by the spirit and other times perched in a flowery garden, representing Paradise.

A woman emerging from an inanimate body.

The spirit in other cultures

Oriental meditation for the purification of the soul.

In other cultures such as Asian, African, and American, we find a spirit concept analogously similar to the concept developed by the religions of the Judeo-Christian group (including Islam) and European philosophy.

The spirit from the Vedic or Veda point of view, is The Self (Atman), which by nature is eternal (without birth or death or without beginning or end) of substance different from that of the physical body and which has its own consciousness.

From this perspective, material science, or that which studies physical or material phenomena, is limited because it cannot study spiritual phenomena since its nature is different from physical.

Spirit in Ancient Egypt

The human being, according to the ancient Egyptians, has seven degrees in his personality:

a. "Ren", that is "the name", being able to remain existing according to the care of a correct embalming.

b. "Sechem" is the energy, the power, the light of the deceased.

c. "Aj" is the unification of "Ka" and "Ba", in view of a return to existence.

d. "Ba", what makes an individual being what it is; it also applies to inanimate things. It is the closest to the western concept of "Soul".

e. "Ka", the life force. Supported by food offerings to the deceased.

f. "Sheut" is the shadow of the person, represented by a completely black human figure.

g. "Seju" designates the physical remains of the person.

h. "Jat" is the carnal part of the person.

Buddhist beliefs

One of the three marks of existence, Anātman is the "Insubstantiality of things". Nowhere does the scripture speak of an intrinsic essence of being or something inner with which to connect. It is normal to confuse the "Ultimate Reality" of the mind which is the indestructible "Buddha Nature" like a diamond (Vajra Sattva); however, on a philosophical level that indestructible nature is the emptiness of things and is completely different from the concept of Atman, soul, Being, etc. Those concepts are considered to arise from the ego and confusion of the mind.

The Buddhism teaches that all things are changing in a constant state of flux. Everything is temporary and there is no something perennial. That applies to the entire cosmos and therefore to humanity itself. There is no permanent "I". Anātman expresses in essence the Buddhist idea of that continuous change.

The mistake of believing in a permanent "I" is the source of human conflicts and worldly desires. Attachment to the defects of cyclical existence, samsara, brings about rebirth.

When it comes to rebirth, in Buddhism, it is the ego and the manifestation of the confused mind, of the stream of consciousness. The concept of reincarnation is also used, although it is not as correct as the previous one; however, there is no exact translation for the concept so far.

The Buddhism believes that there are three levels in the consciousness of the person: very subtle consciousness, which does not disintegrate in the incarnation-death, the subtle consciousness, which disappears with death and is a consciousness-asleep or non-consciousness, and gross conscience.

Hindu beliefs

The religions that speak about the spirit such as the Hindu, which arose from the Vedas, which are sacred texts for the Hindus, where they speak of life that there is a transmigration of the soul, that is called the wheel of samsara. Death is when the spirit passes from one body to another according to its actions or how it leads its life; This process of the soul was given changes and it became known as Dharma, which is the result of a good life or doing well and karma is everything that must necessarily live to learn from life so that in another life it can become better person.

Buddha, who to some extent has been considered one of the representatives of Hindu culture, says that to save the soul one must reach the state of nirvana, which is the highest state of harmony.

Meditation helps purify the soul and food is very important to achieve nirvana, since life is sacred. Nirvana is also achieved by having a life of holiness, for example, not committing impure acts that can affect the soul and learning to control vices and bad influences.

Iconology

The butterfly was among the ancients the emblem or image of the spirit. The artists of antiquity represented Plato with butterfly wings on his head, because he was the first Greek philosopher who dealt with the immortality of the spirit. An ancient fragment from Stosch's cabinet represents the meditation of a philosopher with a butterfly placed on a skull in front of which the philosopher is reflecting.

The purification of the soul by fire is expressed in a small sepulchral urn in the city of Mattei, through Love that has a butterfly in its hand to which a lit torch approache. A butterfly flying over the mouth of a comic mask seems to indicate that the wearer is alive or animated.

Sometimes Cupid is seen taking by the wings a butterfly that is crumbling, a symbol of the torments that love makes the hearts it dominates suffer.

Chapter Three

The good, the bad, and the spirit

Don't get things twisted. Spirituality does not mean religiosity. Religions aim at strict beliefs (dogmas), following certain rules and sometimes even power games to control people, their members or even other people while spirituality is about the question of the meaning of life in a larger context.

Ultimately, nothing else is meant by the term esotericism. Of course, there is a common intersection between religion and spirituality. Any positive form of religious orientation should be spiritual, but not every spiritual way of thinking and living is religious. That is infinitely important.

Spiritual vs. material existence

There are now two extremes: those who do not want to deal with spirituality and only think in terms of worldly parameters. The others who flatly reject worldly views and want to devote themselves exclusively to their spiritual existence. This form of duality is out of place. The society of the future will have to manage to integrate both aspects of its incarnated self into everyday life.

Why not live purely materially?

The properties that we want to develop further cannot be fully described rationally. If we still want to try: it is about the qualities of energies as modern quantum physics must grudgingly assume in order to be able to describe all properties of the behavior of elementary particles. Examples of these qualities are bliss, humility, lightning ideas, and ubiquitous love. In a purely material mindset, we will not experience these things and waste our incarnation.

Why not live purely spiritually?

We made a conscious decision for an incarnation. An incarnation is by definition tied to a material existence. This material formation may, can and should help us to further develop certain characteristics of ourselves in a way that we as purely spiritual beings would otherwise not be able to do. A denial of our material world is therefore not expedient for our spiritual existence.

How do we integrate a spiritual attitude into our everyday life?

We have all arrived very well in the purely worldly world. The question arises as to how we can integrate our natural spirituality into everyday life. To do this, we have to check what people have been doing wrong so far in order to precisely prevent that.

Human problems in everyday life

Unfortunately, people generally like to differentiate. It starts with the separation in work and personal life. A very misleading distinction. If we mark out an area of our life in which we are not ourselves but surrender to a world that deliberately exposes us to malaise as a means to an end (money), we purposefully create an environment that is not good for us.

Free and creative

It is important that we find the expression of our inner love in everything we do. However, this is about a basic form of love, different from the popular vernacular. It's about effortless kindness, compassion for everything that happens. The result is an opening of the heart towards wholeness (not only inward, not only outward). Dissolving negative beliefs is a symptom of this heart integration, an increase in vibration and the rejection of drug abuse.

Confidence and devotion develop, which serves everything that surrounds us - including our "work", if we let it become part of it and do what corresponds to our passion.

From matter to spirituality

Today's top-heavy people begin their journey by wanting to understand. The questions are "Who am I?", "Where do I come from?",

"Who was I in my previous life?", and "Where should I go?" These questions are a good sign. The nature of creation is then explored with a changed view of nature and all incoming experiences examined with regard to their origin, content and purpose. Everything is questioned. Material reality is no longer seen as an origin, but as a symptom of a superordinate structure. One pursues such thoughts more intensely, the other more superficially.

Gradually, we are looking for what is hidden from the simple self. The everyday life of spirituality is characterized by the perception of unchangeable processes of worldly existence (seasons, sleep rhythms, metabolism, etc.). This perception is an important part of becoming aware. It is like slowly waking up from a sleep that has arisen from our personality, which has been programmed by various influences. This perception is considered the most basic form of meditation in Buddhism.

From the spiritual world towards matter

Just as we slowly (again) begin to be interested in the spiritual world, the openness to influences from this very spiritual world grows in our direction. We are not on our own while we want to contest our development. Strictly speaking, we have a whole team of spiritual helpers who we can ask for help. They do not serve to relieve us of our tasks. On the contrary, they will (at our former, specific request) do nothing that stands in the way of our learning task, ie our development.

However, assuming a sufficiently mature consciousness, they will be available to us with a multitude of answers to various questions of existence - because we already know all this, but we just weren't able to take it with us into this incarnation. Our higher self is ultimately more than our simple self, only "unfortunately" does not incarnate the higher self.

Spiritual helpers consist, for example, of our spirit guide who had incarnated himself once and who accompanies us throughout our entire incarnation. Another helper is our guardian angel, who is with us our entire soul life, never had to incarnate, but also does not protect us in the conventional sense (ie not our body), but ensures that we can cope with our learning tasks here. He ensures that our constantly changing circumstances meet our learning task.

It is amusing how our spirit guide alone supports us in some of the simplest everyday tasks, for example opening a can ("Be careful! Other side!"), or before opening someone else's refrigerator ("Slow down, something is about to fly towards you!"). We should accept this help. But we can also ask specific questions to which we may receive an answer that we will understand. If not, we can always ask for signs that we can understand.

The limits of personality

We can already see that the world is not perceived as a whole in the ego. All areas of life are perceived and described separately. At best we can explain how these supposedly separate aspects work together. All of this can be seen in the division of the sciences into physics, biology, psychology, etc. We separate everything.

At the same time, we still see ourselves exposed to high influences. Both are due to the same problem. Our ego manifestation enriches the need for energetic protection (click here) and positive boundaries, which on the one hand is important for one's own integrity in our current society, but on the other hand is also precisely part of the overarching problem that characterizes society.

In any case, it reinforces the fragmented perception in parts, away from the whole. A first step to serve both the development of society and oneself would be to reduce the speed with which we deal with this world through thinking, feeling and acting.

This will also do the area of our interpersonal relationships very well, and it will also allow our consciousness to mature through more honest, relaxed and easy acceptance of honest feedback from the partner.

Spirituality in everyday life; Enjoyment in the now

Life should become meditation. It starts with conscious breathing in every moment. We can also:
- Walk consciously
- Be more aware of your own movements
- Eat more consciously

and so on.

It is of central importance to get to know yourself, to dissolve your own blockages, to experience your own hidden talents and abilities. All of this is possible from within, but can also be done through external aids - the "book of your life", for example, can help you to get to know your soul. However, the natural maturation of the empathic sense can only take place from within.

With everything that can be achieved in this material world, however, the golden goal is to always live in the here and now, no matter how difficult it is to keep. Otherwise, we practice so much with cramped goals - that would be a really worthwhile one. If you want to choose the most direct route, you can try DMT. The experience with an ayahuasca potion comes very close to deep meditation. But generating the frequencies yourself is always the more sustainable way.

Ultimately, however, the question is, how do we still achieve what we have to do here on earth? After all, we don't want to develop a split personality? To live in the here and now is in apparent contradiction to the material existence in which one should live out one's abilities. But that's not a contradiction in terms. Planning and acting does not mean that you cannot enjoy the journey to your destination - and vice versa.

If we make regular friends, that means not just planning and chasing goals that we assume that our life will only begin afterwards, something exciting will happen. The result is a deep phase of cleaning up contaminated sites. Old emotional or mental blockages in the form of trauma or thought patterns, beliefs or automated actions that have become irrelevant slowly dissolve. Mindfulness sets in.

One comes to naturally being in the here and now. But not in the sense of intoxicating, lasting pleasure satisfaction, but in the sense of centered liveliness. We get to know a stream of life that goes from above into the head, through the entire body and into the feet. Our consciousness will increase exponentially. We are becoming clearer, more permeable, more sublime - and even more creative.

Sublime task completion

Increased awareness creates an inner calm in us, with which we do our tasks. We are considerate of ourselves and others, and thus, in a slower way, we may even manage more than before. In any case, we are less carried away and less lost in frequent courses of action and activities. Thus, we are also less charged with external energies, which makes energetic protection just as less necessary as the processing of stressful everyday experiences through the psyche (for example during sleep). If you are part of the described stream of life, you are on the one hand more part of everything, but at the same time the whole is also much more in us, which not least also increases our (real) self-confidence.

People are very fond of, and extremely quickly, differentiating between "good" and "bad". He can classify good people and good deeds just as quickly as he can classify bad people and bad deeds. Society has trained itself to use thought patterns that are predefined by supposedly clear moral concepts and kept stable by literature, film and media reports. This article is intended to critically examine the perspectives on "good" and "bad" and end in a conclusion as to whether and when these attributes make sense. In order to approach these questions, each reader should be as open in mind and heart as humanly possible.

Evil from the point of view of society

Let's first clarify what the vernacular thinks is good and bad. Good people obey moral standards. You have a conscience and you use it. But this is where the differences begin. What is considered moral and what is not is subjective. One perceives a white lie with the boss as a necessary means to get ahead in life, the other perceives it as very reprehensible. So the first problem is already the basis of what we see as a reference for good or bad behavior.

The second problem is valuation. If we assume clearly defined foundations for moral behavior, if we equate morality with legal texts, the question still remains of how I evaluate a situation against this (for the moment, uniform) basis. Let's make a rough distinction here between the rational and the emotional view.

The rationally thinking person judges coolly and on the basis of facts, weights the available information about the behavior of a person perhaps using a key along criteria and finally comes to a result: 92.5% moral. The heart-centered person may take into account the particular circumstances of the person(s) involved in the particular situation. It does not come to a value, but to a tendency, a qualitative demarcation. So he could only compare two differently acting individuals against our moral basis from the beginning: Person A acted more morally.

For example, is it good or bad to help a homeless person? The rational person can argue: with a donation I promote the laziness of the individual, and thus the fact that people sabotage society. The heart man can argue: it is a different being, it may not be to blame for what happened to it, it is my duty to help it. Who's Right - Nobody? both? And finally: who should finally assess this and make a decision? Only society as a whole can do that.

No matter from which direction we come, whether mind or heart have priority, or we try to incorporate both as best as possible (subjectively), there will be no really stable evaluation scheme, so no moral police makes sense. Even with actually uniform requirements, the laws, there is still a lot of leeway for legal disputes depending on the situation and circumstances, why should it look better with far more subjective things such as human morality.

Nevertheless, people will always agree on very specific points: if I help an old woman across the street, it is "good", if I kill someone else, it is "bad". Is that generally true, or are we still making it too easy for ourselves here?

Evil in Humans: Society vs. the view of psychology

No psychologist will say that murder is a defensible thing. Also, no psychologist will say that certain women should not be helped across the street. But if we take a look at how the topic of criminal therapy is dealt with, one discovers, among other things, the following, very consistent trace of prejudice along the supposedly enlightened society:

- "Therapists only see the good in people, even if that doesn't exist"
- "As soon as someone feigns repentance, he is pardoned"
- "Therapy for offenders is just pointless pampering"

Society is certain: good people don't kill anyone, only bad people do that, and they should be locked away or killed.

- *Evil people as an incarnation of horror?*

First of all, one could immediately object to the fact that if we keep criminals locked up or even killed, we as a society can never learn what they did and how it could be prevented from other potential perpetrators in the future. However, this already implies an understanding of what many people lack: people are not simply born bad, they are made to commit acts that the majority of society considers evil through certain abuses that are perpetrated on them.

There is absolutely no question that certain acts should not have any excuse. Nevertheless, psychology sees each person as the sum of different character-building blocks that are formed by various factors. Certain intensities and constellations of these characteristics make a person more likely to commit "bad" deeds than others in certain situations.

From this, it can immediately be deduced that many people who could actually be potentially very dangerous simply never experience a situation in which they have to commit a crime. Example: Husbands are killed by their wives far less often than in the past, since divorces now result in an equal separation of property. Many potential murderers simply no longer have to commit murder - due to a lack of social "necessity."

Other people, on the other hand, may even have less potential to become criminals, but have a sufficiently strong situation that they trigger certain "bad" actions. Fortunately, many others have neither the necessary building blocks in the necessary mature form nor a situation in which they could prove their "malevolence."

So we are slowly starting to see that psychology deals much more sensibly with the subject of "good" and "bad". It simply excludes these terms as attributes of a person. A kind of modular principle prevails here, an attribution that provides a certain potential for certain actions, the execution of which requires a trigger.

Whether the respective action is then classified as less good or even as malicious is up to (a) the viewer and (b) the applicable assessment basis. We should ask ourselves whether we ourselves don't do something once a week that others would classify as "bad" in a certain way, but which we ourselves can excellently justify. Just as it happens all the time around us in small, hopefully insignificant situations around us, it can also be the case on a large scale.

Psychology sees not only the symptoms of an action, but judiciously to their cause, of course, with the aim of repairing act on these (and not about sweeping assumption that without exception every person would be treatable and cannot be more today so easily deceive as before). Above all, however, it does not expose an action to an ad hoc vote in the form of "good" and "bad."

Curse and blessing of reason and the question of justice

The perspective of psychology is very positive here and on the one hand should be anchored much more deeply in society. This would make the topic of offender therapy much more mature and, last but not least, simplify the work of psychologists. The social benefit is ultimately more than obvious: if we learn to understand, we can learn to treat, and if we learn to treat, we can practice prevention. Initiatives like "Don't become a perpetrator" consist of the results of psychotherapeutic research.

But you quickly make a jump here. You might think to yourself that if there is no such thing as good and bad, then there is no real justice either, right? If people simply perform certain actions, each of which is a consequence of their legacy plus the triggering situation, everything is subject to chaos, right? The idea of a god or the like would also be off the table or he would be pretty disinterested or sadistic.

Here we come up against the limits of pure reason. As nice as it is not to be able to easily classify "good" and "bad", "justice" is still conceivable here on a completely different level.

The view of spirituality

A question that psychology does not ask itself in any way - and that is certainly not its task - is that of the origin of the contaminated sites. This is not intended to mean the influence of one person on another, for example a pedophile educator, whose victim later becomes the perpetrator himself. What is meant is why a soul gets into exactly such a situation in which it is exposed to such an educator.

When we talk about karma, it is important that we discuss legacy assumption. Contaminated territories are not tied to physical life. In a previous life we made certain experiences, but also made certain "free" decisions, which on the one hand expanded our own treasure trove of experiences and on the other hand also had an impact on other people/souls.

We are allowed to experience the consequence of this influence, assuming no honest repentance based on understanding/empathy, at the latest in a subsequent incarnation, which we indirectly choose. This is how the topic of justice can also be described: from a purely psychological point of view, it is not fair if a person falls victim to another person just because they call certain circuits their own, no matter how well they can be explained psychologically.

From a spiritual point of view, however, we can rely on the fact that the big picture has a meaning and that there is - outside of the closed incarnations - a generally applicable justice. Of course, this initially eludes our understanding. However, there is evidence in the literature that raped women have been regressed to see how they molested other women in a previous life as a man.

Just as psychology does not want to find an excuse for the perpetrators' decisions, spirituality should not be understood at this point as a free ticket for negative actions, this does not have to be emphasized. Only one view should be motivated, which makes justice explainable in the absence of objectively definable malice.

But what about the terms "good" and "bad" themselves? What is exciting here is that, based on this superordinate view, benevolent (light) energetic influences can very well prevail - and always when they specifically neutralize lower - frequency areas. In terms of a generally valid origin of certain energetic patterns that influence everything that is, we can of course speak of "good" and "bad". Yes, there is a devil, demons, goblins and more (if we want to call these beings that). There is also black magic and "bad" witches - people who use their conscious connection for malicious purposes.

Evil as a means to an end

But here on earth we are always exposed to both influences: the positive and the negative, and it is up to us to develop towards the light. It is important to bristle with the negative influences, and this is exactly why these low-frequency influences are so important. "Lucifer" means Bringer of Light.

On the one hand, of course, energetic protection against these negative energies is important. On the other hand, learn above all to vibrate higher than what is opposite you. Evil has an important divine mission, if we will.

The psyche as a breeding ground for pattern processing and action initiation is an instance of our brain that becomes relevant much later. It regulates how we deal with certain influences and of course we can help our psyche, which is not exposed to a certain situation for nothing, to align with our own ideas of "good" and "bad". Psychology can help us with this - just like psychologists can. Some people just need it more than others - and that has to do with their karmic pressures, previous actions, and general mental maturity. If you feel that you are evil or subject to constant evil influence, then you need to engage in mental hygiene exercises.

We know that on a spiritual level, we have the eternal law of resonance. So is it "good" to wish a murderer death?

Let's say it depends on how important your own karma is to you and how long you want to experience the supposed duality of good and bad here on earth. Strictly speaking, the earth is probably even a negative form of exception in the universe. A lot of "bad" happens here, but that's why this planet is so special. Here we experience a limitation that is rather atypically high in the universe. If we manage to dissolve them anyway, any species can.

Chapter Four

Spiritual Enlightenment

Since the dawn of humanity, humans have raised questions and ideas about what spirit is and what it isn't. Some say that the Spirit is God – the beginning of all things. Some say it is the soul – the true self. The truth is, this spirit is your state of consciousness. It is the ability to accept changes (feelings, thoughts, actions, and behavior) in your life.

The perfect one is like water
Water provides life for all things
Without competing with anything
Water lives where people hate
Therefore, it can be compared with the Way
Chapter 8 – The Book of Ethics

A state of consciousness or spirit that follows the Way is flexible (like water). It swells and shrinks. Some events bring joy and goodwill, causing it to swell; others bring pain and sadness, causing it to shrink. The Way is a state of enlightenment first mentioned by Lao Tzu in the Book of Ethics.

Humanity also has a spirit that contracts and expands. When it expands, humanity experiences growth; civilizations flourish, and development occurs. When this collective spirit contracts, the opposite occurs. The most common example of this is the Dark Ages. The church, for whatever reason, felt that its truth, its way, was the only way. However, their way was not the true Way. It was not a state of enlightenment, a state of being and non-being.

The highly virtuous people do not pray for virtue; they already have virtue.

The lowly virtuous people want virtue, so they don't have virtue.

Chapter 38 – The Book of Ethics

Why Does Spiritual Enlightenment Matter?

When one's spirit reaches a state of flexibility, a state of being and non-being, we say it has attained spiritual enlightenment. But does spiritual enlightenment matter? Why bother with spiritual enlightenment?

An enlightened spirit won't bring about riches because it is neither rich nor poor. It won't make you have plenty because you are neither full nor empty. Instead, the enlightened spirit shows you how to live a happier, longer, and better life.

Searching for happiness

In man's eternal journey, he is always searching for happiness. But the search for happiness is the pursuit of the Way - of spiritual enlightenment. Still, so many people fail to find happiness; why? They look for happiness in the wrong place, and in doing so, they further stray from the Way. You need the discipline to follow the Way.

There is no mystery in finding the Way. All that's required is to keep calm and empty your mind and yourself of every action and desire. When you are empty, you become self-contained. You become valuable to everyone around you. A pot is useful because it is empty. It is what holds our food and lets us cook. We can live in a new house because of the space. If it were full, it would have no value, no use, so like the pot and the new house, we must first empty ourselves. Only then can we find the Way.

As easy as it sounds, finding the Way is almost impossible for most people. The chances of them finding the Way are almost as impractical as seeing pigs fly. Their state of consciousness, their spirit, is yet to expand and attain any form of enlightenment. All they care for is eating and playing.

Life is like a dice game for most people. They place their hopes, dreams, and talents on the dice and hope a roll of the dice will give them all the fortune they desire. That is as far as their spirit has expanded. Their happiness depends on their luck as far as they are concerned.

For some individuals, the Way is something they can almost taste because, on some level, they are aware of this enlightened spiritual state. The problem is they don't know how to achieve it. So they turn to one form of prayer or the other to better tune themselves to the Way. Their true desire is to achieve spiritual enlightenment and embody the way. Yet, it is this desire that keeps them from gaining what they want. Instead of emptying themselves, their thoughts and actions are clouded with desire. They try to reach this enlightened state, so they fill their minds with prayer, but like the pot, they are full, so there's little else they can take in. Until they learn to empty themselves, the Way will remain out of their reach.

The Way is the eternal breath. It is the beginning and the end of all things. If the Way is the beginning and the end, then the Way is in everything, and everything is the Way. The Way is in the sound of nature, the gentlest of breezes, the first light of the morning. To be one with the Way, you need stillness and calm. Stillness, to listen, to hear, and to understand. Prayers and mantras can only take you so far; they often cloud your mind and keep you from the Way.

Close-lipped, breath held
Life is full
Open-lipped, always busy
Life is futile
Chapter 51 – The Book of Ethics

The search for happiness is the search for the Way. Money, fame, wealth, and all worldly desires bring only temporary happiness. True happiness is found in the Way.

An Exercise to Try: learning to listen

The sages of old had to seclude themselves in caves and meditate for years on end before gaining enlightenment and becoming one with the source of all life, the Way. Unless you plan to give up on civilization and become a hermit, that's not possible today. Still, you can try this simple exercise to help you connect with the origin of life.

Find somewhere quiet, sit, or lie down comfortably. Listen to the sounds all around you. Like a rabbit, your mind will wander – let it. The goal is to empty your mind of all thoughts until you are one with the sound surrounding you. Do this for twenty minutes every day for several weeks.

This exercise requires patience. It'll take a while before you can let go of all the thoughts that cross your mind. But pretty soon, you'll find it easy to reach that state, and you will have taken your first steps towards enlightenment.

Chapter Five

The Way to Inner Peace

Peace is a precious thing
Victory is not something to rejoice about
The one who rejoices in victory is a ferocious man who likes to kill.
By enjoying killing, one cannot satisfy people.
Chapter 31 – The book of ethics

We have never been more connected than we are today. The internet age is often praised as an age of growth and expansion, yet we have never felt more disconnected as humans. Anxiety, stress, depression, even internet-induced ADD (attention deficit disorder) are issues most of us are familiar with these days.

Most of these issues exist because of an imbalance somewhere in our life, be it a chemical, emotional, or physical imbalance. The most practical solution is therapy for some of these people, but for others, the search for inner peace to quell anxious thoughts and dispel stress.

But is inner peace something you can order from Amazon? Or turn on like a light switch? Inner peace is simply another form of spiritual enlightenment; like all that is part of the Way, attaining inner peace is a lifelong journey that requires your full commitment.

So how do we attain inner peace, and what does inner peace even mean?

Does the Internet leave room for inner peace?

Whether we choose to acknowledge it or not, the internet takes a toll, often a heavy one, on us. The internet never sleeps, and because of that, there's this subconscious pull on most users to stay plugged in for as long as possible. This leads to increasing cases of insomnia, stress, anxiety, and even depression.

The internet can also be rather unforgiving. People are praised for being savage, for dragging others, so much so that it even gave birth to a new form of violence, trolling.

Some might say the internet isn't real; you can just plug it out whenever you feel like it. But the reality is, a huge part of our lives relies on the internet. Our jobs need us to stay connected. We pay our bills on the internet; we get the news on the internet; it feels like there's no room to breathe and slow down. For many people, trying to keep up with the internet traps them in a self-destructive cycle.

One reason for this trap most people have found themselves is that few people are aware of the Way. They are either consuming everything and everything the internet has to offer or giving too much of themselves to the Internet, which leaves no room for the Way.

Does this mean today's society can't find inner peace? No! It simply means it's harder and will require a conscious decision on your part to get it. The search for inner peace must be consistent and active part of your life. You must work for it. It is the only escape out of the chaos of the internet age. As we proceed, you'll learn a few tips that'll help you attain inner peace. You'll also learn how inner peace relates to the Way.

Defining Inner Peace and Its Importance

Whenever people hear the term inner peace, they assume you're referring to something spiritual and relate it to Eastern religions such as Buddhism and Taoism. But inner peace can be practiced by anyone regardless of their religious beliefs.

The reason inner peace is associated with Eastern teachings is that understanding the Way originated in the east. Remember, practicing the Way means embracing inner peace (peace with yourself) and outer peace (peace in your environment). One cannot fully grasp the Way if he/she lacks peace.

Unfortunately, outer peace is something you can't always have control over. As for inner peace, that is completely in your grasp as long as you choose it. Before you can understand inner peace, you have to understand what it isn't.

Inner peace is not:

- Turning down opportunities to try new things, grow your life, or expand your spiritual consciousness.

- Staying passive and watching life pass you by.

- Becoming timid, quiet, meek, or a reserved individual. A lot of people confuse being meek with having inner peace. It is not. The Way is not for the meek.

In other words, inner peace is not about how people see you; just because an individual appears humble does not mean he or she has attained inner peace. Can inner peace influence or change how others perceive you? Absolutely. But first, you need to have reached a state of inner peace. When you reach this state, others will subconsciously recognize that you are becoming one with the Way.

Now that you know what inner peace isn't, it is time to understand what it is. A seeker, one who yearns for the Way, is said to have achieved inner peace when his spiritual and mental bodies are in harmony (more on this later). You may recall that the Way is in all things; the Way is nature, and to hear it and tune into it, you need to calm your mind and empty yourself. Inner peace is this state of calmness. The thoughts in your head slow down and go quiet; the tangled threads in your spirit begin to unravel. Soon you'll be able to sense the state of oneness that is the Way.

The world is a loud place. It's no wonder very few people are even aware of the Way. But when you gain inner peace, the constant noise gradually dims, leaving only silence.

Why does inner peace matter?

Inner peace is important for all sorts of reasons. It is an important foundational step for those seeking the Way. Even if you're not interested in enlightenment, inner peace is still quite useful.

By achieving inner peace, your thoughts grow silent, allowing you to examine yourself fully and discover the problem areas in your life (be it physical or mental)? Those battling stress and anxiety can slowly unravel the thread causing them anxiety or stress. As you cleanse yourself of these burdens, you'll find that your mind is clearer and that your view of life has changed. The journey to inner peace can be a saving grace for millions if only they knew its value. Lucky for you, you've gotten your hands on this book. You've taken the first steps towards becoming a better you.

What does inner peace look like?

I'm sure right now you're asking yourself if inner peace is something internal and not external; how do I know if I've achieved inner peace? You know you've attained inner peace when:

- You don't rely on material things and achievements to be happy and content. Your happiness comes from your connection with your spirit. The stronger the bond, the more content you'll be.

- You've become a complete version of yourself without any new gains.

- You let yourself be whoever you want to be, and you always strive to be the best version of yourself – one that has mental clarity and calm presence that comes with connecting with your spirit.

- You're not bothered, but superficial plans or weighted down by physical worries.

- You accept everything that comes because you know that the Way is everything, so everything that happens is preparing you for the Way.

Six habits Blocking You from Attaining Inner Peace

The road to achieving inner peace is long, the journey is solitary, and some may find the path much easier than others. How you choose to travel on this path varies from one individual to another, not to mention the mental and psychological blocks you need to overcome before you can reach a state of peace as well.

Regardless of how your journey goes, some obstacles are common to anyone looking for inner peace. Most of these obstacles exist because of the age we find ourselves; others exist because the collective spirit of humanity often manifests itself in the same form to everyone (even though most people are ignorant of this global consciousness). Let's take a look at some of these obstacles and how you can overcome them.

1. *Tying your happiness to material gains*

Thanks to capitalism, people end up measuring their happiness by the number of things they have. This book isn't here to criticize capitalism as far as economies go; it is one of the most successful. However, there's no denying that capitalism has its problems.

Unfortunately, the happiness that comes from material items is fleeting. Human wants are insatiable, so to tie your happiness to something like that is a recipe for disaster. You may tell yourself I'll be happy when I get this promotion, so you work towards it, and you get it. Soon enough, your lifestyle goes up because of the increase in your income. Before you know it, that moment of joy that came from getting that promotion is gone. This is where anxiety and stress start to come in, and you start waiting for the next promotion before you're happy again.

True happiness comes from within, and yes, that sounds like a cliché, but clichés can be truths. The first step is to connect with your spirit consciously (see the previous exercise); then, you can figure out what you can offer life and get back from life in return.

2. *Running from your emotions*

Growing up, I heard from everyone around me how men don't show emotions because showing emotions made you weak. Sadly, I was an emotional kid, so I ended up burying my emotions because I wanted to be seen by the world as a man, as strong. But, of course, that only caused problems along the way. The emotions I bottled up kept erupting at the worst times.

It wasn't until I discovered the Way that I realized that emotions are a part of us, and to deny them is to deny part of who we are. By denying your emotions, you're creating disharmony within yourself. Society tells us that certain feelings are good and others, such as anger, fear, jealousy, sadness, are inappropriate, and we should hide them. If you truly want inner peace, you have to accept all your emotions, both the "good" and the "bad." Understand why you're feeling those emotions, accept that they're there, but don't let them rule you.

Of all the emotions, the one people struggle with the most is emotion. When people get angry, they deal with it in two ways; suppress it and channel their thoughts positively.

Thinking positive thoughts is an understandable gesture. Many self-proclamation gurus claim the power of positive thinking as the response to anger and other "negative emotions," but why should you have to suppress your anger? The Way is everything, and everything is the Way, which means anger, happiness, sadness, fear, all of that are part of the Way.

Feeling anger on its own isn't a problem. The problem is letting it control you and lashing out because of it. The best way to let go of anger is to understand the source. Once you understand the reason for your anger, you can develop a solution to deal with the problem. The same goes for jealousy, fear, and any other "bad emotion" you might be feeling. The emotion isn't the problem. It's how you deal with it, that is.

Once you've gotten the hang of working your way to the source of your emotions, you'll find that you're one step closer to getting inner peace.

3. Constantly comparing yourself to others

Theodore Roosevelt once said, "comparison is the thief of joy." Comparison is also a major obstacle on the road to inner peace. Modern-day culture is obsessed with comparison. People don't just compare physical items anymore. They compare the number of likes and followers on their social media pages. Some even go as far as crafting fake likes to boost their following and number of likes.

Teenagers fall into depression and become unhappy because their posts on social media are doing fewer numbers than their friends.

Unfortunately, there are no exercises that can help you overcome this obstacle quickly. You can only overcome it when you learn contentment.

4. *Placing your self-worth on productivity*

Everywhere you look, you'll see articles, blog posts, and videos on how to increase productivity or how such and such made $10,000 in three days. So it's no surprise that we've gotten the idea stuck in our heads that only when we're productive does our lives have meaning.

The problem is, you can't be productive every minute of the day. You also can't let the achievements of others pressure you and have you believe that your life has no meaning if you're not productive.

Half the time, this idea that we should always be productive stems from being scared of looking like failures to others. So we try to fill up time with activities that end up causing unnecessary stress.

5. *Having low self-esteem*

We can often be our own worst enemies. One major obstacle that hinders us from attaining inner peace is our self-esteem. Self-esteem refers to your sense of self (value). Low self-esteem arises when you lack confidence in yourself and feel bad about yourself. It often causes you to criticize yourself harshly and can even negatively impact your physical and mental wellness.

Low self-esteem will make you feel like you're not good enough and don't deserve the wins in your life. Left unchecked, it can affect our psyche and cause one to start having suicidal thoughts.

No matter who you are or where you're from and regardless of your socioeconomic class, always remember that you matter and you are enough.

6. *Running from our past*

We all have a story to tell, and it's not always a rosy one. It's filled with heartache and pain, regrets, and skeletons in the closet. When you run from your past due to shame or fear, you end up getting chained by memories of your past. You may not feel the effects of these chains, but they are there, constantly affecting your spirit and hindering your growth.

How can you achieve inner peace if you're ashamed of your past? Unless you acknowledge whatever action you did back then and accept that it happened, you're never going to make any progress on this journey to inner peace.

Inner peace means being at peace with all parts of you, including your strengths, weakness, and everything in between. If you try to hide some parts of yourself, it'll be impossible to find inner peace.

The road to Inner Peace

What does the journey to inner peace look like? What does it feel like walking on that road? Is it something you can start and finish in a single day? Is achieving inner peace as simple as flipping a proverbial button?

Inner peace doesn't exist on its own; you can't go to sleep with troubles and wake up the next day content and peaceful. While miracles do happen, they are called miracles for a reason. Ninety nine percent (99%) of the time, you have to work and earn this peace for yourself. Inner peace is not a dial you can just turn anytime you want; it's a process.

Because of the perceived difficulty in achieving inner peace, most people believe you'd have to be spiritual and practice your spirituality for years before attaining inner peace. But inner peace has nothing to do with your level of spirituality.

The reason it's so hard for most people to achieve is they're not willing to accept every part of themselves. There's good in everyone, but there's also much ugly in us too, and for most people, they are unwilling to accept that part of themselves. How can you be at peace if you deny yourself?

We tend to indulge in many self-destructive behaviors that block us from progressing on the road to inner peace. These habits reduce our mental and spiritual energy and redirect our focus on the wrong things, creating disharmony and imbalance within us.

The good news is it takes very little to readjust our energy and daily behavior and put our focus back towards striving for inner peace. Here are some adjustments to change your thinking whenever you feel like the journey is becoming too difficult.

- *Stop blaming yourself*

To achieve inner peace, you need to accept every action, both good and bad, that you've taken in life. This means taking accountability and accepting responsibility for your past and present actions. It does not mean blaming yourself for every little thing. You'll only end up appearing self-righteous.

You need to balance accepting responsibility for your actions and recognize that some things are beyond your control.

- *Let go of the victim mentality*

While some excessively blame themselves, others constantly see themselves as a victim. They are always on the lookout for a reason to justify their actions or someone else to blame. These people find it hard to take responsibility for their actions.

Victim mentality causes one to be self-conscious, leading to self-esteem issues, thereby hindering one from finding inner peace. Instead of thinking and acting like it's you against the world, re-examine your actions and take responsibility for situations you caused yourself.

- *Stop people-pleasing*

Another bad habit that you need to let go of if you want an easier time on the road to inner peace is people-pleasing. If you spend your whole life trying to please everyone, you'll end up pleasing no one and lose yourself in the process. Seeking praise and admiration from others prevents you from being your true self and acting with your own will.

Instead of spending all your time and energy trying to gain admiration from others, you're better off learning more about the Way. One with the Way is one with everything. When you know the Way, everything follows.

"By keeping the great Way, the people will follow.
Because the Way is a comfortable and peaceful place
Chapter 35 - The Book of Ethics

• *Let go of past grudges*

Holding on to past grudges is a way of consoling ourselves against the hurt we feel. But by holding on, you're only stopping yourself from healing and growing. When we're mad at people and carry a grudge, in some way, we think we're punishing them, but we're only punishing ourselves.

Why waste your energy on someone who isn't thinking of you nor cares about what you think of them? Resentment stops you from achieving inner peace because it locks you in the past. If you're unable to move on, how will you be able to see all the new opportunities and experiences waiting for you?

• *Stop trying to be perfect*

Perfection is another excess that stops you from achieving inner peace. When you strive for perfection, you train your mind not to settle for anything else, so you're never content until you reach whatever level you consider perfect. Because of this, they easily give up and only work towards things that offer assured self-gratification.

Some lucky few can use this need to be perfect for motivating themselves. They understand that perfection cannot be gotten in one go. So they keep on trying, developing themselves, working towards perfection. I was not one of the lucky ones. My struggle with perfection also created self-esteem issues for me. I'd start a project, and no matter how good it was, I was unhappy because I could not achieve this ideal image of perfection I had in my head. Soon I started feeling like I wasn't good enough; I started attributing my achievements to luck, and I ended up giving up on many things.

It took a while, but after I started on my road to inner peace (and believe me, my journey was not easy), I understood that the idea of perfection I had did not exist. I understood that the only reason I wanted perfection was that I secretly craved the admiration of others. Deep down, I believed I was better than people, and only through creating something perfect could I make everyone see it too. I was small-minded and wanted to feel superior to others. It was only when I stumbled on the teachings of the Way that I could understand all this about myself and take the proper steps to correct this imbalance, find inner peace, and begin my journey to living a better life.

If you also struggle with this, ask yourself why it has to be perfect. Is it for praise? So others will look at you in envy? Why do you chase perfection? If you can't find an answer that isn't toxic, why would you want to spend your life chasing toxicity?

Practical Exercises to attain Inner Peace

Inner peace is like a muscle. It is not a trophy you get and leave on a shelf. Like a muscle, you need to exercise it before seeing any gains and continue exercising to maintain those gains.

Every single person can achieve inner peace. You don't have to be a member of the clergy or a Buddhist monk, or a high-level Wiccan to achieve inner peace. All that's needed is the will to see the journey to its end. Here are some exercises you may find useful on your journey.

• *Train yourself in the act of mindfulness*

Being mindful is the process of focusing on a particular thing per time. On the other hand, multitasking is doing several things at the same time. The practice of mindfulness enables you to be fully active, focusing entirely on a single action.

Besides focusing on a particular thing, mindfulness requires you to be dead to your senses. Being aware of them only leaves you in a constant state of consciousness that is momentary. The Way teaches a state of inner consciousness that is not based on the happenings influenced by external factors. Our inner state controls the outer appearance. As such, being empty in mind with no thoughts preoccupying the inner state is also being mindful. The advantages that are gotten from mindfulness are paramount to our day-to-day activities.

Mindfulness is the ability to live in the now. It's the ability to be aware of where we are and what we're doing without getting overwhelmed by the external activities going on around us.

Mindfulness is a great way to learn how to control our actions and emotions, as the state of awareness keeps us from reacting impulsively to whatever is happening.

You must practice Mindfulness at least twice daily if you want to achieve inner peace. To learn how to practice mindfulness, refer to the nature exercise from earlier. To recap;

Find somewhere quiet

• Pay attention to what's happening in the present

• Make a mental note of the thoughts that arise, but let them pass by

• Go back to observing the present

• Don't judge or criticize yourself regardless of the thoughts that pop up.

When you lose focus and wander while practicing mindfulness, don't let it stress you. When it happens, forgive yourself, put a smile on your face and relax. Check if the wandering brought information or clarity. If it is significant, change your angle, take it that your mind needs a break, readjust your breathing, and continue.

• *Foster Healthy Relationships*

No one exists in a vacuum, so it's impossible to find inner peace if toxic relationships surround you – and no, I'm not referring to only romantic relationships. Although inner peace happens within, you also need to have a relatively stable and peaceful environment, or you'll find it hard to achieve peacefully.

• Having healthy relationships around will help you limit the noise and the distractions you're sure to experience daily. So how do you cultivate healthy relationships?

• Remove toxic people from your life. Anyone that distracts you or directs your thoughts towards unhealthy habits needs to go.

- Establish healthy boundaries in your personal and professional life, and don't feel bad about holding them.

- Learn to communicate effectively and let your family and friends know that you're trying to make changes in your life so you'll no longer be able to indulge in certain things.

- *Practice Detachment*

Detachment teaches you not to take everything so personally. It doesn't mean you don't care; it just means you let go of the idea of trying to force or control a specific outcome. Instead, you surrender yourself to the process and are satisfied with whatever the results are.

Detachment has nothing to do with being unemotional or distant. It's a state of mind that should be more accurately called "non-attachment."

"The root of suffering is attachment." - Buddha

By practicing detachment, you'll be able to sit back without fear or worry over a specific outcome because you understand that whatever happens was meant to.

How to Preserve your Inner Peace

Everyday living comes with many distractions and interruptions. One way to shield yourself from all of the chaos of today's society is by practicing inner peace. But achieving inner peace is only one-half of the journey. Recall I said inner peace is like a muscle, and like any muscle, it'll atrophy if you don't strengthen it every day. How do you strengthen inner peace? Through constant meditation. You also need to safeguard yourself. Otherwise, you may end up falling into old traps and habits.

Watch out for these four mind demons even after you've achieved inner peace.

- *Greed*

As you get more attuned with inner peace, you will find that the thought bubbles up in your mind to cause a little trouble. This is just greed manifesting itself, and wanting more will only disrupt the level of contentment that you have achieved.

- *Vanity*

A key concept on the road to inner peace is acceptance. You need to accept who you are, including your failings. It also means accepting criticism when it comes without blaming yourself or trying to play the victim.

- *Fear*

Achieving inner peace will help you understand the importance of living in the moment. However, you should still be open to whatever the future brings. Fear of the unknown, of uncharted territory, will only cripple all your achievements.

- *Attachment*

Attachment is what leads to control. You try to control every little detail of your life and the love of others. The only way to preserve your inner peace is to accept whatever comes and realize that there will always be things you can't predict or control.

Nowadays we are constantly being influenced by different sorts of stimuli, and it is very easy to get distracted by superficial things that really do not give us anything but a waste of time. This is why it is very important to know how to distinguish and identify those things or stimuli that give us energy. They give us something positive or something that we need at the moment. On the other hand, the stimuli that wear us out and take away our energy do not give us anything positive other than wear and tear; energetic, physical and emotional.

Chapter Six

Meditation

Today's society has taught us that material things are the only reward in the material world. But as you learned earlier, no material item can give you true peace. Sure, it'll hold your attention for a bit, and for a while, you'll feel like you've achieved something, but eventually, you'll get bored of the item, and it'll lose its appeal. This is how people get stuck in the rat race.

So what's the alternative? Give up on all life? No! You can try meditation instead.

Meditation is about finding peace, love, happiness, and joy within yourself. We all have our inner demons (you can call them inner blocks if you prefer), and these blocks are constantly fighting to tear us apart. With meditation, you can break free from these blocks and the unnecessary wants and desires that keep you trapped in the rat race. In time, meditation will also teach you balance as well as compassion and wisdom. It'll also teach you to let go of your attachments, fear, greed, and whatever mind demon troubles you.

Nobody wants to be a hater, and nobody wants to be in a state of constant anger. Anger is a natural human emotion. Sadly for most people, it makes them miserable and poisons their bodies. Meditation can free you from their clutches. Finding peace today can be harder than finding a needle in a haystack, especially for those without proper guidance.

Meditation helps to connect with your Spirit while clearing out whatever chooses to block this connectivity. One of the primary concerns of the Way is allowing you to connect to the sense of nature and the universe (the Spirit of heaven and earth).

Can you remember the last time you stopped to appreciate the vast sky? We're merely a speck in our universe, yet some people have never thought to look beyond themselves because they've let themselves be trapped by their egos. They're not connected to their innermost self, the Spirit. Since its inception, one of the purposes of meditation has been to connect you with your true self, your Spirit. Some call this connection filled with the Holy Spirit, awakening your soul, or attaining the Buddha state. Whatever you want to call it, it's all about connecting to the inner core with you. The more you meditate, the more your ability to connect your Spirit increases.

The initial goal of the internet was so people could share resources. With time, it grew to become a global connection hub. Yet, people have never been more disconnected from one another. The way you experience life is determined by the lens through which you view it, and for a while, the internet was a new lens that let us view life in different and exciting ways.

But like all material things, it has become shackles on most people. Meditation helps you release whatever inhibits you from experiencing life to the fullest. This doesn't mean you have to disconnect from the internet fully. Like it or not, you're a part of this physical world, so you have to interact with it. Meditation simply lets you take back control. It also gives you a sense of clarity you may have been missing, allowing you to interact with the items of the material world without getting influenced by them.

Many people can't find happiness because they don't feel this connection to their Spirit. They know sometimes it is missing but can't recognize what it is. Connecting with your Spirit, finding the Way, can turn a fool into a wise man. Meditation allows you to relax at the center of your being, allowing you to find balance and learn compassion for others.

Fusing Your Life Experiences to Become a Better You

How many notifications did your phone get today? Add to that the number of random information you come across, and you'll agree with me that we often experience an information overload daily. What happens when you overload a computer? First, the processing speed slows down; it warns you to close some applications, and if the overload remains, it starts overheating and may eventually shut down. The same thing happens to us. The only difference is you do not hear the warning signs because there's so much noise in our consciousness that we can't tell what's important and what isn't.

Humans are complex creatures. Our experiences are horrible and wonderful. For every joyful experience, there's a stressful one. To center ourselves, we need to fuse these experiences. In order words, you need to accept both the horrible and the wonderful if you want peace, and this is where meditation comes in. Not only does it help you sort out all the noise and clean up our system, but it also helps in allowing us to accept every part of ourselves.

We may live in a more civilized society today, but the people of old were more in tune with the Way, the natural breath of life. Today, society is constantly in a rush that people don't even know this breath exists. This constant rush means your mind and body are always active. When your mind can't rest, it goes wild, and when your body can't rest, it gets agitated, further stressing the mind. Before you know it, you're stuck in a negative feedback loop, and your body reacts with a full-blown stress response. When this happens, you may find yourself losing sleep.

Eventually, your emotional state crumbles, and you start having emotional outbursts with no warning. The people around you start asking how this happened, and the sole reason for that is because your bodies – mental and physical – are out of balance. You failed to let all the noise coming from the outside digest, which in turn caused your mental body to be overstimulated. To digest all of this new information and new experiences, you need to meditate.

What Is Meditation?

People say they're meditating, especially new-age yogis, but as wonderful as it sounds, hearing it doesn't exactly describe what they're supposed to be doing. It's like when people say they pray. You don't ask if they're praying to God, an angel, the Devil, or the owner of their favorite restaurant. You just smile, nod, and say, "Oh, that's wonderful that you pray." Just hearing that they meditate or pray is enough.

Many forms of meditation do indeed exist, but Westerners mix up meditation with contemplation. They think meditation is when you place all your thoughts on something. So if you think about an idea, westerners say, you're meditating on the idea. But from an Eastern point of view, thinking about an idea isn't meditation; that's an analysis.

True meditation looks more like philosophy to those in the western world. But even then, while they appear similar on the surface, they're completely different. Philosophy is defined as the study of the basic ideas about knowledge, right and wrong, reasoning, and the value of things. Eastern philosophy looks at ideas like reincarnation and karma, while western philosophies examine ideas about good and evil, specifically God, heaven, and hell. Meditation isn't concerned with examining ideas. It is a process of connecting with your Spirit and releasing the blocks accumulated in your mind and body.

The reason most people fail at meditation is that they come at it with the wrong mindset. They start meditating because they expect to get something from mediation when meditation is the ability to let go. As long as you start meditating only so you can obtain something, you'll never get anything out of it. Expectations have no place in meditation. Buddha never meditated to get something. He did it to get free of the need for things, and that's the key. Meditation isn't to help you get things. It's to free you from those desires.

As we proceed, we'll look at the Water method of Taoist meditation as described in the book of ethics – the teachings of the Way. Spiritual enlightenment starts with improving your body, hence the first part of this book. Once you become fully relaxed and your physical health is in peak condition, you can then start working to connect with your Spirit.

Making Sure Your Expectations are Balanced

One who acts fails
One who holds loses

> *Therefore:*
> *Sage doesn't act*
> *Thereupon he doesn't fail*
> *Doesn't keep*
> *Thereupon he doesn't lose*
> *Chapter 64 – The Book of Ethics*

Another aspect of meditation that is crucial for spiritual enlightenment is that it relieves you of the weight of expectations. We've been conditioned from a young age to keep up with external expectations constantly. It gets to a point, and you can't even remember why those expectations matter at all. Expectations don't lead to inner peace or longer, better life.

Expectations are rooted in power, and like everything else in life, they have their pros and cons. The physical world is filled with all kinds of scientific marvels and inventions, and your expectations help you take advantage of them. However, having expectations in your inner world can create conflict within yourself. Meditation helps you manage your expectations. The meditation method that we will learn will help you let go of expectations. You can move from where you are to where you want to be by casting off those burdens. With enough practice, you may eventually arrive at the goal of Spiritual Enlightenment or, as the Christians would say, directly commune with God.

The Water Method of Meditation

> *Under the dome of the sky, nothing is softer than water.*
> *But the hard-hitting attack is nothing more*
> *So nothing can replace it*
> *Chapter 78 – The Book of Ethics*

One of the main tenets of the Way is fostering spontaneity. Most people have lost the spirit of spontaneity because so many expectations tie them down. People care more for how they look on the outside yet spend little time taking care of their inner selves. The Way considers humans as being one with nature, even though they're unaware of it, so the first step in learning the way is connecting with your true self, and this is where meditation comes in. The Way does not believe or promote any God. If anything, it celebrates all God as one with nature. The only concern is freeing people from their internal struggle and helping them reach spiritual enlightenment.

Inner versus Outer Wealth

There are more churches, alternate religions, and spiritual practices than they were a decade ago. Thousands of years ago, religion wasn't as mainstream as it is now. People were free to practice in whatever and whoever they wanted. Yet, with so many religions around, people today seem to be far from spiritual enlightenment and inner peace than people of old.

Sadly, most religions today prioritize the gospel of prosperity over one of spiritual enlightenment. They preach the story of wealth and say that by joining them, you'll unlock your riches, get powerful, basically feeding into your desires. They address the issue of external riches. Meditation is concerned mainly with enriching the inner and using that to make your outer life better.

We live in a physical world, so of course, external wealth is important. You need money to get access to food, clothing, shelter, a good education, and a host of other things. But developing your inner self, your Spirit, is more important than chasing external wealth.

It is the strength of your Spirit that will allow you to ride the ups and downs that litter the road of life. So how do you cultivate inner wealth? Through the meditation of course. In time you'll find that you're happier, not because you're richer or because of any change in your external circumstance, but because you can finally sense the connection with nature that you've been missing all this time. You can use the water method of meditation to find clarity, connect with nature, and attain spiritual enlightenment.

What is the Water Method of Meditation?

Ancient Chinese had a philosophy that described the nature of all things. They called this philosophy the yin-yang philosophy. The philosophy states that the universe has a dualistic nature composed of two complementary and competing forces, dark and light, male and female, hot and cold, hard and soft. The ancient Chinese also created meditation techniques based on this philosophy, namely the fire meditation method and the water meditation method. The fire method of meditation corresponds with the Yang force; it is a hard technique where one changes and attempts to connect to their inner self through hypnosis.

The water method is based on the Yin philosophy and is a soft method of meditation. It teaches release, that is, releasing everything harmful and unnecessary from your life. It preaches letting go.

Lao Tzu first introduced the water method of meditation in his Book of Ethics and, since then, has gained popularity both in China and across the globe thanks to the growth of Taoism (the practice born from the book of ethics). Part of why the water style of meditation is so popular maybe because we yearn to be like water, soft yet powerful deep down. Water is so powerful that mere sound, sight, and even touch is enough to bring most people into a peaceful state.

Water as a style of meditation may be so appealing because deep down, we yearn to be more like it. Its effects are so powerful that the mere sight, sound, or touch of it alone is enough to bring us into a peaceful state.

Another reason it's so popular is that we're water bodies. The average human is 60% water; even the earth we live on is made up of water (about 70%). There's no doubt that we're connected to this life-giving liquid on a fundamental level.

Water also plays an important role in various religions and cultures. It signifies purity, clarity, and calmness.

The Christians use water when carrying out baptism to symbolize purification and being reborn through Christ. In Islam, water is seen as sustaining and life-giving. Giving water to another living is seen as a noble and greatly rewarded act. The Japanese Shinto religion uses water in its purification rituals. They view water as a symbol for the flow of life. The Hindus also view water as a means of purifying and washing away sins.

In Taoism, the Chinese tradition founded by Lao Tzu, the writer of the book of ethics, water represents dissolution. That is dissolving blocks, negative emotions, and connecting with nature.

How Does Water Meditation Work?

Water provides life for all things
Without competing with anything
Water lives where people hate
Therefore, it can be compared with the Way
Chapter 8 – The Book of Ethics

The water method of meditation works by stilling the mind and focusing on the inner. It is a yin-based meditation method that uses awareness to dissolve or wash away all the blocks and negative energies that have accumulated in our bodies. This form of meditation allows you to awaken your Spirit (sometimes called soul, life-energy, or chi). By practicing this water meditation regularly, you'll be able to:

• Calm the mind

• Harmonize your body, mind, and spirit (more on harmonies later)

• Release physical and mental traumas

• Free yourself from anxiety and stress.

• Relax your nervous system

• Be more open-minded to all that life has to offer

• Become more productive

• Live a longer life

• Become more adaptable

Benefits of Water Meditation?

Water meditation is a straightforward practice if you know what you're doing. Most of the benefits have already been stated earlier.

However, to emphasize the importance of water meditation, here are some more benefits.

- It helps to improve concentration and focus.

- It helps in improving your mental state.

- It'll leave you feeling healthier and full of energy.

Exercise to Try - 3 Breathing Techniques

One way to develop an awareness of the energies inside you is through internal breathing. You can practice this technique while standing or sitting. Remember to always breathe through your nose unless you need to breathe through your mouth due to some medical condition.

There are three breathing techniques for you to try. They can benefit you in so many ways. Before you get started, you should remember to:

- Stay relaxed, especially in your face, neck, jaw, and shoulder areas.

- Use the tip of your tongue to gently touch the roof of your mouth while practicing any of these breathing exercises.

- Go with an attitude of curiosity and patience. Try to stay focused on the practice without creating any tension.

- *Abdominal Breathing*

The first breathing technique is known as abdominal breathing. Start by finding somewhere comfortable to sit, preferably in an upright position. Close your eyes and pay attention to the movement of your breath. Observe your inhalations and exhalations without trying to alter their natural rhythm. Follow this breath for ten cycles.

Next, form a triangle with your fingers over your navel. Taoists call this area the lower tan tien (or dantian). To form the triangle, gently place your hands on your lower abdomen. Let the tips of your thumbs touch each other directly over your navel while your first fingers do the same a few inches below.

To practice the abdominal breathing technique, let the lower portion of your abdomen, the part beneath your fingers, gently expand with each inhale, and relax back to its natural position when you exhale. That's all there is to it. You inhale, expand, then exhale, and relax. Repeat this process for ten cycles.

- *Reverse Breathing*

As always, sit upright in a comfortable position, then follow along with the natural rhythm of your breath. Repeat this for ten cycles without trying to change its rhythm or quality in any way.

Form a triangle with your hands (see abdominal breathing technique) and place it over your lower abdomen. As you inhale, let your lower abdomen, the part beneath your fingers, contract inward towards your spine. Reverse breathing is the opposite of abdominal breathing, hence the name. As you contract your abdomen, you may feel a gentle inward and upward scooping sensation. Take note of this sensation. As you exhale, allow your abdomen to expand outward to its natural position.

Once again, you contract your abdomen on the inhale and expand on the exhale. Repeat this for ten cycles of breath.

- *Vase Breathing*

Vase breathing is a variant of abdominal breathing with some reverse breathing added to the mix, and to top it off, a visualization technique. The vase starts the same as the other two by following the natural rhythm of your breath for ten cycles and placing your hands over your lower belly in a triangle shape.

As you inhale, allow your lower abdomen to expand outwards and touch your hands (see abdominal breathing). While inhaling, picture your torso as a vase, and every time you inhale, the vase is being filled with fresh, clean water. The water fills the base (your lower abdomen) first and then gets to the brim (your collarbone).

Allow your abdomen to relax back to its natural state as you exhale. Since vase breathing is more complex than the other two, your best bet is to get familiar with those two first. Also, instead of doing ten cycles, you can do two, three, or four cycles till you're comfortable and familiar with the practice.

How to Calm the Monkey Mind

Most people that are trying meditation for the first time usually have the same complaint. Their minds keep wandering, and they can't stay focused. This is a common problem today. We live in a fast-food society, meaning we want everything immediately. Our mind gets addicted to this instant gratification that comes with living in such a society.

Your mind can get you in plenty of trouble if you start using it to think instead of just observing; in other words, you've allowed the monkey mind to lead. The monkey mind gets us into trouble because it always seeks stimulation, jumping from one thought or idea to another. As a result, we get involved in things we're not supposed to because of the monkey mind and our egos.

But the mind isn't the villain here, and we certainly can't destroy it. It's a part of us. So what do we do with it? How do we get the monkey mind to sit still? There are many ways to handle the monkey mind. We'll be looking at one of the ways you can get the monkey mind to go where you want and do what you want. The monkey mind loves stimulation, so that's what we're going to use. We'll give the mind what it loves; an activity to focus on. Soon it'll get lost in the activity, and before you know it, the monkey mind will finally quiet.

Instead of trying to empty your mind, which is almost impossible, the trick is to let the mind participate in the mediation. This won't be easy; we're already conditioned to letting the mind get its way. But little drops make an ocean, and practice makes perfect. At first, the mind will resist and try to jump elsewhere, but in time it'll come to accept meditation as one of its favorite activities. By getting the monkey mind to do many things at once, it'll end up losing itself. You'll find the yin (the emptiness, the connection to the way) through the yang (activity). This is how to calm the mind. You slow it down with various activities to connect to the energy inside, the emptiness, and nature.

Once you learn to lead the monkey mind, you'll stop thinking with your mind and start thinking with your inner self, the heart. Letting the monkey mind lead is like driving a car a hundred miles per hour. If you were to look outside, all you'll see is a blurry landscape. But if you stop the car and walk, you'll be able to take in everything. This is what meditation teaches, and it's what you get when you calm your monkey mind. You'll be able to see the big picture, observe all that's happening around you instead of letting the monkey run around. When the monkey leads, you end up living a reactionary life, and you'll never really accomplish all that you want in life.

What makes the monkey mind so interesting is that it loves playing tricks, which is how it traps you all the time. But if you know how, then you can turn the tables on the mind. Instead of chasing the monkey, you let it come to you. There's a saying, "to catch a monkey, stick a banana in a jar, and the monkey will come for the banana." The monkey mind functions in the same vein; it'll stick its hand in the jar and reach for the banana. So now the monkey has a banana in its hand but can't get said hand out of the jar. It can easily take its hand out if it lets go of the banana, but the mind won't, and that's how you end up trapping the monkey mind.

The monkey mind is associated with the ego, and the same way you trap the monkey with the banana is the same way we get trapped when the monkey, the ego, leads. The monkey mind will rather hold on to the banana than let go even for its freedom. As you're reading this, I'm sure you can recall situations that could have been solved easily if only you had let go, but you refused because of your ego. Now you know why that is; you were letting the monkey lead.

This is how you get the monkey mind to relinquish control. You get it focused on an activity, and it'll forget where it is, what it was doing, and finally, it'll forget why it was leading. And just like that, you have tricked the monkey mind into becoming dormant.

This is exactly what the ancient Chinese sages did when they practiced meditation. They give the monkey mind what it loves most – activity. Then they trap the mind in one area with the activity. Soon enough, by giving the mind all that activity, it'll forget itself.

The sages used to keep the monkey mind busy by getting it to try and trace the thirty-two energy channels in the body. You can try something different and have the monkey mind focus on the rhythm of your breathing, or you could picture a ball of light at the location of your third eye (also known as the inner eye or mind's eye) and have the monkey swim towards it. You'll soon see that the monkey mind easily gets lost in its activity. That is how you get the monkey mind to participate in your meditations actively.

Calming the monkey mind is good for more than just meditation practice. You'll find that you can focus more on your regular life. You can think clearer, but more importantly, you'll realize that you're one step closer to the Way. As the monkey mind starts to lose itself, it'll enter into the void (the Way). When that happens, you'll be able to observe the nothingness of nature and communicate with your Spirit. So next time the monkey starts jumping all over the place, just smile and direct it where you want it to go and watch as it leads you into the Way.

The Way of Tao

The Way is empty but not used up
The deep Way is like the root of all species.
The Way blunts the sharp
The Way unties the trouble
The Way softens the glare
The Way harmonizes with the dust
The Way is dark, but it seems to exist
I do not know who the children of the Way are.
But the Way appeared out before heaven and earth
Chapter 4 – The Book of Ethics

Becoming one with the Way requires our mental, emotional, and physical bodies to be in harmony. This harmonization occurs through three stages; concept, desire, and manifestation. The Way is simple, think, and it happens. But how do you harmonize your bodies? What do concept, desire, and manifestation mean?

We are made up of three bodies: the physical body (the one everyone is aware of), the mental body, and the emotional body. These bodies follow a sort of structural hierarchy. The mental body manages the emotional body, while the emotional body controls the physical body. So when we talk of concept, desire, and manifestation, we mean using our mental (to create a concept), emotional (to desire that concept), and physical (manifesting the desires) in tandem.

Here's how it works. Any action you take starts with an idea or a concept, and the concept (the mental body) controls the emotional body. The emotional body is the desire to make it happen, while the physical manifests that desire.

Although you may not be familiar with the idea of three bodies, the idea isn't new. Mainstream media marketers and self-proclaimed gurus call it the power of positive thinking. What is positive thinking of not creating a concept and generating a positive thought to produce the desired result? The difference is most people didn't know how it worked, which is why they found it hard to apply it in the first place.

Like Napoleon Hill once said, "What the mind can conceive and believe, the mind can believe."

When your mental body gets the concept, you'll gain understanding, and from there, your emotional body creates desire, giving you results. Without this process, you'll not be able to accomplish anything. This manifestation can take a while, and it can happen almost instantly. It all depends on how good you are at conceptualizing your mental body and activating the emotional body to get what you want. The more your practice, the better you'll get, and you'll be able to get your results faster.

This is how you practice the Way. Because the Way is nothing and everything, you'll find that most people already do this, only, they are unaware of what they're doing.

Human creations and technology all start as a concept, then a blueprint is created, and that blueprint goes into engineering and manufacturing. Finally, the components are assembled in a factory. We do the same thing in our daily lives but without the awareness of what we're doing.

When you become conscious of the Way, you'll find that manifesting becomes quicker. All manifesting is, is connecting to the Way. One with the Way has everything and nothing. So the more you practice, the stronger your connection becomes and the better you'll be at manifesting.

The Value of Nothingness

The softest thing in the universe
Wins the hardest in the universe
Emptiness can get into space because there is a gap
So one knows the value of nothingness
Chapter 43 – The Book of Ethics

What is nothingness? Nothingness is the Way, and the Way is everything. So nothingness is everything. When you stand in the middle of nothing, you're actually in the presence of all things. Everything comes from nothingness.

"In the beginning was the Word, and the Word was with God, and the Word was God." - John 1:1

The Bible verse above tells us that everything came from nothing. In this case, nothingness is considered the word, and the word was God, and God created the world. You can also see it in science with the big bang theory, the explosion that birthed all life. To go into nothingness is to return to this nothingness (because we all started from nothingness). This nothingness is God, the Way, infinity. Words are not enough to explain it.

The Way – cannot be told.
The Name – cannot be named.
The nameless is the Way of Heaven and Earth.
Chapter 1 – The Book of Ethics

Trying to use words to explain this nothingness (sometimes known as the infinity God) creates limitations, so you see why nothingness is beyond all words. Lao Tzu called it the Way because he knew the monkey mind would obsess over calling "it" a name, so he called it the Tao (meaning Way).

The Taoist version of creation sounds similar to the big bang theory. A concept thrown into the empty space of the universe was reflected out, hence the bang. A collective thought (or energy) was formed, and this thought was sent into the nothingness, the universe, and it was reflected like light reflecting from a mirror. Creation, and the big bang, is the first known manifestation process. This is how we can manifest everything from nothing because we came from nothing in the first place.

Once you can understand and master this, fully connect with the Way, you'll be amazed by what you can accomplish. All of life is connected; all of life is one. When we form a thought and send it into the universe, we're simply borrowing energy from the collective to manifest it in the physical. You can practice this for a few minutes each day, and with time, it'll manifest in the physical plane. It'll appear when you least expect it. Whatever we want, you can manifest it, whatever the thought, concept, or configuration.

The original act that led to the creation of the universe is something we put into practice, at least subconsciously, through thought every day. But with a clearer understanding of what we're doing and why we are doing it, our focus increases, allowing us to send stronger thoughts into the universe, which it sends back and manifests here in the physical plane. The more we practice, the faster we'll be at manifesting our desires. When we practice every day, we are honing our awareness, making us more conscious of this manifestation. Without practice, we are blind to what we manifest. It never looks like what we want because our monkey mind has confused us with too many distractions, and we lose sight of what we wanted in the first place.

You must be careful with your thoughts, especially when you are conscious of this ability. Whatever thought you send out to the universe will be reflected in you. Ignorance will no longer be an excuse as you are aware of your ability to manifest anything. As you think, so you will become.

When people pray to God (in whatever form they believe in), they're sending their energy out to the heavens and expecting an answer to their prayers. Sometimes their prayers are answered, but for different reasons than what they think. Prayer is asking God for something, a solution to your problems, money, a new car, a new job, a house, whatever it is. In reality, when people pray, they're sending out their energy. Some prayers are answered because the person sending them has a strong desire to reflect the energy and manifest it here. If you understand how and why prayers work and focus properly, praying will be more effective for you.

If nothing is everything, and God is everything, then we are God. The ability to manifest is something we all have within ourselves, and we just don't know it because we forget who we are. Some people don't think prayers work; others think it's ineffective or depends on something arbitrary, like luck when they don't understand the concept. It's not enough to just send a thought out to the universe. You have to put your energy into it. It is this energy that the Christians call faith. Without this energy, nothing will happen.

The same thing happens everywhere, even with black magic practices. People fear witches and wizards because they believe these witches or wizards have power over them when they're the ones feeding it their energy. They strongly believe that a witch/wizard has power over them, so they send that energy out to the universe, and so what happens? It reflects back, and that belief is manifested as black magic. All prayer, all manifestation happen because of you. You are the creator and the one manifesting, it's all our energy. When you send your energy out, the universe multiplies it and reflects it to you, but it's still your energy, just supercharged so it can manifest your desire in the physical.

Chapter Seven

Self-Realization: Discovering Who You Are

Self-realization is the process of fully connecting with the Spirit. It is rediscovering what we already know but are not conscious of. The road to self-realization is a slow one due to the fact the road leads nowhere. There's no destination because what you need to discover lies within. It is the journey into nothingness, into infinity. Infinity is never ending but a continuum. For the unaware, it means continuously becoming. It's like climbing a mountain, and your motivation is getting to the top. But on getting there, you realize there's another peak, and on and on, you continue climbing, reaching for peak after peak. This is the nature of infinity - having no beginning and no end.

Those who have discovered their true selves and reached the goal of self-realization are aware of one truth; if infinity has no beginning and no end, then there's no point in that never-ending climb. Wherever you are is where you need to be.

The rat race is another name for this continuum. People get trapped in this rat race because they're always trying to get to the next peak and the one after that. They say to themselves, "Oh, I just need this car, and I'll be happy, or I just need to finish this project, and I'll spend more time with my family." The monkey mind keeps creating peaks for them to reach, and they fail to realize they're stuck in a continuum.

Another truth the mind tries to keep from you is that whatever you want from life will always chase you, especially if you understand how to manifest. But you get so busy running the rat race that your wants and desires can never catch up to you. If you stop running for a moment and take some time to discover yourself, find inner peace, or even do some meditation exercises, you'll find that things you want from life come to you.

The highly virtuous people do nothing
Yet nothing is undone
The lowly virtuous people always do
Yet many more things need to be done
Chapter 38 - The Book of Ethics

This is the secret to living in the Way. It is an effortless way of living. As you become more comfortable with meditation, you'll get one step closer to self-realization. As you learn to tame the mind, you'll slowly start to recall all you have forgotten about the Self. This process of self-realization can only happen when you meditate and find inner peace.

There's a popular saying in the West, "No pain, no gain." It means you can only achieve something through hardships(pain). But the Way teaches us that if there is pain, then there's something wrong. Pain is the body's alarm system. It tells us that we're going against the flow - the natural order of things. We learn to go with the flow on the road to nothing to achieve equilibrium with nature. The Way teaches you to swim on your own, it shows you the path, but you must walk on it yourself. The journey into nothingness is one of self-discovery, so how can anyone teach you? You know yourself best; you know what is inside you, what you're feeling, and what you're going through. No instructor will have that knowledge, so you can only get direction from your lessons.

Teaching yourself also has its benefits. You become more self-sufficient and energetically independent in all aspects of your life. You'll have clarity in all you do because you know what you're going through and can tell what you need to solve it. As you progress in your journey of self-realization, your connection with your mental and emotional bodies also improves, and so does your ability to manifest.

According to Taoist religion, there are three paths to enlightenment. The first is through prayer and worship, the second is through good deeds, and the third is the Way. The first and second can help people reach enlightenment, but you won't know why it'll happen, when it'll happen or how it'll happen. The third path is self-discovery, and you know the why, the when, and the how.

We have mentioned the monkey mind several times in the last chapter and this one. The monkey mind is your greatest obstacle on the path of self-realization. You are part and parcel of the divine, of infinity, but you don't remember who you are. The monkey mind (your ego) draws you away from your true self and traps you in its system of thinking. It draws you away from the path of self-realization and interrupts your connection with the Way. But the monkey mind is not an enemy; it is a part of you. On the path of self-realization, you first have to acknowledge the monkey mind and learn to work with it.

Once you understand how the monkey mind works and realize that it is only your ego, you can take power from it. Remember, nothing happens if you don't give it power. The reason the monkey mind can run amok is that we empower it. The moment you take back that power, you'll be able to direct it to work for you and not against you.

Becoming Your Own Teacher

The beauty of the Way is that it helps you understand that enlightenment is in your hands. Spiritual independence is encouraged as you progress and get closer to nothingness (the Way). You are your own teachers. The exercises and formulas are only there to guide you. You are the only person that can understand what you're going through. Your friends cannot, your parents can't, and no Guru on the internet promising you enlightenment for a monthly subscription can understand. The journey into nothingness is an individual one, and only you can lead yourself to self-realization.

Every individual is unique. You had a one-in-six-trillion chance at life, and you won. There is no one else in this world with the same combination as you. The journey into nothingness also teaches us that there are no enemies or friends in life, only teachers. They are in our lives to teach us what we need to learn, just as we are in their lives to do the same. Everybody around you and every situation you go through teaches you something new about yourself.

There are many roads in life. The Way teaches us that the path to enlightenment means following the middle path. But we must pay attention to what's happening on the left and the right, or we will end up getting lost. If you don't know where the left and right are, how will you know you're walking the middle path? The left and right paths are the two extremes of life, our greatest teachers, calling them friends or enemies, fail to describe their role in our journey to nothingness accurately. The extremes teach us what we need to know about ourselves because they only reflect what we need to learn. This is why we're our own teachers. Everything we need to learn is already around us, and all that's needed is the awareness and the discipline to take the first step. The thing with religion is you're giving your energy to someone else, meaning you lose some of your energy. Although you may learn some new information, you don't learn anything new about yourself. When you give out your energy, you're putting your growth in someone else hands, and it is up to them to use your energy to take care of you or not. You don't lose the energy, but you're giving away your freedom and responsibility to someone else.

If you learn to take care of yourself, then there's one less person to take care of, and that's how you help everyone else. As you learn to take care of yourself and learn how to take responsibility for yourself, there will be no reason to give your energy to anyone else. If someone comes to you in an earnest, respectful, and sincere way, seeking the truth from you, then it's perfectly okay to share the concepts and ideas. When you give out your energy to a master, guru, or religious teacher, you're leaving your spiritual growth in the judgment and mercy of others. Their limited understanding will be what determines your fate. This is not a position to be in, it makes you codependent and leaves you relying on others for discoveries and understanding you can get yourself. The worst part is they can never truly figure out what's best for you because they can't see inside you to know what you need. The only one who knows what's best for you is you.

The Little Pine Trees

The sages of old likened our progress on the Journey into nothingness to the growth of a little pine tree. At first, it seems like the pine trees aren't growing, but if you give it time, you'll find that they are fully grown - bigger and taller than a two-story house. Because you kept looking at the pine trees, it felt like they weren't growing. But after some time, you could see the whole transformation and appreciate the time it took to get there. This is what happens in the journey into nothingness. By practicing the meditation and manifestation techniques slowly over time, the transformation will happen. This change is often so subtle that you don't even realize it's happening until one day, you take a look, and there are two big pine trees inside you.

When you keep up with the practices, your life will change even without you noticing as you connect with your Spirit and achieve self-realization. Since it happens so subtly, you won't even realize the changes are occurring. If you plant a tree and every other minute, you're digging it up to check up on it, it'll never grow. It's the same thing that happens on your journey. If you are constantly looking for changes, you are "uprooting" all your progress. Next thing you know, you're wondering why it isn't working. This obsession with monitoring your growth comes from the monkey mind doing what it does best, causing mischief.

 The pine tree didn't do anything special to grow as big as it did. It simply went with the natural order of things, absorbing water from the rain, sunshine and going with the universe's flow. This is what the Way tries to instill in us. To connect with your inner self is to go with the flow of the universe. If you do only that, you'll see that anything else you may ever want will follow you.

In the first chapter, we practiced an exercise to help us listen to nature because the answer to all your questions about the Way can be found in nature. A forest can reveal the natural flow of the universe. As you look at the tree, a seed drops down, burrows itself into the ground, and disappears. At first, it seems like nothing is happening, but the seed is flowing into the universe. It is rooting itself in the soil and then after six months it breaks the surface of the soil and becomes a little pine tree. In six months to a year, it becomes a pretty-good-sized tree. It becomes a big tree in ten to fifteen years; then after thirty, forty, fifty years, it is a huge tree; and in seventy to eighty years, it is a gigantic tree. A hundred years later, that little seed becomes a big pine tree that everyone can see from miles away. No one sees the hundred years that led to its growth; all they see is a big pine tree.

Spiritual enlightenment is similar. You may not show any outer progress, but there's a little seed growing. Like every seed, it needs nurturing, and this particular seed gets its nurturing from the practice we do each day. A little bit of water, some sunshine, and before you know it, our seed of enlightenment turns into a big pine tree.

What happens if you expose a seed to too much sun and give it too much water? It dies. Moderation is key, so we say that progress on this journey to self-realization, to nothingness, only requires a little bit of practice. Five to ten minutes of practice every day is enough to turn the seed inside you into a big pine tree.

Chapter Eight

The Way of Happiness

What is happiness?

It is to be satisfied with what you have, accept things without trying to force them and change the consequences, and find beauty in anything.

It's a state you can reach right now, without having to move, do or say anything. It comes from understanding the Way and knowing oneself.

Happiness is an inner state that is easy and simple and requires just a little change in your mindset and the way you look at things.

Happiness is right here, at this very moment. It's in you and everywhere around you. It's in the things you love doing, in the things you have but take for granted, in being kind to others and sharing what you have. From this, we can say that happiness is contained in the Way.

The Road to Happiness

If someone walked up to you right now and asked, "Are you happy?" Will you be able to say yes? Happiness, like everything else, is a personal journey. No one can tell you if you're happy or not, it's something you know for yourself. Happiness, like inner peace, is not something you can win in a lottery. It's not something you stumble into. It is a conscious decision that you have to make constantly.

If you're not happy with someone, then there is no point in keeping that relationship. If you're not happy with your job, quit. If you're happy with the body, you have and don't want to do anything to change it, okay then. It's all about whether it makes you happy or not. That's the ultimate technique when in doubt or have to make an important decision.

The problem is that most of us don't know how to be happy. We may try to find happiness, fix our current situation, or change things. But eventually, we find ourselves in the same old state - wondering if we're happy. This happens because they are stuck in the continuum, so they keep repeating the same mistakes over again.

Here are the three mistakes and how to overcome them:

* *Trying too hard*

People think they need to do something to be happy, so they start working too hard, pushing themselves to the limit, expecting too much, waiting for happiness to come, and so on. While most people can't recognize this trap for what it is, those of us practicing the Way can tell it is just another trap by the monkey mind to lure you into the continuum.

At some point, you begin to realize you've spent a lifetime trying to reach a certain state when it was in front of your eyes the whole time. What's most beautiful about being happy is that you feel perfect because you're okay with everything, it's like being in sync with everything. Most importantly, you're grateful. You find that things have become easy and they are just the way they should be, so you don't need to make any extra effort, put too much pressure on what you do, or make it harder and more complex than it should be. Look around you and really reflect on how you've gotten to this point. Let go of the pressure you've brought into your life, and things might just get better.

* *It's a place*

What many people think is that happiness is a goal, a destination, or something out there, or they will reach it in the future. They think it's a goal to be accomplished and they will feel great when it's done, and everything will be fine. This is wrong and never happens, because the future never actually comes. What's even worse is that if you had some kind of a deadline, when you reach it, you would be grossly disappointed because things just wouldn't be the way you expected. You will then begin aiming at something else, trying to find a satisfaction that will never come.

You cannot find happiness anywhere else but right now. Happiness is now. It is right here, and nothing will be different even after a decade if we remain blind to what you presently have. Happiness is not dependent on what goals you accomplish, so when you connect it with something you are looking forward to in the future, you are denying that it's now.

You need to stop making so many goals and plans, spend less time in the future, and live more in this present moment, because happiness is right here and right now, and it's your up to you to decide if you'll enjoy it or let it go.

- *It is in material items*

Some people try to raise their level of happiness by either buying stuff, going to different places, hanging out, having one relationship after another in the bid to find the perfect one. Or worse - by over-eating, drinking alcohol excessively, using drugs, getting immersed online etc.

It may work for a while, but later you'll realize you've created a much larger void inside of you. Now the only way to fill that void is to keep indulging in those excesses. This is a self-destructive behavior, and you will never feel better for real unless you realize you need to make some changes from the inside out.

Happiness is an inner state. It doesn't matter what we have, what we do, who we meet, and how we fill our time. The only crucial thing that defines our happiness (or the lack of it) is how we react to things and our attitude towards life. Do we actively enjoy our lives, are we in harmony with ourselves, and are we full of appreciation for all of life?

Finding Happiness

If the Way is happiness, does that mean anyone not following the Way will never be happy? Of course not. You can still find yourself even if you don't devote yourself to the Way. The difference is in your state of awareness. By reading the rest of this chapter, you can still find happiness (whether or not you're a seeker of the Way).

The 4 Step Plan to Finding Happiness

Many people often ask, "how do I become happy?" Such a simple question with an even simpler answer: *just be.* Be one with nature, with the universe, with life.

That's all it takes to be happy. That is how it works. And yet, we know so many people that have everything they want, everything it takes to be happy no matter what your definition of happiness and success is, but still don't feel satisfied, don't feel like they have a reason to be grateful for, take everything for granted and just aren't happy.

Some people have less than the average person, but it's more than enough for them. And they are way happier than those who have more. It's simply because they appreciate it and are thankful for it every single day.

Then what does it take to become one of them? If most of the nation hasn't quite found the way to do it, there probably must be a specific way, steps to follow. Here is how to become grateful and thus bring satisfaction and contentment into your life.

- *Be aware*

First, you need to become aware, not necessarily of the Way, especially if you're not ready for that, but be aware of the things you have. Contrary to what you may think, you do have many things you are probably unaware of. Think about the people in your life - family, friends, people who have helped you and supported you through hard times.

Remember every person in your life, even those who have insulted or betrayed you. And thank them for having the chance to learn the lesson they were meant to teach you. Every person we encounter on our way is meant to be there. They teach us something we can understand only if we are aware of that and are willing to learn from it.

Become aware of the things you have. Your home, job, places to go, clothes, technologies, the toys you played with, your books, and so on. Even if you don't live a luxurious life, you still have things that you use daily. Be aware of them, and don't take them for granted.

Be conscious of the things you do every day, which we don't even think of, and forget that they are a gift. Each day you eat a couple of times, most often food you love that tastes and looks so good, you take a shower whenever you want and use the amount of water you wish. You have electricity, and it allows you to do so many different things.

- *Appreciate the little things*

To appreciate is to see that there is beauty in everything, notice little things and be thankful for them, and realize that what you have or do right now is amazing because others would give everything to have it.

Appreciation comes from within, because everything beautiful comes from in there. It is important for you to practice it until it becomes a habit, and once it does, everything will seem different to you, and you'll be much more content with life.

Appreciate things as they are now. Because they are perfect, all the circumstances, no matter how bad you consider them to be, all the people you meet, things you do, whatever you have or don't have, everything you experience and think of, is perfect just the way it is. And even if you'd like to change it, you first need to accept it as it is.

- *Slow your pace*

We live in such a hurry that not only do we not notice the beautiful things surrounding us, but we also start to miss what matters - the people, events, and things that are right in front of our eyes. We rush through life, doing the daily tasks we consider important, working a job we can't stand, spending our free time in unconscious activities that only distract us from our purpose and journey (such activities are watching TV, browsing the net, and socializing online, using other technologies).

Sometimes you need to stop and take a breather. To stop means to take a moment now and then to look around, forget mundane things, problems, daily worries, selfish desires, fake goals, and current events, and focus on the essentials. Like your family, the things you love doing but never find time for, nature, opportunities.

- *Be Grateful*

In a nutshell, you need to be thankful for everything around you every day. A good way to do it is to say it out loud. Make it a habit. Gratitude jars have become popular, and there's no reason why you can't try them out. It's a simple practice that includes writing down things you should be grateful for and putting them in a jar. Soon it will be full of notes and you'll realize how many reasons you have in your life to be happy.

Another way is to make it a part of your morning or evening routine. Every day before bed or right after you get up, say everything you're grateful for in the mirror in the bathroom out loud. Try to feel excited about having it, smile, breathe deeply, and fill yourself with appreciation.

You can also put sticky notes in different places in your house. This way, you'll remind yourself of a thing to be grateful for whenever you enter a room. Keep a gratitude journal. Write down everything that happens to you for which you are grateful.

Choose the way that works best for you. And don't forget to enjoy the whole process. Becoming grateful is a big step in your personal development process and can work wonders. It will also have a positive influence on every other aspect of your life.

The final goal is to become mindful of everything you do, to do it with joy and excitement. It's time to be thankful and happy wherever you are.

PART III

The Harmony Of Body And Spirit

Chapter One

Inner Peace

L earning to protect body and mind, closing the door to the noise outside, helps us to recognize the importance that the spirit has in our life. We are not made of reason alone and even less of matter; our spiritual part, if nourished and developed, forms a solid ground on which to grow certainties.

To find ways and solve problems, the school teaches us from an early age how to use reason, helping us to develop our rational system. While this method penalizes emotions, it still seems the best way to prepare future generations.

But when we have to make an important decision, what do we make reason or heart prevail? Reflecting calmly, to better understand if it is an opportunity or something else, would be the best way to face important decisions, but finding moments of tranquility is increasingly difficult, because our thoughts are constantly interrupted by the noises of external confusion that they confuse and disorient us, postponing what we have to do.

Learning to protect body and spirit, closing the door to the noise outside, helps us to recognize the importance that the spirit has in our life. We are not made of reason alone and even less of matter; our spiritual part, if nourished and developed, forms a solid ground on which to grow certainties. To protect our spirit, we must take care of it as the gardener does with his garden, keeping it alive and luxuriant. Pauses of silent prayer or meditation make the flowers of awareness bloom and the branches of intuition grow that help us see the path to take.

In this sense, spirituality is also a practical technique for annihilating stress and daily fears that open the doors to many ailments that are harmful to our health. Spirituality helps us increase our focus, allowing us to give our best during decision making and making us more empathetic with others.

It also helps to achieve a deeper inner peace, transforming many negative beliefs with simple truths. Permanent physical ailments heal because the quality of life improves, we are more centered and objective, perceiving an inner wisdom that does not come from simple knowledge. By consolidating this lifestyle, it replaces uncertainties and anxieties with greater balance and consequent emotional stability which at the same time favors the body and mind. For some, they prefer to call it, 'inner peace.'

But then, isn't it all talk and nothing more?

Without mincing words, inner peace is not easy to find these days. The hectic pace of life we lead makes us stressful because we don't have the time, we wish we had for ourselves.

There comes a time when we need to stop, put an end to unnecessary worries, and embark on the search for our inner peace.

Achieving inner peace means having a feeling of well-being, of happiness, which envelops us in immense tranquility.

It is about making a special connection with ourselves, making a connection between our body and spirit, as well as with the world around us, to be able to perceive details that we did not have, not aware of it before and, at the same time, to appreciate them.

In this state, we manage to isolate our mind: any fear, worry, negative thought or feeling that might bother us will be beyond our reach.

The benefits that come with inner peace

Let's focus on our goals.

Spirituality makes us more aware of what we want to achieve. If we know what our goals are and know exactly what we want, we will focus on achieving those goals.

a. *Avoid bad habits*

By making a spiritual connection with ourselves and the world around us, we learn to differentiate between what is good and what is bad for us and for others. It will help us change our bad habits.

b. *The way to happiness*

Inner peace allows us to channel our energy towards the positive aspects of our life, towards what makes us feel good. It will help us to be happier.

c. *Reduce stress*

When we achieve spirituality, we learn to put aside all our concerns, which increases our level of psychological well-being. As a result, all the accumulated stress will begin to disappear.

Is this then, a strife toward perfection?

"Perfection is not attainable, but if we aim for perfection, we can achieve excellence." - Vince Lombardi.

Despite all the drawbacks associated with possibility of turning perfectionism into a force without it compromising your health or your life in general? But then, it is possible.

For this, read these 8 tips that will help you find a harmonious and balanced life.

* *Be a balanced perfectionist, not neurotic*

Perfectionism can be quite a healthy trait. Problems only appear when we live it to the extreme.

The vast majority of the problems exposed among the negative aspects of perfectionism are actually extreme and toxic forms of perfectionism. Perfectionists who do this are neurotic and let their accomplishments define who they are. They often feel a deep discomfort in front of their goals and the future seems rather gloomy to them.

They always aim higher, to the detriment of everything, whether it is their relationships or their personal health. Unfortunately, this form of perfectionism is glorified in the media, where the focus is on the end result and not the sacrifices that led to the development of some innovation, or the achievement of a feat.

On the other hand, there is healthy perfectionism. This allows you to stay motivated while constantly seeking to improve. It does not focus on failures, but allows you to stay focused on the end goal.

By discovering the difference between these two forms of perfectionism, the healthy form and the neurotic form, you will be able to recognize the times when you slip into the dark side of perfectionism and moderate your behavior.

For this, let's move from perfectionism to optimalism and adopt the behavior accordingly.

• *Stop thinking in all-or-nothing mode*

The "all-or-nothing" mentality is a big deal with perfectionists. Perfectionists have a very binary outlook on life. For them, it is either "White" or "Black", "All" or "Nothing", "Success" or "Fail", "Complete all" or "Start nothing".

Yet such a thought is self-defeating or at best, unreal. In the real world, no one achieves success without hiccups or failures. No athlete wins a competition without going to the trouble of training. No entrepreneur succeeds without first failing in some way or another.

And no one has produced great achievements without struggling with their tools, and without producing infamous drafts along the way. In reality, everything follows a progression, the all-or-nothing does not exist.

In Silicon Valley, there are thousands of companies including large multinationals like Facebook, Apple and Google who are encouraging failure. Countless successful entrepreneurs share the stories of their failures. There is even an annual conference called "Failcon" which encourages people to come to terms with their failures.

This is because they see failure as part of success, and by failing quickly you quickly learn what works, what doesn't, and grow from there.

Therefore, get rid of this all-or-nothing state of mind. When you think in all-or-nothing, what you get is more or less nothing-or-nothing. Allow yourself to do things incomplete, imperfect, and imprecise. Only then will you be able to progress in achieving your goal. Focus on recording your progress every step of the way, and use experimentation and failure lavishly, as this is the surest way to guarantee your future success.

- *Use the Pareto Principle*

The mind of the perfectionist is a complex labyrinth. He is able to absorb large amounts of information, analyze details, and establish elaborate procedures for each task.

At the same time, you need to be careful not to fall into the vicious cycle of perfectionism, that is, the ability to drown yourself in countless information and parameters. Because a perfectionist is detail-oriented and able to store up mountains of information, this often prevents them from taking action.

For them, everything is important and everything must be done. In the end, they end up overwhelmed by the magnitude of what there is to accomplish. Some perfectionists procrastinate, others get stuck in analytical paralysis. Some give up, while others spend a lot of time just doing the most basic tasks.

Do you also tend to set yourself an extremely high bar for every task you do? Unfortunately, this expected level of quality often puts a damper on you, to the point where it prevents you from moving on. If so, here are some questions for you:

1. What are you trying to accomplish?

2. Who are the people who have succeeded in achieving this goal, or who tend to achieve it excellently today? What did they do to be successful?

3. Based on your answers to question 2, what details are you obsessed with ... Are they critical to the success of your goal? If not, is it time to put them aside (or reduce your investment on them)?

Focus on the 80/20 law and identify the few factors that are helping you the most in moving towards your goal. Beware of the law of diminishing returns, which occurs when you try to perfect every detail, especially those that have no influence on what you are trying to accomplish.

Chapter Two

Harmony with oneself

We need to know that not everything is black and white, but that there is a whole range of grays. We have to accept that there are, and there will be, situations and experiences that we cannot control that will cause us to feel negative emotions, which are inevitably a part of our life. Achieving inner peace is synonymous with balance. There is no doubt that there will be unnecessary burdens that we can let go of, but we have to learn to deal with many others in our daily lives. That is why we must learn to balance our life, so that the mind stops fighting and ends up finding complete peace.

Simplify, you will conquer

We often complicate our lives and, as much as we find it hard to admit, it's up to us to make the most of every moment.

If we reset our mind and let it get rid of unnecessary ideas and negative thoughts, then we can focus on our zest for life. By simplifying things, we will achieve inner peace, then we will be happier.

Listen to your inner self

With all these worries and thoughts flooding our minds, it is very difficult to talk to yourself. To be able to penetrate deep inside, we need a lot of calm, a silence that allows us to coexist with our own loneliness.

Listening to yourself in order to live in harmony with yourself is essential. If you don't listen to yourself, who will? Indeed, listening to your body, your mind and your emotions, you are the only one who has this super power:

The body is through ailments, bodily sensations, the 5 senses.

The mind by the thoughts and the fluidity of the information that we receive which naturally influences the mental load.

Emotions are manifested to guide us in our satisfactions, our choices and indicate to us if we are on our right track. Listening to yourself is also being anxious to respond to your needs, which are reflected in your emotions.

So listening to yourself means paying attention to what's going on inside you. A pleasant feeling symbolizes that all is well, a feeling of unease signals that something is not right for you. Finally, listening to yourself means being in agreement with your values, your desires, your personality and your aspirations.

In addition, it is a question of responding according to oneself and not according to what others expect (in an effective or supposed way). It is daring to know how to say "no" or to position oneself even though that would not suit everyone. Listening to them means trusting yourself and following your intuition, opinion and moods in order to live fully in harmony with yourself.

We have to learn to let ourselves go so that we know what our real internal concerns are. With a lot of patience and by slowing down our breathing, we can gradually achieve inner peace.

Keep the critics out of your life

Empathy is fundamental to moving forward on the path of inner peace. We have to put ourselves in other people's shoes.

Negative criticism towards others and ourselves makes us uncomfortable, it hurts both the recipient and the sender.

Get to know yourself. This process is not easy. In particular knowing that we are beings who evolve and we adapt to each age, to each event and each experience that arises. Some people will get to know each other while others will go through their lives without even thinking about it. It depends on our personality and our life course.

Knowing yourself means being aware of your strengths and resources as well as your weaknesses and limitations. Knowing yourself involves knowing what you want, what you aspire to and what you don't or no longer want. It is knowing your needs, your emotions, your capacities, your talents. It is also accepting his past, his good as well as his bad experiences, his relations, his ruptures, his personal/family/school/professional journey!

In addition, it is also about knowing its qualities and its faults. Even if some people advocate that we have the qualities of our faults and the faults of our qualities, it is nonetheless to be aware of who we are in our most beautiful imperfection is a source of well-being because a source of progress! When we know each other, we know who we are, what we are worth and what direction to take for our future.

We must learn to see the positive side of things and to avoid all negative thinking, including criticism. The further we remove criticism from our life, the closer we will come to inner peace. We provide more details of this in the subsequent pages of this chapter.

The importance of meditation and reflection

To achieve inner peace, it is essential to calm our mind. For this the ideal is to carry out meditation exercises, which will help us to face the daily life better, with a more relaxed mind.

We have within us the capacities to know if what we are experiencing is good or not for us. It is possible for us to make choices, to remain in these choices or to modify them. We can't go back but we can always adjust to stay true to our own path. It is a wealth that we all have, regardless of the experience: we all have the choice and understanding each other allows us to experience them in harmony with oneself. It is very important for his well-being.

This power involves our ability to also understand our emotions, identify them and understand their signal. It is knowing the meaning that we put behind our actions, our ideas, our changes and our difficulties. Highlight our values and principles in our general behavior.

Understanding oneself includes the relationships we have, those we build and strengthen, but also those that we break or avoid. It is therefore to understand our expectations and our aspirations in the bonds that we form, in all areas: love, family, professional, friendly and social.

You should devote part of the day to regaining tranquility through meditation. In this way, our body and mind will be more predisposed to reflect and find the long-awaited inner peace.

In full consciousness, accept your strengths and your flaws, your qualities and your faults, your positive and negative emotions, etc. Everything that constitutes you and that makes you a unique and exceptional being! Living in harmony with yourself goes through this step! It is about respecting yourself in your entirety in order to achieve feelings of well-being and satisfaction.

Accepting yourself implies that you assume yourself as you are. It's knowing yourself, understanding yourself and not being afraid of it! Not afraid of not being accepted or being judged or criticized and fully asserting yourself in all awareness of who you are. It is possible for this to change vocabulary ("I am sensitive to injustice" for example rather than "I am angry", or "I have the character that I have" instead of "I have bad feelings character" - anyway what does "having a bad temper mean ??), change your attitude (no longer de-value yourself or fall into a box), change your view of things (practice positive communication) and work on your emotions negative social (such as shame).

You have to be thankful that you are well born

Recognizing life and all the positive things around us is fundamental to finding the path to inner peace. It helps us to be happier and to achieve balance.

There is always something to be thankful for, even if sometimes it is hard to believe it. When we reduce our complaints about what we don't have and begin to be grateful for what we have, we will regain our internal balance.

You have to love yourself. is to cherish yourself, to take care of yourself as a close friend or a member of your family. It's loving who you are and what you have. To love oneself is to adore what makes us up in our finest flaws.

We are indeed different: be it tall, short, fat, skinny, white, blue, black, neon or glitter, what does it matter? We are human! With our qualities, our faults, our experience, our family history, our desires, our dreams, etc. Everything that constitutes us makes us rich internally, to become aware of it with gratitude and benevolence: it is to love oneself. You really think you can live in harmony with yourself without loving yourself first?

To accept oneself is to accept this difference in a positive light. It is not because we do not think like everyone else, that we do not find ourselves in our place, that we do not fit "the mold" that it is a bad thing. The greatest geniuses of this world have often been "different", yet they have marked history.

We all make mistakes, no one is perfect and fortunately! This is what allows us to move forward and tend towards a "better", towards a change in order to love each other even more. Noticing who we have become despite the pitfalls and obstacles or even failures, isn't that self-love? Tolerance and mercy towards us?

 To love yourself is to accept yourself fully with the best possible compassion and care. And it is by learning to love ourselves that it is possible for us to love others "healthily" (without emotional dependence, excessive jealousy, fear of abandonment or rejection, etc.) and to build relationships with all kinds that are fulfilling.

When you love yourself, it is easier to love others. So there is no question of accepting toxic and devaluing relationships. Or not to accept violence, mistreatment; whether physical, mental or emotional. We only seek to build and move forward with positivity and serenity in the Love of oneself, others and its environment.

Generosity, giving without receiving anything in return, is linked to gratitude. We must move away from selfishness to come closer to peace and serenity.

The power of forgiveness

The act of forgiving and asking for forgiveness has a therapeutic effect which is fundamental to achieving spiritual peace. Through forgiveness, we trade destructive behaviors towards the person who hurt us for constructive behaviors.

Forgiveness is also, for ourselves, probably the most difficult thing to give. It is precisely at this stage that we must insist on achieving inner calm.

The act of forgiveness is complex because it is not an isolated moment, on the contrary. It is an ongoing process that can be deepened and completed over time.

Chapter Three - Connection Between The Body And Spirit

As established in the previous chapter, the body is composed of flesh and bones. It is a physical container that houses the spirit, while the spirit is your state of consciousness. It is the ability to accept changes (feelings, thoughts, actions, and behavior) in your life.

Understanding The Connection Between The Body And Spirit

Man is always searching for happiness and, as such, pursues mundane things to fulfill their thoughts or consciousness. For instance, due to the desire as humans to be loved, valued, and needed, some people participate in social media activities by posting pictures and engaging in contests. Doing this helps them feel noticed and validated as they receive recognition from strangers that fool them into thinking they are loved and accepted.

Great Virtue of practice is with the Way
The Way cannot be touched or captured
It cannot be felt or captured
But there's an image inside
It cannot be supposed or captured
But there is a category inside14
The Way is dim
But inside has substance

This substance is genuine
Which contains belief
From the primitive to the present
The Way is eternal
The Way is the creation
How do we know that Way is the root of all creatures?
Chapter 21 - The Book of Ethics

Receiving recognition may satisfy that craving for validation for a short while. One may even be happy for a while; however, as the world moves on to the next exciting thing, the feelings of dissatisfaction with oneself returns. It is an insatiable feeling that is due to the entire state of one's mind. In life, the search for happiness is in the Way-which is Spiritual Enlightenment. If you were wondering, Yes, the body and spirit can be harmonized.

The Way does not act
But nothing is not done
If the king notices this
Then everything will change itself
If one wants to do
Be simple and rustic
Be invisible without desire
When there is no desire, then you will be undisturbed
This is the path to self-healing.
Chapter 37- The Book of Ethics

The body and spirit are interrelated, closely connected, and reciprocal in action. It simply means the issues of life steams from within. As understood from the story, a change in heart was responsible for the difference in appearance. Spiritual strength/enlightenment yields physical well-being. To find true happiness, it is necessary to be in a state of spiritual enlightenment - The Way.

To a school of thought, the body is a hindrance in living purposefully and finding happiness. Why? The body is perceived as a lowly nature, full of sin, evil, and actions contrary to our desire. Looking at the life of a kleptomaniac, these individuals pick petty items too ridiculous to be stolen by the will of their bodies. How can the body move without the permission of the spirit? The act of theft is carried out in a state of unconsciousness. Perhaps, could it be an imbalance in the spiritual enlightenment needed for the body to vibrate at a specific frequency? Cases like these and more make it difficult for one to understand the balance between spirit and body.

Nevertheless, being a physical being does not imply evil and sin. The purpose of the body is to serve the spirit. The relationship between the two elements is beautiful. Interestingly, the spirit cannot be made perfect without the body. Only with the body can the spirit find purpose.

What does this mean?

> *People with profound Virtue like babies*
> *Bees and snakes cannot spit poisonous nibs*
> *Wild beasts cannot grab*
> *Birds can't peck*
> *Soft bones and weak tendons*
> *But hold firm*
> *Don't know how to have sexual intercourse between men and women*
> *But perfect vitality is living in abundance*
> *Screaming all day but not hoarse*
> *That is called Harmony*
> *Knowing the Harmony is invariant*
> *Knowing invariants is bright*
> *Greed is catastrophe*
> *Being greedy is not Harmony*
> *Disharmony is the opposite of the Way*
> *The opposite of the Way is soon destroyed.*
> *Chapter 55 – The Book of Ethics*

It simply means:

When one is indeed in the Way, Harmony is achieved. Being in a state of consciousness is a character only possible with a body. As much as the spirit's will wants to be expressed, it is limited to a living body. That is to say, the body without the spirit is dead. Wow! What harmonization. The body, spirit relationship is directly proportional to each other, whereby the body's functioning is dependent on the spirit, vice-versa.

The correlation between the spirit and body can be said thus: The purpose of our spiritual enlightenment is to bring Harmony through our body. Our spiritual strength influences physical well-being. Our thoughts and feelings trace their source from within and translate into physical experiences, which become our actions and behavior.

Feel opposed, suffocated, excited, satisfied, valued, etc., is the inter-relationship between spirit and body. Our noble feelings are expressed in the physique.

Victor Hugo said, "No external grace is complete unless vivified by internal beauty."

Let's take into cognizance an account of a trip you embarked on with your family to a resort center. On your arrival, you had a glance at the environment. It was picturesque, serene, scenic, and a sight to behold. However, after you showered and had lunch, with slow strides around the resort, you began to notice imperfections in the structure. Even though the flaws saw, the peace, calm, good energy you felt at your arrival was not lost. That is true beauty springing from a state of Harmony. True beauty is the purity, radiance, Harmony, light that emanates from a person's inner light, which actualizes in the bodily form.

After an accident made him blind, French writer Jacques felt like the world had come crashing down against him. However, as he journeyed in life, he saw the light never seen throughout the days; his organs of sight were functional, and he concluded, "To be blind meant not to see but, I saw." The testimony of this young man and others who have lost their sense of sight, perception, or one thing or the other is an eye-opener that indeed, spiritual enlightenment is what brings balance and harmony to our body; what you see within translates without.

Do not go out but know the world
Do not look out the window but see the Way
The more one goes, the less one knows
So, a sage does not go out but knows
Do not only look but see
Do not only do but accomplish.
Chapter 47 – The Book of Ethics

Your manner and Way of life affect balance. One needs to be careful of the physical image he paints to the world. Live a life that portrays your spiritual enlightenment to yield proper balance. As you notice imbalance and lack of Harmony, it is proof that you lack enlightenment and you will need to work on this.

Chapter Four

Balance And Harmony

Many of us wonder about the essence of harmony between the body, spirit, and soul. The foundational pillars of harmonious life are based on these components. The body and spirit have to be in constant relationship and balance to attain harmony. The energy generated within our inner state of consciousness, the actions that this energy produces outward to the seeing of others, and the channeling of power from the cosmos (the Earth and its components) have to be perfected as one sound, united together to sustain a peaceful life.

We have experienced several situations in life that are easily relatable to understand what not living in harmony entails. Some examples are:

1. In most cases, we find ourselves thinking, overworking, and beating ourselves up concerning adverse events that happened in our lives than the good times we had. For instance, if you are offered a position, or you relocate to a new school, nation, etc., your initial response to this situation will be negative. You think of how difficult it is to cope, feeling alone or left out, the hardships, contrary to how that circumstance will profit you greatly. If we are sincere with ourselves, we discover that we are designed to be full of negatives. Sadly, this is interpreted as your spirit (state of consciousness) not being in harmony with itself.

2. Using the body as an example, what we experience all comes down to your self-perception. Just as a lot of our young ones face today, the craze to have an image everyone appreciates on social media is on a high. However, suppose we confront most of them to know how they see themselves when they look at the mirror

or, better still, do a practical test of each one facing the mirror and telling us whose image they see reflecting. In that case, it will amaze you to know that a significant percentage of those smiling, gorgeous, cute, well-dressed ladies and gentlemen do not see advancement into what they aspire to become or beauty in themselves. It only means you are not in harmony with your body.

3. Regarding the spirit, if you look carefully, some of your neighbors, friends, or acquaintances who are spiritually enlightened have a defined way of life. One notable thing about them is the desire to learn, being knowledgeable, and the ease they offer the knowledge gained over time. Either way, a life of giving and receiving is their culture. In plain terms, they are not inflexible, living in a box; they have stretched their body and spirits beyond and grown drastically by their and others' experiences and knowledge.

Ponder on these questions: do you believe you understand everything? Do you show interest in learning anything that arouses your curiosity? Do you judge the source of what you are learning? After your honest evaluation of these questions and your answer to any is NO, it is disheartening that you are not in harmony with your body and spirit.

What is Harmony?

Harmony is a powerful Chinese expression describing the chase for balance between a man, his atmosphere, people, and spirit. The concept of harmony is as such wise and philosophical.

Harmony exudes diversity first, then balance. It is how a lot is combined with being balanced. When diverse thoughts, concepts, colors, and actions are balanced, it produces a harmonious event. For example, imagine a group of persons singing in the same tone. What do you see? Beautiful singing without melody or richness. However, when other techniques are added to the singing group, we experience a rich, refined blend of tones producing a harmonized sound. Now, the various styles we heard singing came together to create a balanced effect. This is the theory of harmonization.

Fundamentals of Harmony

The theory of harmonization exists because of some particular truths, which makes for Its foundation and strengthens its convictions.

1. **Yin-Yang Oneness:** Taoism is greatly influenced by the Chinese theory of Yin and Yang opposites. Yin is dark, and Yang is light. They are both intertwined and connected, representing balance and harmony. When your yin and yang are in harmony, it is possible to prolong your life, and otherwise, your life is shortened and susceptible to diseases. Hence, harmony is based on the yin-yang oneness.

You need to understand the 'oneness' principle because you are part of it. To attain this level of oneness, a rich connection with nature, the earth, and its elements are required. By learning to be an observer of nature, you take note of its rhythm and interconnection amongst all elements. You must become like water.

2. **Wei-wu-Wei:** This means swimming with the current, stooping in to conquer, etc. It is the flow that makes it possible for an individual to achieve harmony with all things. Wei-Wu-Wei means to follow or without acting on, allowing things to be within nature. It is not passive or living to chance. It is flowing with Earth (nature) as it flows with Heaven and feedback of Heaven as Tao (nature). Just as it rains, Heaven and Earth are seen uniting. The showers that fall upon the Earth are responded to naturally by humans without a command or instruction. That is Wei Wu Wei; Flowing freely with nature as it communicates with us.

3. **Water characteristics:** In the Book of Ethics by Lao Tzu, water was used severally to communicate the water features of Taoism. Water moves swiftly and is always serving others, humble, transparent, etc. This is therefore understood as the water characteristic of Tao. The main features that make up the water characters include:

   A. Altruism is the ability to pour yourself, serve others entirely without any form of expectation. Water is an essential need of life that all organisms depend on for survival and habitation for another. Taoists should be just like water.

B. Modesty and Humility; As rightly explained, water maintains a low profile after its great acts of service. If we all are altruistic, possessing the heart of service and humility, the numerous conflicts we face in the world would drastically reduce. The Way teaches a nature that does not show off but is ready to learn and remain low amidst the applause of men.

Modesty and humility are virtues that help a man harmonize with himself, others, and influential leaders. Like the sea that births numerous streams and rivers, humility makes a leader accept the visions of others as theirs and work towards achieving them. Such people attract others to themselves and work in unity for one purpose.

C. Adaptability and flexibility; Water can take the shape/size of any container. Humans are also known to be able to adapt to any situation. However, we do not see this in full expression. Adaptability is a skill required for exceptional leadership; the ability to handle any situation. Also, rigidity hinders you from flowing freely with nature. To be in a harmonious state, you have to be flexible.

D. Transparency and Clarity; When an individual is honest and transparent in his ways, they are said to be a person of integrity. If no one makes water unclean, it remains fine. Yet, it is made clean by allowing the impurities to settle. Likewise, as humans, external factors tend to make us muddy and unclean, which differs from our true nature.

E. Soft but persistent; Gentle but powerful; Taoism teaches us to be soft in embracing the uniqueness of others yet constant in flowing freely with nature. Water is a subtle yet powerful tool whose traits should be emulated. What about the negative features of water, you ask? Whenever Yin and Yang are not in harmony, disasters like floods and water-related disasters occur solely due to external factors (acts of man).

4. **Love for peace:** Lao Tzu- the founder of Taoism, lived in an ancient time of the Zhou Dynasty when people and states were at war with each other. His utter dislike for violence made him resign as a historian in the Imperial city to live as a hermit on

the mountain. In opposition to war and its likes, he has been an advocate of peace from the onset.

Taoism is firmly against acts that lead to the detraction of lives and properties. As such, harmony boasts peaceful living.

5. **Tolerance and appreciating differences:** Openness and tolerance are critical aspects of Taoism that foster harmony with nature and other individuals. The world is a complicated place; being open and tolerant is necessary to harmonize with nature and one another. It is against The Way to aspire to be like someone else. Everyone is created uniquely with differences, and that is what brings harmony to our world.

Harmony, therefore, means tolerating, understanding, and appreciating human differences.

Balance in the Body and Spirit

Meditation and spiritual enlightenment are essential in obtaining inner harmony. Physical harmony is dependent on good health. A healthy body is not just fit or built but in tune with the spiritual vibrations from within and responds accordingly. Sometimes, the body's immune system gets weak, and we fall ill. During those moments, the body does all it can to restore balance and fight. You are expected to help your body maintain that balance by taking medications, eating the proper diet, taking fluids frequently, etc.

Also, when you conform to the consciousness of the spirit by maintaining inner beauty, frequency, and vibe in a manner that only allows the inflow of pure/godly thoughts, it is a state of spiritual balance.

According to Chinese philosophy and medicine, yin and yang (female - moon and male - sun attributes) need to be in harmony for all life to flow through it. Fill the heart (spirit) with harmony and balance. It will lengthen life - Guan Zi. The yin and yang symbol mean homeostasis and self-maintenance; it brings to remembrance the importance of balance.

A skilled plant is difficult to eradicate
A skilled grasp is difficult to slip
Virtue will be honored from generation to generation
By fixing Virtue in oneself, Virtue will be real
By fixing Virtue in the house, Virtue will have redundancy
By fixing Virtue in the village, Virtue will grow
By fixing Virtue in the country, Virtue will be in abundance
By fixing Virtue in the world, Virtue will be everywhere
So, by oneself that considers others
By one's house that considers other houses
By one's village that considers other villages
By one's nation that considers other nations
By one's people that consider other people
How do we know what people are? Thanks for that!
Chapter 54 – The Book of Ethics

Balance versus Harmony

Balance is the way humans behave. An average person is to act in a balanced, law-abiding manner concerning the environment. Normalcy is a static form that humans find hard to relate to because they are dynamic.

Unlike balance, harmony is not static; that is, fixed in a place. It is a flexible term that connotes locomotion. Every individual is a product of his decisions, passions, and thoughts, not his circumstances. The way you think has a significant role to play in your reaction or response to events. Situations do not make men instead; men make situations, especially if the state of consciousness is not beclouded.

Hence, finding balance is objective and rational, while harmony is subjective and visceral. Harmony is a better concept than balance due to the ease of being flexible and adaptable.

It is easier to maintain harmony than achieve balance. When we feel joy, insight, wisdom, euphoria, they are subjective ideals making it more practical for internal harmony to be sought.

Harmony is felt when we accept our nature, who we are present. It is a perception of both positives and negatives towards our identity. What you consider your:

- Strengths and weaknesses

- Achievements and failures

- Talents and defects, etc.

You build a harmonious nature when you accept yourself wholly, flaws and all. The challenges that self-rejection causes are more significant than we can imagine; low self-esteem, personality disorders, thieves, verbally and physically abusive individuals, panic disorders, and bullying. It is difficult not to feel wronged concerning our limitations. However, that is what makes us unique. They are the yin and yang tones, expressions that join together to form harmony.

Light and darkness in Christianity is a group of morals. Light is seen as being morally upright, worthy of emulation, while darkness is evil, to be defeated.

Make it all empty
Keep your mind calm
All species born also pass away
Then they go back to the original source12
Returning to the origin is stillness
It is according to the law of nature
The natural law is immutable
Knowing the circulation of heaven and Earth is lucid
No knowing the circulation of heaven and Earth is dark
Knowing the circulation is lucid
By being lucid, then the soul is exuberant
By being exuberant, then the soul behaves fairly
Fairness is everywhere
Everywhere is suitable with nature
What is suitable with nature is suitable with the Way
Being one with the Way is the accurate Way

Even when the body dies, the Way remains.
Chapter 16 – The Book of Ethics

However, the Taoist approach states that darkness is a natural flow and rhythm of the universe and should not be overcome. Achieving balance from the Taoist view aligns yourself with the cosmos (world) and a life of harmony with nature resulting from the belief in natural order or The Way.

The Way is the eternal breath
The Way is a woman
The woman is the mother of the beginning stage
The mother's gateway is the root of heaven and Earth
Like a veil very hard to see
Using the Way will never dry out.
Chapter 6 – The Book of Ethics
How to Achieve a Balanced Life

A balanced life is paramount for oneness and harmonious living in society. The following are methods to achieving a balanced life:

• *Be objective in your approach*

As the Way, there is no discrimination between light and dark, good and evil. It would be best if you accepted everything and everyone. The perspective of good and evil must be blocked from your mind, paying no attention to personal preference. Defining circumstances, individuals, and others in our environment cause conflict.

Examples:

If you see modesty as good, you will most likely paint whatever is perceived as indecent to you as bad.

A lady who greets persons is homely and respectful; ladies who do contrary to that are disrespectful and cannot manage a home.

1. *Accept the natural course of life than defining its qualities*

A lot of us like to think things through thoroughly. Why ponder over things again and again when you certainly have no control over the situation. It is healthier and beneficial not to try to make sense out of it. Giving meaning to a natural progression only makes the process painful.

2. *Move on to the past or think of the future. Live your life in the now, making wise use of what life offers to you.*

The past is past; it is behind, and you cannot turn the hands of time. Stop sulking and enjoy the flow brought to your doorsteps.

Examples:

You are at the beach, unwinding and sipping a cold drink with the provision of a coconut shade to obstruct the sunlight rays and keep you cool. But it begins to rain suddenly. Usually, this unforeseen circumstance should ruin your mood; however, instead of feeling miserable, dance in the rain and enjoy the moment.

3. *Allow the universe to introduce your school of thought*

Your ideologies are not forcefully passed worldwide. At this age, everyone has something to say, even when it's sensible or not. They crave relevance, and their influence is overwhelming. There is an excellent population of people who claim to be teachers/scholars. The only thing they do is give out advice, teachings, information without a desire to listen to another's perspective.

Benefits of Maintaining a balanced Lifestyle

- *It alleviates stress* - by taking time to exhale and inhale, it slows down your pace, allows you to relax and be more objective in your decisions.

- *It enhances your mood* - the noise that comes from the cares and worries of this life will most likely weigh you down. However, taking breathing exercises will help you brighten up.

- *It aids in boosting energy* - energy is the ability to do work. The balance, therefore, helps in channeling the flow of energy to the right places for productivity.

- *It betters your state of mind* - we are in constant war with our minds, affecting the quality of our inner state without our conscious knowledge.

- *It increases longevity and reduces aging* - the simplicity of balance takes away stress, bodily fatigue. Aging is caused by numerous stressors that take a toll on the physique. Remember, our inner consciousness produces our physical form. Therefore a troubled inner state will yield a troubled and worn-out physical form.

- *It prevents health-related diseases* - the issues of life are from within. Too much of everything is bad for your health. You should take life step by step. Excess activities stimulate the production of body hormones resulting in a hard time for the body to pick up with it and maintain homeostasis.

- *It boosts your self-worth and confidence* - performing at maximum level is only possible when you maintain balance. Your words, steps, and even inactions exhume confidence.

- *It gives you an understanding of life* - In seeing life from a more straightforward angle, you realize there is no rush in life; you take things slowly and live in the moment!

- *It enables you to be selfless* - true satisfaction is obtained from helping others become better versions of themselves or providing the platform on which they can become empty individuals who pour themselves into humanity without expectations or commendations.

- You master how to handle life issues and challenges without affecting your inner state.

- You attract positive energy and abundance from the flow of life.

My sayings are simple to understand, simple to practice

But people do not understand
Therefore, people do not practice
My words have the root
My job is well-structured

Because people do not understand me
So, they don't know me
People who understand me are tiny
People who follow me are rare
So, the sage wears the rough cloth
But the heart embraces precious jewels.
Chapter 70 – The Book of Ethics

The Importance of Harmony in Life

Harmony is a spice of life that spurs togetherness among individuals and Nations. It is the capacity to handle different areas of our lives. Individual harmony must be attained to have a free flow of energy with nature. Hence, every individual must effectively cope and provide solutions for areas in our lives that seek to stress and frustrate our inner peace. Chinese culture takes harmonization seriously. Through harmony, people share their perspectives without conflicts.

The Importance of Peace in Life

For every human and even society, desiring a peaceful environment to thrive and succeed is essential. Violence affects the harmony and balance of society. To live a balanced life, our inner peace should be undisturbed to channel energy flow properly. We have to understand situations that cause disturbances and handle them, such as anger, fear, insecurity, etc. We appreciate and honor each other when we live in peace despite our religious, social, and cultural differences.

A peaceful person orchestrates harmony and maintains such relationships amongst others and society.

Peace and Harmony are interdependent and related. It is a fundamental necessity for living.

Living in harmony fosters community building and development. The power of Harmony amongst individuals cannot be under-emphasized. The crisis, wars, violence, hardships, and other mishaps in society result from individuals or groups of persons who refuse to understand the uniqueness of man forcefully desiring others to accept their way of life.

The mindset of peace and Harmony is endorsed by a healthy way of life as resolving conflicts, tolerance, adaptation, empathy, etc.

The perfect one is like water
Water provides life for all things
Without competing with anything
Water lives where people hate
Therefore, it can be compared with the Way
Accommodation is humble
Thinking is deep
Treatment is forgiven
Talking is genuine
Assertiveness is fair
Working is competent
Action is timely
When there's no contest, then there will be no mistakes.
Chapter 8 – The Book of Ethics

How to Live in Peace and Harmony

Since we have established the importance of peace and Harmony in our daily lives, we would look at some steps to take in achieving a peaceful and harmonious life:

- *Make time for yourself daily*

Our present generation keeps us glued to social media, work, extra-curricular activities, etc. With such trends and a sense of busyness, it is easy to lose ourselves and get carried away by one thing or another. Creating a time for yourself to unwind and relax is something we need to balance yin and yang. A time for activities also requires a time to be still, calm, and flow with the energy within you. Do not forget, the imbalance in yin and yang causes diseases that shorten your lifespan.

- *Live your life intentionally each moment*

Don't linger on memories. Instead, learn from your previous mistakes, apply the solutions to your present. Worrying about the future is futile. The decisions you make now will give you the future you desire.

• *Ensure that your choices and decisions are carefully thought of before making a move*

Don't make decisions you will regret. As much as The Way advocates going with the flow of nature, it does not imply living your life to chance. An actual state of oneness would make you so harmonious that it extends to your outward appearance, which involves your actions. Actions are products of your decisions - a mental and physical balance yields productivity. Make sure the principles of the Way back your choices.

• *Think before reacting to situations*

The Way is against violence and its acts. Making rash decisions has led to outbursts of anger, regretful decisions, death, wars, and so on. Hence, follow the Way of peace and harmony at all times. Flow with the equilibrium of your inner state.

• *Meditate*

Meditation is a necessary means of attaining peace and harmony. It has been rightly discussed in the previous chapter. Meditative practices foster stillness and focus. This aids inner peace and harmony. Make sure to engage in reflective exercises, often even for 10-20 minutes daily.

• *Engage in selfless activities*

By giving your time and effort to a worthy cause to harmonize the environment, society will assist you in living a peaceful life. Activities like global warming, giving to the needy, anti-pollution campaigns, etc. A faithful follower of the Way seeks to empty themselves for the betterment of nature. Engaging in such enhances your inner state of peace and balance.

- *Make sure to surround yourself with peaceful and harmonious people or things*

Spending your time watching, reading, or listening to violent/disturbing content, including video games, will make you lose harmony. Get healthy materials that will help you attain harmony. When you have the right company around you, it helps to strengthen your faith and boosts harmonious living. The best company to keep are those who are on the same path as you.

Eliminate learning and worry less
What differentiates good and evil?
Why are we scared of what others are afraid of?
So immense, it is impossible to know.
Everyone is as cheerful as when enjoying a buffalo feast
Like spring on the hill
I am silent alone
Like an infant who cannot yet laugh
Hanging down, walking like a homeless person
People have become redundant
I am destitute alone
My mind is like a fool
How dumb!
People are all bright and sharp
My own is dark and dull
People like the ocean's waves
I do not know which way the wind is blowing
People are busy
My own boorish
I am different from people
I'm unlike other people
I trust in mother's milk to feed all species.
Chapter 20 – The Book of Ethics

Chapter Five

How To Get Financial Harmony

G reed, corruption, and envy seep into your heart when you do not live a harmonious life. The beauty of Harmony is in satisfaction. As humans, the tendency to get jealous and covetous of others is excellent. Most times, we feel bad when our counterparts have attained a height we are yet to reach. This is not the way.

Great Way spreads everywhere
It moves to the left and moves to the right
It is depended on everything
It creates without holding back
Work is accomplished, yet taking credit
The Way fosters all species without mastering
Without desire, it is called small
All species come back without mastering
And so are called great
In the end, the Way doesn't receive as marvelous itself
That is why it accomplished a great thing.
Chapter 34 – The Book of Ethics

Harmony regarding finances is achievable when you channel all the negative thoughts into the proper flow of life. Block the bad energy, check your heart, ponder on the reasons why you are stuck in a stagnant position, rather than envy, appreciate the people who have attained the height you desire.

The law of honor states that you attract what you celebrate. In appreciating your superiors and those at the same level as you, you channel the proper flow of energy to yourself.

Too much noise in our inner selves is responsible for the bad decisions we make. It is possible to live a humble, satisfied and appreciative life.

Often, life circumstances push us beyond limits exposing us to the imbalance that causes chaos. No man was born evil. The state of their consciousness and spiritual enlightenment was relatively poor that it could not contain their body; hence they made choices contrary to the Way.

Asides from the circumstances we are faced with, a specific career path we take pushes us towards internal Imbalance and chaos. Having a work and life balance is essential.

It is no doubt that you have heard of situations where rivalry in workplaces, government offices, marketplaces, etc., has pushed others into evil. The competition produces bad energy that leads to chaos and violence amongst us. People no longer see eye to eye; arguments, misunderstandings, threats, and even death become the order of the day.

Skilled walker leaves no footprints
Skilled talker does not miss words
A skilled mathematician does not need a comparison
Skillfully closed needs not locking
But no one can open it
Skillfully knotted needs not tied
But no one can remove it
Sage takes care of everyone
Not missing one
Sage takes care of everything
Nothing missing anything
That is called bright-hearted!
Who is a good person?

The teacher of the bad person
Who is the bad person?
Someone meant for the good person to teach
If the teacher is not respected
And the student does not love
Then there is confusion in talent
That is the pivotal point of the mystery.
Chapter 27 – The Book of Ethics

The path of Harmony is the solution to the chaos the world is facing. Our inner selves require this harmony to help us be at a state of equilibrium and peace. Satisfaction is harmony. A man who is content and satisfied with his resources is so blessed that life he issues have no hold on him. There is no room for hatred, mischief, lies, and all sorts.

Steps to take in achieving financial harmony

- Choose a career path you are satisfied with: The problem is satisfaction. Choosing a career path should not come from greed; instead, to help society and man at large. Making an impact and creating balance for a peaceful world is the responsibility of every man. If you are satisfied with yourself and what you do, no man will push you to the wall.

- Be peaceful with yourself and others: Yes! We want to be better and achieve greater heights. However, every man has time to attain a peak in life, finances, influence, and relevance. Be at peace, be diligent, and the right moment will come to you. If there is no peace in the world, even the height you hope to attain would be snatched from you.

- Practice meditation: Positive affirmations and hearing motivating speeches will translate to your spirit. Meditating daily shapes your thoughts and innermost desires. You are what you listen to. Take time to invest in your meditations. Ensure to have these solitary moments day and night

- Be vocal about appreciating others: Emptiness makes you reach out to others without restrain, pretense or pride. Relate with others because you want to know them genuinely, not for ulterior motives. Search your heart daily, think about what your innermost heart contains. Don't hide your true motives, it only takes a moment for your spirit to be known by all men.

The highly virtuous people do not pray for virtue; they already have virtue

The lowly virtuous people want virtue, so they don't have virtue
The highly virtuous people do nothing
Yet nothing is undone
The lowly virtuous people always do
Yet many more things need to be done
The humane person works without letting the job go unfinished
The righteous person works, but the undone jobs are many
The polite person works, but no one responds
When the Way dies, the Virtue is born
When the Virtue dies, humanity is born
When humanity dies, the righteous is born
When the righteous die, the polite is born
Politeness is a shell of disloyalty
The clue of chaos
Using the mind to foresee flashes the Way
The clue of foolishness
Highly virtuous people live faithfully
They do not respect politeness
On the fruit, neither in the flower
One chooses this but leaves that.
Chapter 38 – The Book of Ethics

Chapter Six

Harmony And Health

Health by the Way is based on allowing the Tao to flow with ease and maintaining the harmony of the universe. In previous times, health was defined as Harmony and balance. The purpose of the Way is to grasp nature and live in harmony with it through the understanding gained. When mental or physical ailments/illnesses occur, it just implies that harmony is lost in the inner state. The Way provides solutions to the world's current dilemma: balance, harmony, relaxation/peace, and moderation.

Since the way is directly in tune with nature, it is expected that the standard approach to health will require natural methods.

The following health care practices for Taoists are described:

1. **Palliative care** - For people in the Way, natural sources of alleviating pain are the most practical choice. If medication serves its aim of recalibrating the body's natural ability to function, drugs are not out of bounds. The flow of nature will take its course when treatment has stopped being responsive.

2. **Self-decisions and Patient's authority** - The family has a significant role in the end-of-life decisions for Taoists.

3. **Death and Beyond** - Death is Natural. However, Taoist believes that it does not cut ties between the dead and the living.

By keeping body and soul together
Is it possible to keep them apart?
Pay attention to breathe
To be soft

Can one become an infant?
With spiritual cleansing
Can the stain be gone?
Love people and rule country
The heaven gate opens and closes
Through everything
Can't we do anything?
We are born and raised
Instructions without possessions
Made without merit
Instruction without ruling
Such is the root of the Way
Chapter 10 – The Book of Ethics

Lifestyle Practices for Longevity

1. Live life fully

Life is lived to its fullest daily, as it is loaded with experiences and richness. This manner of living creates a means for one to be healthy, flexible, and robust. Pursuing means to elongate one's life artificially leads to critical shortenings of life. It is against the Way, which advocates a natural flow.

2. Eat good meals

The quality of life one expects to have is directly connected to the diet one takes. For the body to function correctly for a long time, you must eat a well-prepared, balanced and healthy diet. Eating a properly balanced diet is Key. A subtle reason many diets or nutrition is inadequate is that we refuse to change or upgrade our diet according to our respective bodies' needs. There is no particular meal that contains the essential and balanced nutrients required by the body. Instead, it is our responsibility to listen to our body's needs and offer vital mixtures to the body. Green tea, Cabbage, Yogurt, and Brown rice are foods of higher quality than others.

As a follower of the Way, the life cycle of the food we eat and its practices before its death, especially livestock, should be carefully considered before consumption. The Way teaches a habit of respecting food processing and intake with balance and moderation.

3. Obey nature

Our world is incredibly distracted; numerous goals to achieve, a lot of ideas to implement, a list of desires to accomplish, other factors trying to influence, compete and lead you with a belief system they consider higher than yours. You can never attain a long life with all these distracting sounds. However, bringing all sound together is advantageous; harmony gives you an edge over others because of the Way.

The Way advocates Nature. As you get older, you begin to walk with nature dutifully. Adulthood changes like menopause, reduced energy, loss of sight, etc., are not ignored but used for personal expansion.

4. Exercise regularly

Physical fitness is not optional. You have to keep your body in perfect condition and functioning. Qigong is an exercise practice that is beneficial to keep the body agile and in good shape. The fact that physical fitness is essential does not mean that you overwork yourself and overstretch your body. Dance through life; do not fight life or your body. None is the enemy - the Way.

5. Attitude

Treating your body as the opponent or a container that should be subjected at all costs limits your life. The rate at which you resist the world is directly proportional to the rate the world restricts you. This is already a lost battle because, in comparison with the world, which is bigger and larger, one entity is nothing and will be easily swallowed. Fighting back excessively would only wear you down. Are we saying don't fight back? Allow yourself to be tossed by any and everything? No, stand up for yourself but not against the world ruthlessly. It will wash you away.

The proper lifestyle of the Way is a good sense of humor, low stress, and a positive outlook.

6. Have a spiritual practice

Spiritual practice is a mixture of intentions with actions and the discovering of mysteries in life. It is highly advised to engage in spiritual activity to keep harmony between your mind and body as a boost, mind, and spirit. Think of this as the practice by which an individual discovers peace with nature.

A healthy, sound spiritual practice is a component of the Way. Many of the techniques are related to Shamanism. Everyone is expected to establish his practice. These practices are a source of inspiration for leading a lengthier happy life. There are diverse kinds of training based on philosophy, science, religion, magic, etc. One thing, however, that strikes a balance amongst these numerous views is the acceptance of the Way.

7. Avoid addiction

The Way describes addiction as a redefinition of the space with an external factor to nature while living is to be yourself. Life is a push, and the struggles we encounter are a means to sharpen us. Usually, addictions seem like a means to make life easier, which is false . It is a dead-end.

Be open to humiliation
What does "be open to humiliation" mean?
Accept bad luck like its human destiny
Reception is not important
Do not worry about loss or gain
This is called "be open to humiliation."
What does "accept bad luck like it is human destiny" mean?
Bad luck comes from one's body
If not, where does that bad fortune come from?
Be precious to one's body
As people believe one's body is everything
Love this world like one's body
Then one can fulfill everything.
Chapter 13 – The Book of Ethics

Chapter Seven

Living A Balanced Life

A balanced life is not restricted to a certain way. There are numerous ways for you to live a balanced life. The ball is in your court; it always has! The simplest way to be balanced is by harmonizing your body and spirit. Keep in mind that the goal of this is to live in harmony, thereby attracting plenty.

Our top goal in this life is to live in harmony with ourselves (body and spirit) and everything in our environment. Harmony is the pathway to balance. Balance yields peace and abundance.

If you are on a path to attain balance, your progress is measured based on your internal flow. When we obstruct a particular flow in our body, it will sprout in a way spiritual, social, or otherwise. Imbalance is caused by the inevitable challenges in life that confront us and hinder our growth. Taoist are of the school of thought that when people apply the concept of yin and yang, they will realize that just as the symbols preach harmony and balance, the interlocking spirals show that life is an ever-changing passage. Hence both light and dark are necessary for balance.

Affirming that you have yin and yang moments that have shaped you into who you are is not all to balance. The functionality of life of credit comes with striking an understanding between these phases.

Living a balanced life is possible by having an objective approach to life. You must be capable of embracing every person without prejudice.

Stillness is easy to grasp
Formlessness is easy to plan
The crispiness is easy to break
Small pieces are easy to disperse
Prevent at, yet present
Treat at, yet chaos starts
Big tree as one hug
They are born from a small seed
A nine-story high floor
It is erected from a crate of soil
Walking thousands of miles away
But starting with the first step
One who acts fails
One who holds loses
Therefore:
Sage doesn't act
Thereupon he doesn't fail
Doesn't keep
Thereupon he doesn't lose
Things often fail when they are about to be accomplished
Because not as cautious as at first
If the following caution is used as before, the job will not fail
So, the sage avoids ambition
Or precious desire
He wants to teach the uneducated
Help bring people back to the Way
Help things grow naturally
Therefore, one should not interfere with anything.
Chapter 64 – The Book of Ethics

Here are some reasons why you may find balance difficult

1. You are yet to recognize that your life needs balance.

2. There are significant pathways to be balanced you do not know (resources, relationships, self-development, self-maintenance).

    •   Resources: If the first thing you think of as resources is money, you are sadly missing out on the value in your life. Resources are values that can be traded or substances you require for day-to-day operations.

    •   Relationships: This is not secluded to a romantic or emotional affiliation. It is how you interact with others, including non-human (plants, animals). As one who is spiritually enlightened, your relationship with the Way is in this category. In addition, as one who seeks to understand themselves, a relationship with yourself is significant.

    •   Self-development: You must invest in making yourself better. Successful individuals make a constant sacrifice for their skills and upgrade. Whatever form of learning that reshapes you is categorized here. If you do not invest in yourself, you cannot be your greatest motivation, and it will be difficult to fall back on yourself.

    •   Self-maintenance: This is grooming and taking care of yourself; food, shelter, water, clothing, etc. It is ensuring your biological needs are met

3. You are ignorant of the problems caused by an imbalance.

4. You have not looked out for a means to get balance.

Here are practices that you should engage in to achieve balance

1. Purity: The Way teaches that the body must be pure for the spirit. To be balanced, there are certain things that you should abstain from, like lust, greed, dishonesty, ego, unforgiveness, amongst others. As established already, the inner state of your consciousness affects your physical outlook.

2. Meditation: This is the process of attaining stillness. It is crucial in creating a mental equilibrium and boosting attention. Meditation enables the person the chance to know the Tao directly.

3. Breathing: It is the most straightforward form of ch'i. The breathing exercises carried out by Taoists are numerous and known as Qui Gong.

4. Energy flow: Ch'i is the flow of life energy. It can be increased, controlled, and harmonized by different meditations, exercises, and acupuncture techniques.

5. Martial arts: Tai Chi exercises are also used in achieving balance.

6. Diet: Some food choices should be avoided in Classical Taoism, like meat, beans, alcohol, and grains.

Philosophy of Balance and Tao of Pooh

In the book Tao of Pooh by Benjamin Hoof, he relates Winnie the Pooh by A.A. Milne to Taoism's principles. The book describes a group of wine tasters as great thinkers; Confucius, Buddha, and Lao Tzu.

The character of Winnie the Pooh is likened to the principles of Wu Wei or the concept of effortless living as well as the concept of openness, unburdened. The characters of Owl and Rabbit exaggerate challenges and think to a point where they are confused, the Eeyore is a pessimist who sees everything negatively. Wu-Wei is just like the flow of water in a stream.

Analyzing Pooh's demeanor is a simple character, a humble view of life, and a high problem-solving instinct.

Hence, Pooh is an example of a person living in the Way. There is no greater way to succeed or be ahead in life than to have such essential features. The simplicity in understanding good and bad and the ease in proffering solutions to others is the balance we all desire. Be the balance the world seeks. Some of us do not fully grasp these Wu Wei principles that are linked to the Character of Pooh.

From the character, we see the following principles:

1. *Simplicity, Compassion, and Patience*

Your greatest treasures in life are the three mentioned above. To be simple in your thoughts and actions, you go back to your source - The Way. By being patient with your friends and foes, you flow with the natural progression of life. Compassion reconciles you with the world's beings.

Lesson to Note: Complications in life occur often but, just like Pooh, do the basics. This did not only help him be balanced but also managed his relationships and actions with the Owl and Rabbit.

2. *Go with the flow*

A short quote that describes the concept of Wu Wei is "When nothing is done, nothing is left undone." Allow things to take their natural path rather than fight it. No matter the hurdles water faces, it passes through effortlessly, carving a way out for itself naturally. Like water, go through situations without painstakingly creating a path for yourself. If you truly merit it, it will find a way to you.

3. *Let Go*

Change is inevitable, and death is no respecter of persons. These are the only constants in life. Letting go is tough, but we free ourselves from hurt, pain, and suffering in doing so. Holding on produces double the pain when compared to letting go. By letting things take on their natural path, we don't hold on to anything, regardless of what it may be; a relationship, job opportunity, or what have you.

4. *Harmony*

The blending of Yin and Yang (femininity and masculinity) brings Harmony; accepting this normalcy and events of things without perceiving it as evil, bad, or dark is balanced.

5. Genuity be true to yourself

You can only deceive others for a while, but you know the truth. Being true to yourself is wholly embracing everything about you. Only in doing this can you achieve success, take giant strides towards the future, and solicit assistance.

Look but not seeing because of formlessness
Listen but not hearing because of soundlessness
Get it but can't keep it because of being inanimate
Those three things cannot be traced
Because they are one
Above, do not illuminate
Underneath, do not overshadow
It is hard to describe something
When you are far away from it
Then back to nothing
The form of the formless
The shadow of the shadowless
That is called indescribable, non-visualizable
By standing in front, one can't see the head
By following, one can't see the tail
Keep the Way of the past in harmony with the present
Knowing primitiveness is the precept of the Way.
Chapter 14 – The Book of Ethics

Chapter Eight

Qigong Exercise

In previous years, the Qigong exercise was known as Tao You, and Nei Kung translated as leading and guiding. The name describes how the exercise movements direct and lead the transportation of Qi/energy through the body, while Nei Kung translates as internal work/exercise. The dance was a basic foundation of ancient times, so the qigong most likely originated from it. They were initially dance movements created to strengthen dancers and ward off physical and mental diseases, which evolved into exercises and were practiced maintaining health and heal ailments. These practices are massages, breathing, movement, and static exercises for health and long life. The significant insight they passed on is that the flow of life resides in everyone, and by developing it daily, all will attain health and longevity. It is created to assist you in preserving your Jing, transform your Shen, and empower your Qi energy. Qigong is a healing practice that involves breathing, movement, and meditation. Qi is translated as life force while Gong is mastery. It is roughly interpreted as a master of one's energy.

Be open to humiliation
What does "be open to humiliation" mean?
Accept bad luck like its human destiny
Reception is not important
Do not worry about loss or gain
This is called "be open to humiliation"
What does "accept bad luck like it is human destiny" mean?
Bad luck comes from one's body
If not, where does that bad fortune come from?

Be precious to one's body
As people believe one's body is everything
Love this world like one's body
Then one can fulfill everything.
Chapter 13 – The Book of Ethics

The Qigong exercise is a set of repeated movements that are easy to learn, and fun to engage in. Its unique practices possess both Yin, being it, and Yang; doing its traits. Therefore, the Qigong Yin exercises are reflected by calm stretches, breathing techniques, and visualization whereas, the Qigong Yang exercises are reflected by aerobics or in a unique manner. This practice is used largely in China for cancer patients.

The practice of Qigong is supposed to generate energy and vitality of nature into an individual's body to boost mental, spiritual, and physical health. Poor physical health is caused by trapped energy in all body sections based on Traditional Chinese Medicine. The qigong practice has a huge belief in boosting an individual's health by allowing energy to flow through the body. Its purpose is to promote the movement of Qi in the body by making specific gates open while energy sources are stretched and twisted. Relaxing and taking deep breaths are significant to Qigong exercises and necessities for the free flow of energy (Qi).

It invigorates and rejuvenates the body within minutes of engagement and strengthens its various systems (digestive, respiratory, skeletal, cardiovascular, etc.). The Qigong assists in giving treatments for chronic and acute illnesses that are common for exercise, physical and mental healing, relaxation, including other purposes like enlightenment and fighting. There is no preference in age or physique.

In the Qigong practice, some movements are calm and others engaging, extensive, and subtle too. These movements vary from each other and possess unique changes on the body and mind. Naturally, as an individual deepens their Qigong practices, a greater understanding of the movements and its purposes will be gained making the practice fun and desirable.

With consistent practice, Qigong will exhibit a great influence on the mind, spirit, and body. The advantages of this exercise include improved wholeness in health and well-being, decreased stress level, and a balanced and positive mindset on the possibilities of life.

In conclusion, the practice of Qigong can be a discipline, in addition to Tai Chi practices or meditation.

Benefits of Qigong Exercise

The importance of Qigong has been established to have numerous benefits in different areas.

- It harmonizes, strengthens, and has a therapeutic effect on the internal organs and body systems.

- It boosts the production and flow of energy in the body.

- It has a calming and soothing effect on the mental and emotional state.

- It stretches and opens the joints and muscles while releasing muscular tension.

- It completely rejuvenates and nourishes the body by boosting the flow of blood and energy.

- It aids sound sleep, which is a product of relaxation and energization.

Based on Chinese Medicine, the Qi is related to the internal organs of the body. It flows amidst the body extremities like the feet and hands. Hence, when you stretch your upper and lower extremities in defined motions, you will enhance the wellness of the internal organs. Breathing in Qigong is key. The breaths are to be calm, slow, and deeply taken from the diaphragm. The benefit of this breathing method is its calming and soothing influence on the mental state, which effectively suppresses the influence of worry and stress. When you are stressed, engage in some minutes of Qigong, and you will be amazed by the level of relief you experience.

The benefits discussed above are just several positive impacts you will attain at the initial stage of your practice. The more you heighten your commitment and get accustomed to Qigong exercises, the easier it is for you to state the impacts noticed on your body.

Fundamentals Of Qigong Exercises

• *Concentration*

This begins and yields from the awareness of Qi energy, its breathing formats, and Qigong practices. It involves paying attention and letting go simultaneously. To focus is to expand your awareness by deep relaxation. Here, you will be capable of creating a mind-frame that is sufficient to contain your whole mental, physical, and spiritual abilities and be attentive to create room for worry, distraction, and daily challenges to pass by. The inward focus that enlarges outwardly to be one with you and the universe symbolizes yin/yang.

• *Breathing*

Lao described the breathing techniques in the sixth century as a means to generate Qi. The two types of breathing are:

The Breath of Buddha: when you breathe in, enlarge your abdomen and fill it with air; to exhale, squeeze your core, expel air from the lung base and push it out until your stomach and chest are relieved from the air. When you inhale and exhale, be imaginative, invite your energy to flow through your body channels freely by using your mind. It should flow with you. Try breathing in for eight counts and out for sixteen counts.

The Breath of Taoist: this technique is opposite from Buddha's. You squeeze your abdomen when breathing in and calm the lungs and torso when you exhale.

As you go through the practices below, do not forget Qigong is to aid awareness.

Warm-Up Practices (1—18 min.)

Qigong Exercise 1: Subtle sway

a. For five minutes, move your arms from shoulders in a calm, swinging manner. This movement originates from your waist:

twist from your waist like your trunk is a cloth you are squeezing. It gives massage to the internal organs with maximum benefits. Don't twist from your knees.

b. To begin, move your arms sideways across your trunk and then forward.

c. Allow your knees to bend slightly, and your hips sway. Clear your mind. Pay attention to free up unnecessary and unconscious stress. Weeks later, your focus should be on swinging the arms and Qi movement.

This exercise gives you an insight into being mindful.

Qigong practice 2: Bounce

For starters, try this for about 4 minutes.

a. Keep parallel feet and shoulders apart; like a wet noodle, hang your arms at the sides and bounce with your knees free. Let them feel neutral and empty. While bouncing, your arms in zero position are to get a jiggling influence.

b. Natural shoulders; do not pull or drag them forward. Use the zero position on the general body to get a feel of deep calmness; internal organs and skin should hang. It fosters consciousness of inner tension to enable you to expel it.

The combination of both exercises massages and tones the organ system gently, which aids longevity.

Awareness Practices

Qigong practice 3: Accordion

Here, you experience Qi by using your hands like a bicycle pump/accordion bellow.

a. Your eyes should be closed halfway. Free your mind and focus on your palms.

b. Make your breath slow, simple, and with ease. You are creating a slight trance.

c. Put your hands together, palms touching, and fingers pointing upward. The Laolong (palm chakra) in the center should connect because they are locations where you can feel the Qi.

d. Move your hands slowly, to keep chakras together. At about 30cm distance, move them slowly together with minimal effort.

e. Reduce the air between them like an accordion.

f. Experience a tingling sensation that may be warm at times at the Laolong points.

g. Move your hands slowly, front and back; go through it again in various directions.

This procedure grows Qi, consciousness and enlightens you. Feeling the Qi energy for the first time transforms your mindset.

Qigong Practice 4: Make the point

Your index finger is an excellent way of channeling Qi energy; right-handed people use their right index fingers while left-handed people use their left index fingers. Point at the palm of the other hand, which is perpendicular to the floor, with the fingers pointing upwards.

Using your index finger as a paintbrush, swab to and from across the palm.

Start with your fingertip about 20cm from your palm; move it near and far slowly, swabbing all through.

You may feel a tickly, cooling, and warm sensation.

Qigong Practice 5: Extend Qi

To gather and generate Qi, engage this exercise with half-closed eyes. Qi practices are powerful while at home, have a teacher supervise you, so your eyes don't leak out.

a. Engage with open eyes for stagnant Qi; breath in fast via nostrils with open or half-closed eyes when breathing out.

b. Channel your intention when you sense Qi; this is the mind/spirit aspect so, use your mind to transport your Qi outwards, enlarging your area of comfort. You can pull out Qi as you exhale and hold it as you breathe in.

c. Move the Qi 1 inch from your body; with an increase of 6 inches, take it outward, push for 3 feet, locate the point you are comfortable with and return it close to your body.

These practices make you relate with your Qi. Increasing the distance at which you can feel Qi from your body enlarges your comfort and the world around you. You will experience less fear/deeper abilities. Bringing your Qi to the skin area makes you extra calm, in tune, and self-confident. By learning to increase/reduce Qi, you become healthier, energized, and harmonized within and without.

Qigong Practice 6: Pamper Qi

This practice is tricky, as it moves Qi along two uniquely connecting channels; Du Mai and Ren Mai.

a. Push Qi down; while your hands push down, your spine and head are straight. As the Qi flows up, your hands rise, elbow bend, palms parallel to the floor, hunch shoulders. Repeat about seven times, breathing in as hands go up and out as they come down.

b. When you are comfortable; you can combine this practice with a slow, deliberate walk forward; left knee bent and raised in an overly stepping mode. As the knee comes up, hands go down, back and spine straighten; as footsteps down, hands come up and back hunches. Maintain a breath pattern, gentle and slow feet movement. Breath in as hands raise and out slowly as you straighten the back.

Qigong Practices 7: Blend Qi

This assists you in being conscious of the numerous reverberations of Qi and how to blend them in harmony.

a. With a shoulder apart distance, stand with your feet, slightly bent knees, let your hand hang at the sides.

b. Move your weight to the balls of your feet slightly. Be conscious of the front body region. Focus on the channels that move along the front of legs and trunk, arms, and face.

c. A minute after, transfer the weight to your heels. Be conscious of the back of your body, head, arms, spine, and legs. This position can be held for 5 minutes or more and carried out for both sides of the body.

d. Be conscious of each part of the body at instances e.g., the side of your head, arm, trunk, leg side, ankle, etc., the exercise becomes meditative this way.

e. Move to a more Nei Dan routine; repeat the first three procedures, without visual movement detection, with your mind, move your weight front and back, perceive your Qi, then try to feel it flow along your front and back together.

Upgraded Qigong Breathing Technique

Through breathing, the Qi energy can be channeled across the body. They can stimulate or relax based on how they are used. Engage this routine (Buddha and Taoist breathing).

-   Sit on the ground with crossed legs in lotus or cross. This helps Qi energy refrain from being static at the lower body.

-   Breath in at counts 4-8 based on preference. For Buddha, enlarge your abdomen, fill it from the base while for Taoists, breath in and reduce your abdomen, breath out, allow your abdomen to relax.

-   Fix your attention on your nose while you inhale. Lead your energy from nose to Dantian (except women on period; on their solar plexus rather) under the navel.

-   Breath out to 8-16 count, shift Qi to your torso, pelvic, and tailbone.

-   Breath in, shift Qi to the back at the shoulder region

-   Breath out, shift Qi to the back at head and nose

Consistency and patience will help you feel the Qi. Increase the rate and finish one cycle in one breath in and out. On breathing in, Qi moves energy from nose to tailbone while breathing out moves from tail to nose.

CONCLUSION

The imbalance caused by the world today proves that humans are in dire need of harmony and balance. The Way is a path that gives insight into spiritual enlightenment, inner peace, balance, harmony, yin and yang principles. Amazingly, it is not restricted to a group of persons or a certain region. All people and nations can practice the Way. It doesn't seek its own glory but rather focuses on achieving peace in this chaotic world of ours. The foundation and principles of the Way are easy to understand and attainable.

Meditation, satisfaction, inner peace, emptiness, and tolerance are the practices one should abide by to connect to mother nature (Earth). As humans, the body, soul, and spirit need harmony. Many of us do not even know that we need the various compositions of our nature to be in perfect sync with each other. Hence the spiritual gap created can only be bridged when we subject ourselves to and are willing to get spiritual enlightenment.

In ancient times, a story was told of a man who had a strange physique that made him stand out from the others. He was sought for within the palace because of the high level of wisdom he expressed. This was all due to his ability to cultivate and maintain his state of consciousness. He was at such peace with himself, balanced from accepting yin and yang, which produced Qi energy enabling him to freely flow with nature and channel its generated Qi to the surroundings and yield outstanding physical attributes. That man was the envy of others who were seemingly normal in physique. He also taught according to the Way - balance is accepting yourself with your perfections and imperfections. It is the beauty of Oneness, yin, and is the beauty of Oneness, Yin and Yang. We cannot all be the same. Life is unique, and our individuality makes it so.

A sage does not have a heart of his own
He gets the heart of the world as his heart
One is good to good people
One is also good to those who are not good
Because the essence of Virtue is being good
One believes those who believe
One also believes those who do not believe
Because the essence of Virtue is believing
Sage in the world is carefree
He's in harmony with everyone
So people look and listen
But sage sees them as children.
Chapter 49 - The Book of Ethics

Diseases, illnesses, issues such as stress, trauma, depression, anxiety, hypertension, panic disorders, bullying, depression, attention disorders, personality disorders, and many stranger medical problems we face today are solely due to our physical, emotional, and mental imbalance. Most of us consume everything the world presents to us hook, line, and sinker, leaving no space for ourselves; instead, we are completely full and probably overflowing with garbage. Does this sound bad? Discouraging? Yes, but do not be distressed. Where there is a will, there is always a way. It is up to you to make a decision, stick to it, be disciplined, take action, and yield results. To be genuinely free, empty, and harmonious, you must work it out.

The Way is the means to escape from the prison the world has put us in because, truthfully, we cannot escape from its violence/chaos. We can only control our response to it. Does the Way teach avoiding situations and circumstances? Does it teach running away from problems? Does it teach one not to confront truth and reality? No, instead, it seeks for you to face your challenges, listen to yourself and thoughts, forget about the past, stop playing the blame/victim card or try to be a perfectionist. Preserve your inner peace by going through the steps mentioned in part 2.

Meditation is a state of stillness that allows you to achieve inner peace and consciousness. Nevertheless, do not forget the first step to spiritual enlightenment is improving your body. The spirit and soul cannot be balanced without a healthy body. The body contains our wills, emotions, insights, etc. When the body is weak, there is little to nothing that can be achieved. The physical (manifesting desire) body, mental (creating the concept) body, and emotional (desiring the concept) body make up the human. The mental manages the emotional, and the emotional controls the physical body.

Accepting ourselves is otherwise known as Self-realization. It is consciously realizing and understanding who we truly are and connecting our personality with the Spirit. Compared to others, individuals who have reached this state are more at peace with themselves and free from the monkey's trap. The monkey's trap is a state when an individual keeps desiring, thinking, and stimulating more to attain satisfaction and happiness. It is a rat race that draws you away from nature, interrupts the flow of the Way, and is the greatest hindrance to self-realization.

The primary purpose of the Taoist concept is humans being at peace with nature and allowing Nature to take its course, that is, handling things, flowing freely.

A story of such goes thus; There was a man who was scared of his shadow and lived in fear of the sound of his footsteps. As he walked alone on a certain day, he panicked and made an effort to run at high speed. However, the faster he ran, the faster his shadow and footsteps caught up with him and made him run the more until he eventually slumped from exhaustion and kicked the bucket.

If he had taken a moment and had only sat at the feet of a tree under its shade, he would not have seen his shadow or heard his footsteps for a while.

Another story is expressed: Once upon a time, a lord wished for a new horse and asked his advisor where he might get a good horse. His advisor pondered for a while and announced that he had a long-time friend who was a professional in the characters of horses and that he would pass messages across to him to get his best horse delivered. Later, a parcel was received from his friend in the country stating that he would be sending a black stallion as a gift to the lord. However, when the horse arrived, it was discovered to be a mare with brown color.

The lord thundered in annoyance, "you said your friend was a professional! Yet, he cannot identify the color or gender of his own horses!"

With a sigh of admiration, the advisor thought aloud, saying, "Alas, has he indeed come this far? A sight so keen that he now cannot perceive things from their outward traits, only the inner virtue matters to him."

These stories have given us a vivid picture with which we can easily connect and understand The Way. It is a simple way of life. The way fosters beauty in all things and satisfaction with everything.

A quality life is attained by balance and harmony. Balance is an all-round thing, it is a combination of emotional, mental, and physical wellbeing. Balance yields a life, ideology, mindset, and a character of positivity. It fosters healthy relationships, a peaceful environment, and a well-developed nation. Harmony works hand-in-hand with balance. Harmony brings all things together, good and bad, to achieve one voice that submits to your inner state. When one aspect of your life loses its balance, it is normal for other aspects of your life to do so too.

A boss once narrated his experience with his employees, particularly the officers, that the stress from work resulted in physical challenges like diabetes, insomnia, high blood sugar, and heart conditions. It is a fact that long periods of stress manifest in depression. Some of the employees were retired athletes, men and women in their mid-forties and early fifties who were expected to be sound physically and mentally due to their previous lifestyle. However, the stress from work had a significant impact on generating and increasing health challenges. The effect of this stress led to a reduction in job satisfaction, frequent sick leave, and prolonged moments from work. In addition to this, there were more complaints and grumbling.

He realized that the problem was that his staff did not understand how they ought to shut off the stress or put a hold on their alertness. It led to the initiation of health challenges related to stress. Their minds were occupied by work; they discuss work away from the office, in their homes, leisure time, etc. They fail to understand that the more you discuss your stressors, the more it takes a toll and stresses you all the more keeping you unbalanced and in chaos with yourself.

By using The Way, this boss took it upon himself to make them conscious of what great future they could achieve if they learned to manage their stressors, alertness, and emotions. The 'Shut the Door on Work' concept was birthed by him to help them leave work at work. A quality life is only achieved when your life is balanced, meaning you have to spend quality time with your family, close friends, have fun doing outdoor activities you love rather than letting work go home with you when you leave work. You cheat yourself and your loved ones from having your company and doing the things that matter.

Discover means to fill your life with positivity; hobbies, fun games, interactive sessions, and activities with family and friends. Take out time alone to unwind and recharge weekly away from the workplace. A mixture of exercise (Qigong exercises, breathing techniques, Tai Chi, mediation), healthy eating, and lifestyle would do great, as discussed in chapter 1 on the importance of the body. Find ways to fill your life with positive activities, fun hobbies, quality time with family and friends, and plenty of personal time to refresh and renew each week when you are away from work. Add to this balance mix exercise, even just walking, and healthy eating.

Furthermore, change how you think about not only work but other areas of your life. The changes, balance, peace, and harmony you want to see will take time, effort, consistency, and practice. Do not relent until practice becomes your way of life.

Act without moving
Do without getting your hands embedded
Taste the tasteless
Increase the small
Make extra the few
Plan the hard work while still easy
Plan the big work while small or not yet present
Hard work in the world
It surely starts from easy
Big work in the world
Surely starts from small
Sages are not doing the big
So, they accomplish the big
Few believe in empty promises
They despise things and face difficulty
Sage considers everything difficult
Therefore, no trouble.
Chapter 63 – The Book of Ethic

NOTES

ON THE SOLDIER'S PATH

PART I: THE FIVE SPHERES

CHAPTER ONE: EARTH - Follow the Map

1. The katana has been an iconic symbol of Japanese Samurai tradition since the 13th century. It is a curved blade of up to 37 inches long with a single cutting edge that faces outward. The katana consists of a handle (Tsuka), pommel (Kashira), hand-guard (Tsuba), and a lacquered wooden scabbard (Saya). Source: "How the Katana Sword Became a Symbol of Samurai Tradition." www.invaluable.com/blog/katana-sword/. Accessed 1 October 2020.

2. "Samurai Swords." www.angelfire.com/dragon/swords/katana. html. Accessed 1 October 2020.

3. The wakizashi is a curved, single-edged blade between 12 and 24 inches long. It is smaller than the katana and offers more ease in close combat fighting. It was also used to behead the defeated opponent. Source: "Samurai Swords: The Wakizashi." *Swords of the East*, www.swordsoftheeast.com/wakizashi-swords.aspx. Accessed 1 October 2020.

4. The wakizashi was used to perform the ritual suicide known as *seppuku*. This ritual was carried out by a warrior who felt that they were living in great shame by disappointing their master or by being humiliated in one way or another. Source: "Samurai Swords." www.angelfire.com/dragon/swords/katana.html. Accessed 1 October 2020.

5. "Samurai Swords: The Wakizashi." *Swords of the East*, www.swordsoftheeast.com/wakizashi-swords.aspx. Accessed 1 October 2020.

6. "The History of Japanese Daisho." www.martialartswords.com/blogs/articles/the-history-of-japanese-daisho. Accessed 1 October 2020.

7. Martin Kelly. "5 Key Causes of World War 1." *ThoughtCo*, 26 March 2020.

8. Blake Stilwell. "The 7 most notorious traitors in military history." *We Are The Mighty*, www.wearethemighty.com/amp/the-7-most-notorious-traitors-in-military-history-2554876440. 6 December 2017.

9. Barack Obama. "Remarks by the President in Address to the Nation on Syria." Office of the Press Secretary, The White House, 10 September 2013. www.obamawhitehouse.archives.gov/the-press-office/2013/09/10/remarks-president-address-nation-syria. Accessed 6 October 2020.

10. ibid

11. "Vietnam War." *History*, www.history.com/.amp/topics/vietnam-war/vietnam-war-history. Accessed 6 October 2020.

12. ibid

13. Cynthia M. Grabo. "Strategic Warning: The Problem of Timing." *Central Intelligence Agency*, 2 July 1996.

14. The first date selected by Hitler for the attack was 12th November 1939, but he didn't attack until 10th May 1940. Source: ibid

15. ibid

16. Between 2007 and 2017, British cyclist won 178 world championships, 66 Olympic or Paralympic gold medals, and 5 Tour de France victories. Source: James Clear. *Atomic Habits*. New York: Penguin Random House LLC, 2018. E-book

CHAPTER TWO: WATER - *Soft As Water*

1. "The Worst War Crimes Ever Imaginable." *All That's Interesting*, https://allthatsinteresting.com/worst-war-crimes-in-history/, 2 June 2016. Accessed 12 October 2020.

2. Two declassified government documents reveal that the United States paid over $2.3 million for the data. The United States also used research gained from Nazi experimentation to improve their own biological warfare program. Source: ibid

3. One of the women, Masika Katsuva, recounting her ordeal to filmmaker Fiona Lloyd-Davies, said that she and her two daughters were raped. Her husband was murdered in front of her, and she was forced to eat his genitalia. Source: ibid

CHAPTER THREE: FIRE - *Fierce as Fire*

1. Kennedy Hickman. "Wars and Battles Throughout History." *ThoughtCo*, 14 January 2020.

2. Books also destroyed included the works of 1929 Nobel laureate, Thomas Mann, a German author whose critique of fascism angered the Nazis; Erich Maria Remarque, whose description of war in her book *All Quiet on the Western Front* was considered "a literary betrayal of the soldiers of the World War"; and Helen Keller, who believed in social justice and championed pacifism, women's voting rights, improved conditions for industrial workers, and the disabled. Works by German literary critics like Erich Kästner, Heinrich Mann, Ernst Gläser; American authors, Jack London and Theodore Dreiser; and Jewish authors, Franz Werfel, Max Brod, and Stefan Zweig were also affected. Source: Holocaust Encyclopedia. "Book Burning." *United States Holocaust Memorial Museum.*

3. United States Holocaust Memorial Museum. "Nazi Book Burning." *YouTube*. https://youtu.be/yHzM1gXaiVo.

4. ibid

5. Julie McCarthy. "Why Rights Groups Worry About The Philippines' New Anti-Terrorism Law." *npr*, 21 July 2020. https://

www.npr.org/2020/07/21/893019057/why-rights-groups-worry-about-the-philippines-new-anti-terrorism-law. Accessed 20 October 2020.

6. ibid

CHAPTER FOUR: WIND - *Enigmatic as the Wind*

1. Bassam Aramin faced similar criticisms from the Palestinians. All they wanted was the lingering enmity between Palestine and Israel. But for Bassam, Rami, and others who understood the path of peace, they knew that "it is not a decree of faith that we should live forever with a sword in our hands." Source: Colum McCann. *Apeirogon.* New York: Random House, 2020. E-book.

2. ibid

3. ibid

CHAPTER FIVE: THE VOID - *In the Void*

1. Source: Imperial War Museums. "10 Surprising Laws Passed During The First World War." www.iwm.org.uk/history/10-surprising-laws-passed-during-the-first-world-war. Accessed 22 October 2020.

2. Other measures included in DORA were regulating the opening times of pubs and reducing alcohol strength, making the possession of cocaine or opium by anyone other than authorized professionals a criminal offence, and issuing fines for making white flour instead of whole wheat and for allowing rats to invade wheat stores. Source: ibid

3. Jack Beckett. "A Turning Point In The Life Of Musashi, The Undefeated Samurai." *War History Online*, www.warhistoryonline.com/ancient-history/turning-point-samuraimusashi.html. Accessed 23 October 2020.

4. Kojiro was the weapons master to the Daimyo of the Hosokawa clan. Source: ibid

5. Kojiro's retinue comprised body servants, friends, students, cooks, and officials who had come to witness the duel and give report to the daimyo. Source: ibid

6. Another account recorded that when Kojiro saw Musashi, he drew his sword and threw his scabbard aside. This action made Musashi to taunt him even more by saying: "If you have no more use for your sheath, you are already dead." Source: Yasuka. "The Duel Between Sasaki Kojirō and Miyamoto Musashi." *KCP International, Japanese Language School*, 26 January 2015.

PART II: WINNING WARS WITHOUT COMBAT

https://libertyanns.medium.com/winning-without-fighting-lessons-from-the-art-of-war-by-sun-tzu-7ac68162831b

https://www.heritage.org/asia/commentary/winning-war-without-fighting

https://www.pambazuka.org/human-security/how-win-war-without-fight

https://www.tm.org/blog/meditation/laozi-and-the-tao-te-ching-the-ancient-wisdom-of-china/

https://hbr.org/2015/12/calming-your-brain-during-conflict

https://blackbeltmag.com/how-to-use-the-combat-concepts-of-legendary-swordsman-miyamoto-musashi-in-21st-century-self-defense

https://davehuer.com/blog/tag/miyamoto-mushashi/

https://cptsdawayout.com/2015/03/20/the-void-the-greatest-samurai-explains-a-devoted-meditator/

https://www.hprc-online.org/mental-fitness/sleep-stress/mindfulness-military

https://www.mindful.org/why-the-army-is-training-in-mindfulness/

https://www.army.mil/article/149615/improving_military_resilience_through_mindfulness_training

https://libertyanns.medium.com/winning-without-fighting-lessons-from-the-art-of-war-by-sun-tzu-7ac68162831b

https://psmag.com/social-justice/a-state-military-mind-42839

http://www.ethikundmilitaer.de/en/full-issues/20192-ethics-for-soldiers/

https://www.militarystrategymagazine.com/article/politics-statecraft-and-the-art-of-war/

https://www.amacad.org/daedalus/ethics-technology-war

https://www.icrc.org/en/doc/assets/files/publications/icrc-0526-002.pdf

https://iep.utm.edu/justwar/

http://isme.tamu.edu/ISME07/Bowyer07.html

https://watson.brown.edu/costsofwar/costs/human

https://watson.brown.edu/costsofwar/costs/human

https://www.e-ir.info/2008/05/22/a-bloodless-war-an-analysis-of-the-weapons-used-by-the-international-campaign-to-ban-landmines/

https://www.peoplesworld.org/article/day-of-the-drone-the-illusion-of-bloodless-war/

https://www.annualreviews.org/doi/pdf/10.1146/annurev-polisci-060314-112706

https://publications.armywarcollege.edu/pubs/2358.pdf

https://www.nytimes.com/1999/01/03/weekinreview/world-war-without-casualties-not-taking-losses-one-thing-winning-another.html

THE ENTREPRENEUR'S BATTLE PLAN

Chapter One: The Drawing Board

1. "Soil Types." *Boughton*, https://www.boughton.co.uk/products/topsoils/soil-types/. Accessed 5 December 2020.

2. "Soil Texture." *Queensland Government*, https://www.qld.gov.au/environment/land/management/soil/soil-properties/texture. Accessed 6 December 2020.

3. "Definition of heavy soil." *Dave's Garden*, https://davesgarden.com/guides/terms/go/443/. Accessed 6 December 2020.

4. *Ut supra*, 1

5. Peter Brodie. "The Four Seasons Of Business: Why Spring Is Around The Corner." Forbes, 18 June 2020.

6. Ibid

7. Ibid

8. Statistics by *Statista* showed that the number of students impacted by school closure rose from about 0.3 billion on 25 February 2020 to 1.38 billion on 23 March 2020. These figures referred to learners in pre-primary, primary, lower-secondary, and upper-secondary, and tertiary levels of education.

   Source: Cathy Li and Farah Lalani. "The COVID-19 pandemic has changed online education forever. This is how." World Economic Forum, 29 April 2020.

9. Ibid

10. Nataly E. Yousef. "Coronavirus Economy: These Five Industries Are Currently Thriving." *NoCamels*, 15 March 2020. https://nocamels.com/2020/03/coronavirus-economy-5-industries-thriving/. Accessed 7 December 2020.

11. "Global Fastest Declining Industries by Revenue Growth (%) in 2020." *IBISWorld*, https://www.ibisworld.com/global/indus-

try-trends/fastest-declining-industries/. Accessed 8 December 2020.

12. The airline cut more than 3,500 jobs to stay afloat amid the pandemic. Source: Dominic Rushe. "Virgin Atlantic files for bankruptcy protection as Covid continues to hurt airlines." The Guardian, 4 August 2020.

13. The companies were Mitsubishi, Mitsui, Sumitomo, Itochu, and Marubeni. Buffett also invested in Barrick Gold—a Canada-based mining company that produces gold and copper—and Dominion Energy's natural gas transmission and storage business.

Source: David Ricketts. "What Warren Buffett's Covid-19 bets tell us about investment in a crisis." Financial News, 4 September 2020.

14. Kimberly Amadeo. "Strategies and Examples of Trading Sideways." *The Balance*, 11 November 2020.

15. People invested their savings into OneCoin. In Britain, people spent over 30 million euros on OneCoin in the first six months of 2016. Between 2014 and 2017, over 4 billion euros have been invested in many countries like Pakistan, Brazil, Norway, Canada, Yemen, and Palestine.

Source: "Cryptoqueen: How this woman scammed the world, then vanished." BBC, 24 November 2019.

16. Nick Statt. "Pokemon Go never went away — 2019 was its most lucrative year." *The Verge*, 10 January 2020.

17. Marty Hudson. "Do You Tweet — Or Is Twitter Just A Passing Fad?" *MedicalGPS*, 8 December 2009. https://blog.medicalgps.com/do-you-tweet-or-is-twitter-just-a-passing-fad/. Accessed 8 December 2020.

18. "Is Twitter a Fad?" Canadian Marketing Association, 20 May 2009. https://www.the-cma.org/about/blog/is-twitter-a-fad. Accessed 8 December 2020.

19. Sam Jordan. "Why Twitter is a Fad." *The Better Blog*, 29 January 2013. https://mediashower.com/blog/why-twitter-is-a-fad/. Accessed 8 December 2020.

20. Commenting on the outcome of his prediction, Stoll said: "Of my many mistakes, flubs, and howlers, few have been as public as my 1995 howler. Wrong? Yep... Now, whenever I think I know what's happening, I temper my thoughts: Might be wrong, Cliff..."

   Source: Sam Parr. "Newsweek in 1995: Why the Internet Will Fail?" The Hustle, 21 December 2015.

21. Merriam-Webster (n.d.). Disruption. In *Merriam-Webster Dictionary*. https://www.merriam-webster.com/dictionary/disruption. Accessed 9 December 2020.

22. Caroline Howard. "Disruption Vs. Innovation: What's The Difference?" *Forbes*, 27 March 2013.

23. "Largest stock exchange operators worldwide as of Mar 2020, by market capitalization of listed companies." *Statista*, 23 November 2020.

24. Warren Venketas. "Forex Market Size: A Trader's Advantage." *DailyFX*, 15 January 2019.

25. Raynor de Best. "Market capitalization of cryptocurrencies from 2013 to 2019." *Statista*, 25 November 2020.

26. Avery Hartmans. "Jeff Bezos just turned 57. Here's how he built Amazon into a $1.56 trillion company and became the world's richest person." *Business Insider*, 12 January 2021.

27. "14 Different Types of Terrain." *Nayturr*, https://nayturr.com/types-of-terrain/. Accessed 10 December 2020.

28. Larry Kim. "5 Entrepreneurs Who Ignored Their Advisers and Became Wildly Rich." *Inc.*, 5 May 2015.

29. Ibid

30. Patrick J. Kiger. "9/11: Six Tech Advances to Prevent Future Attacks." *National Geographic News*, 9 September 2011.

31. Neil Patel. "7 Ways to Prove You're Trustworthy as an Entrepreneur." *Entrepreneur*, 1 June 2016.

Chapter Two: The Attack

1. Betsy Mikel. "1 Personality Trait Steve Jobs Always Looked For When Hiring for Apple." *Inc.*, 11 December 2017.

2. Ibid

3. Ibid

4. Tom Huddleston Jr. "These are Bill Gates' 2 superpowers, according to Bill Gates." *CNBC*, 9 October 2019.

5. Sarah Boseley. "How Bill and Melinda Gates helped save 122m lives – and what they want to solve next." *The Guardian*, 14 February 2017.

6. Stephanie Watson. "2020 Lifetime Achievement: Bill and Melinda Gates." *WebMD*, 4 February 2020.

7. Donna Fenn. "9 Brutal Startup Mistakes That Can Kill Your Business (and How to Avoid Them)." *American Express*, 2 September 2014.

8. Esha Chhabra. "How This Women-Led Ice Cream Brand Shook Up The Industry." *Forbes*, 30 March 2019.

9. *Ut supra*, 7

10. Tim Smith. "Qualitative Analysis." *Investopedia*, 15 May 2020.

11. "Real Life Examples of Qualitative Forecasting." https://small-business.chron.com/real-life-examples-qualitative-forecasting-72990.html, 12 October 2020. Accessed 10 January 2021.

12. Ibid

13. Ibid

14. *Ut supra*, 10

15. Ibid

16. Norman Marks. "Are Your Business Decisions Failing Because They Are Biased?" *CMSWire*, 13 September 2019. www.cmswire. com/information-management/are-your-business-decisions-failing-because-they-are-biased/. Accessed 18 January 2021.

17. "Quantitative Analysis." *Corporate Financial Institute*, https:// corporatefinanceinstitute.com/resources/knowledge/finance/ quantitative-analysis/. Accessed 19 January 2021.

18. Andrew Zaleski. "7 businesses that cloned others and made millions." *CNBC*, 4 October 2017.

19. Ibid

20. Kimberlee Leonard. "Examples of Quantitative Reasoning for a Business." https://smallbusiness.chron.com/examples-quantitative-reasoning-business-30966.html, 5 November 2018. Accessed 19 January 2021.

21. Shaun Snapp. "The Missed Opportunity of Causal Forecasting?" *Brightwork Research & Analysis*, https://www.brightworkresearch.com/the-missed-opportunity-of-causal-forecasting/, 3 October 2010. Accessed 20 January 2021.

22. Chris Morris. "10 iconic US companies that have left America." *CNBC*, 21 April 2016.

23. "The Best and Worst Countries for Business: Ease of doing business ranking." *Wall Street Journal*, 2018. https://graphics.wsj. com/table/DoingBusiness. Accessed 20 January 2021.

24. World Bank Group. "Doing Business 2020–Sustaining the pace of reforms." *World Bank Group*, 24 October 2019.

25. Legal Team New Zealand. "Politics and Business: What Does It Mean For New Zealand in 2019?" *Biz Latin Hub*, https://www. bizlatinhub.com/politics-business-new-zealand-2019/, 25 April 2019.

26. Ibid

27. Endy M. Bayuni. "When business and government mix too well in Indonesia." *The Jakarta Post*, 28 November 2018.

28. Ibid

29. "Economic influence on business activity." *BBC UK*, https://www.bbc.co.uk/bitesize/guides/zjjnnrd/revision/1. Accessed 20 January 2021.

30. Ibid

31. "The economy and business." *BBC UK*, https://www.bbc.co.uk/bitesize/guides/zrwtmfr/revision/2#:~:text=This%20down-turn%20in%20economic%20activity,increase%20when%20un-employment%20is%20higher. Accessed 21 January 2021.

32. "Facebook, Google and Microsoft 'avoiding $3bn in tax in poorer nations'." *BBC*, 26 October 2020.

33. Jemima McEvoy. "Eskimo Pie Becomes Edy's Pie: Here Are All The Brands That Are Changing Racist Names And Packaging." *Forbes*, 26 June 2020.

34. Michael Hogan. "How cancel culture is affecting business." *Smart Company*, 9 July 2019.

35. Jack Kelly. "Wayfair Employees' Protest Of Sales To Detention Centers Could Backfire On Them." *Forbes*, 2 July 2019.

36. Ibid

37. Ibid

38. *Ut supra*, 34

39. *Ut supra*, 35

40. Kweilin Ellingrud. "The Upside Of Automation: New Jobs, Increased Productivity And Changing Roles For Workers." *Forbes*, 23 October 2018.

41. Samuel D. Brickley and Brian M. Gottesman. *Business Law Basics*. http://www.businesslawbasics.com/business-law-basics. Accessed 25 January 2021.

42. "China remains a top investment priority for 60 percent of foreign companies, despite a challenging year for growth and profitability." *Bain and Company*, https://www.bain.com/about/media-center/press-releases/2016/amcham-china-business-survey-bain-2016/, 20 January 2016. Accessed 25 January 2021.

43. "Insights on handling coronavirus from an earlier report on business and outbreaks." *World Economic Forum*, 11 March 2020.

Chapter Three: The Strategy

1. Pauline Meyer. "Apple Inc's Generic Strategy & Intensive Growth Strategies." *Panmore Institute*, 5 June 2019. http://panmore.com/apple-inc-generic-strategy-intensive-growth-strategies#:~:text=Apple%20Inc.'s%20generic%20strategy%20is%20broad%20differentiation.,stands%20out%20in%20the%20market. Accessed 15 December 2020.

2. In terms of safety, it was reported that Tesla's Model S was the safest car ever tested by the National Highway Traffic Safety Administration. It earned top marks across all categories. Source: Michael Kern. "Why Are Tesla Cars So Popular?" *Yahoo! Finance*, 28 March 2020.

3. Tesla owners agree with this. Tesla's technology includes an autopilot feature, over-the-air updates, charger location, almost full driver control of car features, and so on. It has been described as The Car of the Future.

   Source: ibid

4. "Global Smartphone Market Share: By Quarter." *Counterpoint*, 20 November 2020. https://www.counterpointresearch.com/global-smartphone-share/. Accessed 15 December 2020.

5. "Apple's iPhone revenue from 3rd quarter 2007 to 4th quarter 2020." *Statista*, October 2020.

Chapter Four: The Mystery

1. Annie Palmer. "Amazon is on a hiring spree amid widespread coronavirus layoffs and record unemployment." *CNBC*, 9 September 2020.

2. Jay Greene. "Amazon now employs more than 1 million people." *The Washington Post*, 29 October 2020.

Chapter Five: The Winning Team

1. "The Worst War Crimes Ever Imaginable." *All That's Interesting*, 2 June 2016. https://allthatsinteresting.com/worst-war-crimes-in-history/. Accessed 12 October 2020.

2. The United States, in a bid to be ahead of the Soviet Union in global weaponry, chose to give these perpetrators immunity in exchange for the information gathered during the experiments.

   Source: ibid

3. "Trade Secrets: 10 of the Most Famous Examples." *Vethan Law Firm, P. C.*, 11 August 2016. https://info.vethanlaw.com/blog/trade-secrets-10-of-the-most-famous-examples. Accessed 16 December 2020.

4. Chuck Price. "17 Great Search Engines You Can Use Instead of Google." Search Engine Journal, 5 April 2020. https://www.searchenginejournal.com/alternative-search-engines/271409/#-close. Accessed 16 December 2020.

5. *Ut supra*, 3

6. ibid

7. ibid

8. ibid

9. Paul A. Argenti. "When Should Your Company Speak Up About a Social Issue?" *Harvard Business Review*, 16 October 2020.

10. Ibid

11. Data sourced from Yahoo Finance.

Chapter Six: The Early Bird

1. Gary stated that another reason why TikTok became so popular was that it targeted younger audiences.

   Source: Gary Vaynerchuk. "Why The TikTok (Formerly Musical.ly) App Is So Important." *Gary Vaynerchuk*, 2018. https://www.garyvaynerchuk.com/why-tiktok-formerly-musical-ly-app-is-important/. Accessed 17 December 2020.

2. Carl Franzen. "The History Of The Walkman: 35 Years Of Iconic Music Players." *The Verge*, 1 July 2014.

3. Alexandra Appolonia. "How BlackBerry went from controlling the smartphone market to a phone of the past." *Business Insider*, 21 November 2019.

4. ibid

5. Victoria Ahl. "4 Clever Ways These Companies Poached Talent From Their Competitors." *LinkedIn*, 19 July 2017.

6. Ibid

Chapter Seven: The Unpredictable Maneuver

1. Andy Gregory. "Coronavirus: Bar condemned for offering deals on Corona beer 'while the pandemic lasts.'" *Independent*, 3 February 2020.

2. The bar responded to the outrage with a follow-up post which read: "Let's be honest, there are worse things you can catch in Hamilton." John Lawrenson, the CEO of the company that owns the bar, saw the outrage as a good thing for his company. He was quoted to have said, "The great thing about living in today's society is that there is a small but loud minority of people who get offended by everything and I can always rely on them to get triggered. So I'd just like to say thanks to all the snowflakes for the free advertising and thanks to everyone else with a sense of humour who liked the post."

   Source: ibid

3. ibid

4. David Z. Morris. "Coursera offers free online courses to universities worldwide during coronavirus pandemic." *Fortune*, 12 March 2020.

5. These courses taught on how to stay productive, build relationships when you're not face-to-face, use virtual meeting tools, and balance family and work dynamics in a healthy way. Source: Blake Morgan. "50 Ways Companies Are Giving Back During The Coronavirus Pandemic." *Forbes*, 17 March 2020.

6. ibid

7. (1) By offering free courses to universities worldwide, Coursera showcased their vision of creating a future where everyone would have access to world-class education. And this wasn't halted by the pandemic. Despite the pandemic, Coursera achieved its aim of empowering people with education that will improve their lives, the lives of their families, and the communities they live in. (2) Likewise, LinkedIn, by giving out its courses for free, maintained its vision of creating economic opportunity for every member of the global workforce. The pandemic period was a time where many lost access to economic opportunities, but through LinkedIn they were taught how to regain this access, even from the comfort of their homes. (3) Part of the code of ethics of Dolce & Gabbana is Responsibility. And what better way to show responsibility to global health if not by funding research that would look into getting a cure for an incurable disease with a high mortality rate. (4) Giorgio Armani has a corporate social responsibility to support humanitarian projects that are in line with its value.

8. Michelle Greenwald. "20 Ways Apple Masters Customer Touchpoints And Why It's Great For Business." *Forbes*, 21 May 2014.

9. Jeff Wiener. "9 Proven Ways to Beat The Competition in Business and Create a Winning Competitive Advantage." *The Kickass Entrepreneur*, 9 December 2020.

https://www.thekickassentrepreneur.com/beat-the-competi-tion/. Accessed 18 December 2020.

10. "The 50 greatest business rivalries of all time." *Fortune*, 21 March 2013.

11. Devika Pawar. "Nike Air Jordan's Journey From Struggling In The NBA To Making Billions Per Year." *Republicworld.com*, 20 May 2020. https://www.republicworld.com/sports-news/bas-ketball-news/nike-air-jordans-journey-to-making-billions-per-year-the-last-dance.html. Accessed 18 December 2020.

12. Vivian Giang. "3 Keys To Destroying Your Competition." *Forbes*, 24 February 2013.

13. Ibid

Chapter Eight: The Contingencies

1. Daphne Blake. "100 Reasons NOT To Start A Business." *Hub-works*, https://hubworks.com/blog/reasons-not-start-business. html, 2 February 2017. Accessed 22 January 2021.

2. "Famous companies that still aren't profitable." https:// www.lovemoney.com/gallerylist/91226/famous-compa-nies-that-not-profitable, 10 January 2020. Accessed 23 January 2021.

3. Tanvir Zafar. "10 Successful Entrepreneurs Stories About Get-ting Through Tough Times." *Life Hack*, https://www.lifehack. org/837974/successful-entrepreneurs-stories. Accessed 23 Jan-uary 2021.

4. ibid

5. Perrie Kapernaros. "How Competitive Collaboration Can Boost Your Business." *Foundr*, 28 November 2020.

6. ibid

7. Brianne Garrett. "Why Collaborating With Your Competition Can Be A Great Idea." *Forbes*, 19 September 2019.

8. It was commonly believed that human beings have 6 basic emotions—happiness, sadness, fear, anger, surprise, and disgust. But a study led by Alan S. Cowen and Dacher Keltner PhD from the University of California, Berkeley, puts the number at 27. The emotions as outlined by the study are admiration, adoration, aesthetic appreciation, amusement, anxiety, awe, awkwardness, boredom, calmness, confusion, craving, disgust, empathetic pain, entrancement, envy, excitement, fear, horror, interest, joy, nostalgia, romance, sadness, satisfaction, sexual desire, sympathy, and triumph.

Source: Katie Avis-Riordan. "There are actually 27 human emotions, new study finds." CountryLiving, 11 September 2017. https://www.countryliving.com/uk/wellbeing/news/a2454/27-human-emotions-new study/#:~:text=In%20previous%20 thought%2C%20it%20was,is%20as%20many%20as%2027. Accessed 18 December 2020.

9. Gwen Moran. "Are You a Risk-Taker or Just Reckless?" *Entrepreneur*, 7 October 2013.

10. ibid

11. ibid

12. ibid

13. ibid

14. Anastasia Belyh. "Too Much Funding Can Kill Your Business." *Cleverism*, 19 September 2019. https://www.cleverism.com/too-much-funding-can-kill-business/. Accessed 19 December 2020.

15. ibid

16. ibid

17. Kayla Matthews. "10 Ways Greed Can Ruin Your Business." *Business 2 Community*, 7 May 2014. https://www.business-2community.com/leadership/10-ways-greed-can-ruin-business-0875704. Accessed 19 December 2020.

18. "15 Famous Mentoring Relationships." *PUSHfar*, https://www.pushfar.com/article/15-famous-mentoring-relationships/. Accessed 19 December 2020.

19. Neil Patel. "10 Ways You Can Use Your Anger to Build Your Business." *Forbes*, 24 June 2016.

20. Merriam-Webster (n.d.). Self-conceit. In *Merriam-Webster Dictionary*. https://www.merriam-webster.com/dictionary/self-conceit. Accessed 19 December 2020.

21. Merriam-Webster (n.d.). Self-confidence. In *Merriam-Webster Dictionary*. https://www.merriam-webster.com/dictionary/self-confidence. Accessed 19 December 2020.

22. Merriam-Webster (n.d.). Confidence. In *Merriam-Webster Dictionary*. https://www.merriam-webster.com/dictionary/confidence. Accessed 19 December 2020.

23. "End of the line: CEOs who quit their jobs." *The Economic Times*, 28 November 2019.

24. Institutional arrogance. *In Urban Dictionary*, 9 February 2020. https://www.urbandictionary.com/define.php?term=Institutional%20arrogance. Accessed 19 December 2020.

25. The CEOs were reluctant to launch products that could compete favorably with those of Apple and Google. By the time they were ready to take up the challenge, it was already too late. Apple's iPhone and Google's Android had taken a huge chunk of the smartphone market. Source: "Personally Disrupted: 14 CEOs Who Got Axed After Failing To Navigate Disruption." *CBInsights*, 17 July 2019. https://www.cbinsights.com/research/ceo-disruption/#blackberry. Accessed 19 December 2020.

Chapter Nine: The Resilience

1. Oliver Rowe. "How leaders can build business resilience." *Financial Management*, 11 March 2020. https://www.fm-magazine.com/news/2020/mar/how-to-build-business-resilience-coronavirus-response-23121.html. Accessed 26 January 2021.

2. Martin Reeves and Kevin Whitaker. "A Guide to Building a More Resilient Business." *Harvard Business Review*, 2 July 2020.

Chapter Ten: Using Spies

1. Josh Fruhlinger. "What is corporate espionage? Inside the murky world of private spying." *CSO*, https://www.csoonline.com/article/3285726/what-is-corporate-espionage-inside-the-murky-world-of-private-spying.html#:~:text=Corporate%20espionage%20%20E2%80%94%20sometimes%20also%20called,to%20get%20information%20about%20another, 2 July 2018. Accessed 23 January 2021.

2. ibid

3. Tony Tran. "What is Social Listening, Why it Matters, and 10 Tools to Make it Easier." *Hootsuite*, 3 March 2020.

4. ibid

5. ibid

INSIDE THE WAR ROOM

1. Eudaimonia Classical Knowledge, *The Art of War By Sun Tzu*, accessed April 2020 <https://www.obtaineudaimonia.com/taxonomy/term/200>

2. Frank James, NPR, *Christine O'Donnell Makes First Amendment Gaffe* 2010, Accessed May 2021 <https://www.npr.org/sections/itsallpolitics/2010/10/19/130671265/christine-o-donnell-stuns-crowd-with-1st-amendment-ignorance>

3. Gerard Chaliand, *The Art of War in World History: From Antiquity to the Nuclear Age*, The Regents of the University of California 1994.

4. History (2019), *Watergate Scandal*, accessed May 4, 2021 <https://www.history.com/topics/1970s/watergate>

5. Ian Chadwick 2017, *The Municipal Machiavelli: Machiavelli's The Prince Rewritten for Municipal Politicians*, accessed April, 2021 <http://ianchadwick.com/machiavelli/>

6. James MacGregor Burns, *Roosevelt: The Lion and The Fox*, Harcourt Inc., 1956.

7. John J. Pitney, *The Art of Political Warfare*, University of Oklahoma Press 2000.

8. Jonathan Powell *The New Machiavelli: How to Wield Power In the Modern World*, Random House Publishing, 2010.

9. Lawrence Freedman *Strategy: A History*, Oxford University Press, 2013.

10. Michael A. Ledeen *Machiavelli on Modern Leadership*, St. Martin's Press, 1999.

11. Michael Edward Mallet, Britannica *Cesare Borgia*, Accessed April 2021 <https://www.britannica.com/biography/Cesare-Borgia>

12. Michael I. Handel, *Masters of War: Classic Strategic Thought*, Taylor & Francis Book, 1992.

13. Miyamoto Musashi, *The Five Spheres And Other Writings*, Translated by Tham Trong Ma, 2021.

14. Niccolò Machiavelli, *The Prince*, Translated by Tham Trong Ma, 2021.

15. Robert A. Caro, *The Years of Lyndon Johnson: The Path to Power*, Random House Inc., 1982.

16. Robert Greene, *33 Strategies of War*, Penguin Group, 2006.

17. Robert R. Leonhard, *The Art of Maneuver: Maneuver-Warfare Theory and Airland Battle*, Presidio Press 1991.

18. Sun Vu, *The Law of War*, Translated by Tham Trong Ma, 2021.

INSIGHTS TO BETTER LIVING

Part I – The Body

1. What is creationism? - Meaning - Examples- Definition. https://whatdoesmean.net/what-is-creationism/

2. Definition of creationism - What it is, Meaning and.... https://en1.wvpt4learning.org/creacionismo-3788

3. What is creationism? - Meaning - Examples- Definition. https://whatdoesmean.net/what-is-creationism/

4. When your worst enemy is yourself. https://en.psychologyinstructor.com/when-your-worst-enemy-is-yourself/

5. When Your Worst Enemy Is You - Exploring your mind. https://exploringyourmind.com/when-your-worst-enemy-is-you/

6. When Your Worst Enemy Is Yourself | dayspad.com. https://dayspad.com/when-your-worst-enemy-is-yourself/

7. Gut Brain Connection - The Key to Wellbeing - Jo Spies. https://www.jospies.com.au/blog/gut-brain connection/

8. Best 5 Tips To Achieve Inner Peace. | by The Sky Hustle.... https://theskyhustle.medium.com/best-5-tips-to-achieve-inner-peace-6225d4f3c9cc

Part II – The Spirit

1. Lao Tzu (c.605 BC–c.531 BC) - *Tao Te Ching: The Book of....* https://www.poetryintranslation.com/PITBR/Chinese/TaoTeChing.php

2. Lao Tzu, *The Book of Ethics*, Translated by Tham Trong Ma, 2021.

3. Lão Tử, Sách Đạo Đức, Translated by Ma Trọng Thẩm, 2021.

4. Healing Through Nature - Chopra. https://chopra.com/articles/healing-through-nature

5. Philosophy Week 2.docx - *Introduction to the Philosophy of....*https://www.coursehero.com/file/110056520/Philosophy-Week-2docx/

6. Why Mindfulness Is Your Key to Emotional Intelligence | by.... https://medium.com/@ttisuccessinsights/why-mindfulness-is-your-key-to-emotional-intelligence-ca584dbf7eb3

7. Water Meditation: Washing Away the Stress [How-To Guide.... https://unifycosmos.com/water-meditation-guide/

8. The American president Theodore Roosevelt once said....https://forallanswers.com/the-american-president-theodore-roosevelt-once-said-comparison-is-the-thief-of-joy-teroa-discusses-how-constant-comparisons-to-her/

9. Healing Through Nature - Chopra. https://chopra.com/articles/healing-through-nature

10. How to find inner peace: 10 things you can start doing.... https://hackspirit.com/how-to-discover-your-inner-peace-in-4-simple-steps/

11. How to Stay Happy During Social Distancing. https://letsreachsuccess.com/happy-during-social-distancing/

12. 7 Ways You Can Be Healthier At Home - The Spirited Puddle....https://www.spiritedpuddlejumper.com/7-ways-you-can-be-healthier-at-home/

13. Happiness: 5 Mistakes You May Be Making. https://letsreachsuccess.com/2014/05/23/happiness-doing-it-wrong/

Part III - The Harmony Of Body And Spirit

1. A Full Disclosure Of The Mysterious Taoist Diet- Natural Healing Dao https://naturalhealingdao.com/a-full-disclosure-of-the-mysterious-taoist-diet

2. Try the Taoist Standing Exercise to Improve Body Alignment and Digestion! https://bodyecology.com/articles/taoist-standing-exercise-php/

3. Secrets of Taoism Longevity and Living a Long Healthy Life https://personaltao.com/tapism/secrets-of-taoism-longevity-and-lifestyle/

4. What are Dantian? The Energy Centers of Chinese Medicine https://www.healthline.com/health/Dantian

5. BBC-Religions-Taoism: Physical practices https://www BBC. co.uk/religion/religions/taoism/practices/physical.shtml

6. Daoist Harmony as a Chinese Philosophy and Psychology https://www.amacad.org/publication/envisioning-daoist-body-economy-cosmic-power

7. https://www.britannica.com/topic/Daoism

8. https://www.holdenqigong.com/history-of-qigong/

9. https://iep.utm.edu/daoism/

10. https://www.google.com/url?sa=t&source=web&rct=-j&url=https://philosophynow.org/issues/27/Death_in_Classical_Daoist_Thought&ved=2ahUKEwiRrJ6ttPDzAhVDB2M-BHfXjDnEQFnoECCsQAQ&usg=AOvVaw2KUNJqSE-noIq_VYR-pMlOJ

11. https://www.google.com/url?sa=t&source=web&rct=-j&url=https://classroom.synonym.com/what-do-taoists-believe-about-the-afterlife-12086979.html&ved=2ahUKEwiRrJ6ttPDzAhVDB2MBHfXjDnEQFnoECDEQAQ&usg=AOvVaw3Beo2dLC_XfeMv0IqmIOfX

12. https://m.youtube.com/results?sp=mAEA&search_query=The+psychology+of+harmonization